Innovation in Medical Education and Clinical Practice

Summer S. Chahin • Roger W. Apple
Cheryl A. Dickson • Berrin Ergun-Longmire
Editors

Innovation in Medical Education and Clinical Practice

An Exploration of Today's Revolutionary Concepts, Tools and Applications

Springer

Editors
Summer S. Chahin
Pediatric and Adolescent Medicine
Western Michigan University Homer
Stryker M.D. School of Medicine
Kalamazoo, MI, USA

Roger W. Apple
Pediatric and Adolescent Medicine
Western Michigan University Homer
Stryker M.D. School of Medicine
Kalamazoo, MI, USA

Cheryl A. Dickson
Pediatric and Adolescent Medicine
Western Michigan University Homer
Stryker M.D. School of Medicine
Kalamazoo, MI, USA

Berrin Ergun-Longmire
Pediatric and Adolescent Medicine
Western Michigan University Homer
Stryker M.D. School of Medicine
Kalamazoo, MI, USA

ISBN 978-3-032-19115-1 ISBN 978-3-032-19116-8 (eBook)
https://doi.org/10.1007/978-3-032-19116-8

This Springer imprint is published by the registered company Springer Nature Switzerland AG
The registered company address is: Gewerbestrasse 11, 6330 Cham, Switzerland

Preface

In recent years, medical education and clinical practice have undergone a remarkable transformation fueled by rapid technological progress, reimagined learning environments, and a deepened commitment to patient-centered care. *Innovation in Medical Education and Clinical Practice: An Exploration of Today's Revolutionary Concepts, Tools and Applications* arrives at a moment when the boundaries of what is possible in medicine are expanding at unprecedented speed. More than a survey of emerging trends, this book offers a re-envisioning of the future of medical and psychological training, one that is guided by the very learners who will shape that future.

A defining strength of this volume lies in the voices of its contributors. Each chapter is authored by medical students and psychology graduate students who are actively navigating today's shifting educational landscape. Their perspectives reflect lived experience: they are the users of simulation centers, adopters of artificial intelligence tools, beneficiaries of telehealth innovations, and observers of the ways new technologies influence both opportunity and inequity. Their curiosity and desire to improve the systems within which they train infuse each chapter with authenticity and relevance. Every student author is paired with a faculty mentor, ensuring that innovative ideas are grounded in clinical experience, academic rigor, and established expertise. This partnership produces a rich, balanced exploration of emerging concepts in education and practice.

The book opens by defining medical innovation and explaining its relevance across educational and clinical domains. Innovation, the authors emphasize, is not synonymous with technology; it includes new strategies, pedagogies, workflows, and care models that enhance learning and improve patient outcomes. Understanding the foundations of innovation provides essential context for the chapters that follow.

Early sections focus on one of the most transformative developments in modern training: simulation centers. These environments allow learners to practice clinical reasoning, emergency responses, procedural skills, and interprofessional teamwork in realistic but risk-free settings. Simulation now complements traditional lectures and laboratory work, reshaping the preclinical phase of training. Additional chapters highlight innovations in preclinical curricula, such as third-party learning platforms, digital study tools, and approaches designed to promote mastery learning, self-direction, and continuous skill reinforcement.

The book then expands into the rapidly evolving roles of artificial intelligence and distance learning. The global shift to remote education, accelerated by the COVID-19 pandemic, has sparked the adoption of virtual classrooms, asynchronous modules, and AI-driven tutoring systems. These tools have redefined flexibility and access for learners while introducing new considerations around assessment integrity, engagement, and educational equity. Related chapters explore how the pressures of the pandemic catalyzed technological creativity, producing models of education and care that remain influential long after the public health crisis.

Several chapters address innovations in data management, clinical informatics, and healthcare data security. Readers are introduced to AI models capable of processing vast amounts of medical information, supporting diagnostic decisions, predicting outcomes, and streamlining workflows. Alongside these benefits comes an increased responsibility to safeguard patient data. The authors discuss encryption, cybersecurity protocols, and the ethical implications of data-driven medicine.

Training innovations involving augmented reality (AR) and virtual reality (VR) represent another major theme. These immersive tools allow learners to explore anatomical structures, practice surgical techniques, and participate in simulated clinical encounters that mirror real practice. Whether used in early training or ongoing professional development, AR and VR broaden the possibilities of experiential learning.

Not all innovations are technological. Chapters on the education-centered medical home highlight how continuity, mentorship, and team-based care enhance learning and strengthen patient relationships. Another chapter examines technology's role in improving patient safety through enhanced monitoring, error-prevention systems, and real-time decision support.

A significant contribution of this book is its emphasis on health equity and cultural humility. Innovation is most meaningful when it advances fairness rather than reinforcing disparities. The authors demonstrate how telehealth, culturally informed decision-making, and other novel strategies can lower barriers to care, improve communication, and support more just healthcare systems. They argue that cultivating cultural humility is itself a form of innovation, one that reshapes how clinicians understand and respond to diverse patient experiences.

Additional chapters explore decision-making, diagnostic testing, and cognitive strategies that enhance clinical reasoning. Innovations in delivering optimized care, such as interprofessional collaboration, remote monitoring, and patient-driven health management, illustrate the shifting dynamics of modern practice. The expansion of telehealth is examined from both medical and psychological perspectives, not only as a technological advancement but also as a fundamental shift in access, engagement, and continuity of care.

Other chapters investigate cutting-edge applications, including 3D modeling, minimally invasive surgical innovations, and the growing role of lifestyle medicine in long-term wellness. Subspecialty-focused discussions demonstrate how fields across medicine and psychology continue to evolve in response to new knowledge and tools. A concluding exploration of telehealth's benefits provides a comprehensive view of how remote care is transforming the healthcare landscape.

Across all topics, the book delivers a central message: innovation is essential. Medicine is a dynamic, rapidly evolving discipline shaped by scientific discovery, societal change, and technological advancement. Innovation ensures that educational programs prepare learners for a continually shifting world. It accelerates diagnosis, enhances treatment, improves safety, and expands the capacity for personalized, equitable, and compassionate care. Without innovation, healthcare stagnates; with it, the system becomes more responsive, adaptive, and human-centered.

This volume stands as a testament to the creativity and dedication of the next generation of healthcare professionals. The student authors remind us that innovation thrives when diverse voices help shape it. Their insights, formed through both the challenges and opportunities of their training, offer a vision of healthcare that is technologically advanced, educationally progressive, clinically effective, and ethically grounded.

I invite you to engage deeply with the ideas presented here, reflect on their relevance to personal educational or clinical environments, and consider how innovation can continue to transform the future of medicine. This book serves as both a roadmap and inspiration, demonstrating the power of curiosity, mentorship, and collaborative exploration. In celebrating the work of its authors, we celebrate the future of healthcare itself.

Kalamazoo, MI, USA Summer S. Chahin

Contents

Introduction

Linh-Nhu Hoang, Pradnya Joshi, Summer S. Chahin, Berrin Ergun-Longmire, and Roger W. Apple

Goals of This Book

Medical education is constantly adapting, influencing the growth of long-term medical professionals as well as current medical students and residents. While faculty, students, and residents are continuing to teach and learn information around medical concepts, innovations in medical education continue to evolve. Innovations in medical education and training provide an opportunity for improved educational approaches that further contribute to the processes of learning. Research studies around education and training have become a growing importance in academic medicine.

Medical education is constantly growing and keeping pace with innovative developments. Medical students are digital natives who grew up with these technological developments and are bound to encounter more educated and technologically aware patients. In this book, authors will also describe (1) patients who lack health literacy and knowledge on how to utilize technology and (2) innovative ideas to support patients with those experiences. Medical education curricula are growing

L.-N. Hoang
Department of Psychology, Western Michigan University, Kalamazoo, MI, USA

Department of Pediatric and Adolescent Medicine, Western Michigan University Homer Stryker M.D. School of Medicine, Kalamazoo, MI, USA
e-mail: nhu.hoang@wmed.edu

P. Joshi · S. S. Chahin (✉) · B. Ergun-Longmire · R. W. Apple
Department of Pediatric and Adolescent Medicine, Western Michigan University Homer Stryker M.D. School of Medicine, Kalamazoo, MI, USA
e-mail: pradnya.joshi@wmed.edu; summer.chahin@wmed.edu; berrin.ergun-longmire@wmed.edu; roger.apple@wmed.edu

S. S. Chahin et al. (eds.), *Innovation in Medical Education and Clinical Practice*, https://doi.org/10.1007/978-3-032-19116-8_1

to require more research and upgradation of medical knowledge and training. COVID-19 disrupted clinical training but pushed for the emergence of technological teaching methods, such as online teaching, in medical education [1]. Such digital platforms allow medical educators to provide real-time feedback to students to enhance clinical performance. Educators are encouraged to be updated with the technological advances in using digital platforms. It is important to acknowledge that the humanistic aspect of providing patient care is much more difficult to replace with technology. Effective communication and compassion for the patient is important to keep consistent across modalities.

Training medical students in health data science (HDS) can be challenging due to the complexity of teaching both medical and computational concepts to students of diverse backgrounds in education and training. Studies have analyzed students' learning experiences with HDS and artificial intelligence (AI) to better understand learning strategies in medical education [2]. Successful students allocate more time to practical topics to make connections among concepts and through engagement with peer learning in medical education. There is also a call for a balance between medical education and research to improve the quality of training. Psychological support has been found to be a crucial component to medical education research as it addresses emotional safety and well-being [3]. Feedback exchange is also critical in medical and clinical training. There is currently an unestablished set of effective strategies and resources for delivering digital feedback in medical education [4]. This study found that immediate and personalized feedback as well as formative assessment outcomes served as the major facilitators for the utility of digital feedback for students. The incorporation of AI can provide opportunities for personalized and real-time feedback, while ensuring data integrity and privacy.

There continues to be a gap in the literature and understanding of technological curriculum structured for medical education [5]. Despite major advancements in medical education in the last few decades, it is still largely based on traditional curricula. It is important for medical providers to stay updated with the most recent advancements of technology, such as AI, being incorporated into medical education to then use it in practice. There have been efforts globally to incorporate AI within various levels of medical education, though not required in the curriculum framework. As of current, there has not yet been a book published about these evolving innovations in medical education. Further, there has not yet been a book written primarily by learners and mentored by faculty in their respective disciplines. Students are the ones learning about the most up-to-date innovations and likely have thoughts and reactions about the newest innovations, gaps in technology, care, and education, and, thus, are the newest innovators.

Innovative Ideas in Medical Education

Definitions

Understanding innovative ideas in medical education requires understanding the general definitions associated with innovation. Digital health technologies (DHTs) include telehealth, electronic health records (EHRs), mobile devices and applications, wearables, and AI [6]. Technological advancements such as AI, virtual reality (VR), and augmented reality (AR) provide interactive learning opportunities in medical education [7]. VR uses computer-generated and three-dimensional environments to create immersive experiences through the use of interactive devices [8]. VR offers a dynamic platform for medical training through its many forms, such as 3D, screen-based, or room-based environments. AR, on the other hand, is a technology that allows for digitally generated three-dimensional representations to be integrated with real environmental stimuli [9]. AR-based programs have increasingly been adopted in medical schools across the world. The integration of digital health in medicine prepares medical students and professionals for the evolving demands of healthcare delivery. Structured curricula and professional development opportunities must be established to result in the success of the integration of technological advancements. Clinical simulation is defined as a technique that is used to replace or amplify real-life experiences with guided experiences that evoke or replicate aspects of real-world scenarios in an interactive manner [10]. Clinical decision-making (CDM) is the ability of medical or healthcare professionals to gather, evaluate, and interpret relevant clinical information [11]. Clinical reasoning (CR) refers to the cognitive process that medical or healthcare professionals use to understand patient information, recognize clinical patterns, and evaluate evidence to reach a diagnosis and to determine an appropriate treatment plan [11].

One study identified case-based learning (CBL), evidence-based medicine (EBM), problem-based learning (PBL), simulation-based learning (SBL), e-learning, peer-assisted learning, observational learning, flipped classroom, and team-based learning (TBL) as modern learning techniques that have been validated and commonly employed in medical curricula [12]. CBL links theory to practice. EBM focuses on training students to learn, comprehend, and appraise medical literature. PBL focuses on collaborative, integrated, self-directed, and comprehensive learning. SBL is used to mimic real clinical scenarios for training. E-learning includes social media and video lectures to enhance electronic distribution of videos for training. Peer-assisted learning highlights the importance of active help and support of peers or colleagues in the development of skills training. Observational learning is in the form of demonstrative learning and is crucial to enhancing the learning of complex medical scenarios. Flipped classroom is a newer learning method that incorporates a mix of several learning techniques both online and offline. TBL involves a small group of students who engage in various activities and tasks and receive immediate feedback from their educators.

Innovations drive collaboration among professionals and programs. Faculty development that includes competency-based medical education (CBME) using entrustable professional activities (EPAs) is required to improve residency training [13]. Ongoing professional development and scholarly research projects are recommended to enhance the development of residency training. Despite lack of established digital educational curricula, there is a preference for the use of online or hybrid platforms for feedback processes in training. Studies in healthcare professions education (HPE) have found that the use of technology in educational curricula has been as effective as the traditional in-person learning format [14]. The literature has recommended a hybrid or blended format, which integrates both online and in-person learning modalities, to further enhance medical education.

The idea of the technical physician (TP) was developed as an added layer of training for individual patient care through the use of technology. A TP looks at how they can improve their patients' treatment with technological innovations and then adjusts the equipment to optimize patient-specific and individualized care [15]. One study concluded that TPs improve patient care through the integration of their medical and technical competencies [15]. Several training programs have difficulty incorporating technological innovations into their medical curricula and thus struggle preparing their resident physicians for using medical technology. TPs are meant to make patient care more effective and efficient as a result of the innovative ways in which medical technology is used. For example, TPs can optimize treatment for diabetes by assessing how the programming of glucose sensors and insulin pumps can be tailored to a specific patient with Type 1 diabetes [15]. However, there are still some barriers that limit the procedures and interventions that can be otherwise performed by physicians who received a traditional medical degree and can provide direct patient care, as much of the work performed by TPs) involve indirect care [15].

Simulation Centers

Medical education is improving through the integration of skill and simulation-based teaching and learning as supplementary methods to the traditional methods of clinical teaching [16]. A safely prepared and controlled environment with the integration of trained interdisciplinary instructors is essential in providing effective medical education to students and other healthcare professionals. Simulation-based technologies improve students' hands-on learning, knowledge retention, and student engagement by allowing them to practice complex medical procedures in safe, realistic environments [7]. Interprofessional education (IPE) activities, such as interprofessional communication, are important pillars in the delivery of healthcare. Simulation centers have played a key role in providing opportunities for simulation IPE activities to support high-fidelity activities in a controlled environment [17]. However, though it is ideal to achieve higher level learning outcomes with simulation centers, they are not necessary for providing meaningful IPE activities.

Simulation-based training (SBT) has become a transformative approach in medical education through its various types of simulations that are utilized today. Various types of simulation include high-fidelity mannequins, virtual reality environments, standardized patients, and hybrid simulations [18]. SBTs provide a safe and controlled environment for students to hone their technical and nontechnical skills, which ultimately improves patient safety and clinical outcomes. Benefits of SBT include enhanced skill acquisition, error reduction, and the opportunity for repeated practice without any risk to real-life patients. Simulation also allows teaching through guided experiences in safe and controlled environments, facilitating adequate learning and standardized assessment of clinical skills. Simulation centers are located all over the world, including both simulated hospitals and virtual hospitals that mimic actual hospitals. Simulation has become one of the key elements in continuing education with the goal of maintaining and improving acquired skills of medical students and other healthcare professionals [10]. Simulation allows for the training of skills needed for situations that occur infrequently. Simulation scenarios can be repeatable, which allows for the optimal degree of training to be achieved. A social robotic virtual patient (VP) has been shown to help enhance CR training by bridging theoretical learning and clinical practice [19]. The VP has heightened the authenticity and interactivity of simulations being closer to real-life patient interactions. The approach to using VP as part of training is currently most effective in the hybrid format, with the combination of traditional computer-based VPs on the broad level to specific skills development.

Educators should be mindful of the careful integration of technology-driven simulation in medical curricula. The integration of simulation while considering the various learning styles and modalities will help enhance the learning experience of medical and health science students and other healthcare professionals [20]. A review that looked into simulation-related standards through the Accreditation Council for Graduate Medical Education (ACGME) emphasized the need for involving all departments and subspecialties in graduate medical education (GME) simulation and shared curricula [21]. Mandatory curricula should focus on improving and optimizing patient safety and provider competency. Such curricula call for institutional financial support, as individual training programs may not be able to provide such resources.

Artificial Intelligence (AI)

AI is a complex social, cultural, and material artifact that is continuously constructed by different stakeholders [22]. AI has been the focus of scientific, business, and governmental interest. As prototype AI products continue to develop, professional organizations and government agencies are working to maintain regulatory strategies for the use of AI in healthcare [23]. AI has a positive influence on the personalization of medical education training. Structured AI training in medical curricula, such as improving diagnostic skills and fostering critical thinking, is crucial for preparing medical students as future healthcare professionals [7]. AI offers innovative solutions to critical challenges in teaching, assessment, and clinical training. AI supports personalized learning in medical education across several domains, including but not limited to quality and administration, academic guidance, student research, and internship management [24]. AI increases the potential to transform medical education by enhancing personalization, efficiency, and innovation. AI-simulated medical history conversations have been found to help support CDM training [11].

While many web-based resources exist to teach programming skills, the programs that do exist are often restricted to a specific specialty. Very few program curricula are tailored to training medical students without background in data science. Results of a web-based curriculum study revealed that a 1-month investment in AI education during medical school empowered the students to pave a way for AI innovation in healthcare [25]. It is important to note that while AI models generally return high accuracy within the trials in which they are trained, their ability to predict the best course of care for patients should still be considered with caution [26]. A multidisciplinary team should be involved in the contribution of developing policies on the use of AI in healthcare systems.

AI may include a machine learning algorithm (MLA) and natural language processing (NLP) that further amplifies the impact of adaptive learning experiences [20]. AI provides real-time feedback on medical students' decisions, which can highlight missed signs and recommendations to adjust treatment plans. AI-powered patient simulators can further demonstrate high fidelity, realistic physiological responses such as facial expressions, pulse, and blood pressure to allow medical students and residents to practice decision-making in safe and controlled scenarios [27]. Simulation-drive medical education such as this can hold great potential for quality improvement and research in the healthcare field.

Machine learning (ML) is a specific type of AI model that can handle more data than is practical in rule-based systems. These models can also identify meaningful patterns in data regardless of whether those patterns are known [23]. ML has not been deployed widely in clinical medicine compared to other AI models due to its limitations, though the limitations are progressively being improved. There is growing evidence that AI frameworks driven by ML algorithms help make impressive strides in medicine and healthcare [28]. As medical education grows, the development of ML curriculum during postsecondary education may enhance training for the next generation of healthcare professionals. ML can be utilized to help facilitate insights from healthcare data and has been successfully applied to pediatric critical care data [29]. Several techniques and infrastructures for developing and utilizing ML have matured over the years, making its integration more efficient. Building machine learning models requires deep, large data sets in order to provide significant data about each patient [30]. Large integrated databases, such as patient registries, have been the standard approach for building such large data sets in the past few decades. Results of a web-based curriculum study revealed that investment in ML education also positively impacts medical students in the AI and ML innovations in healthcare [25].

Large language models (LLMs), a type of ML model, are generative AI (GenAI) models that create clinical content based on the data on which it was trained to generate [31]. The range of LLM capabilities have evolved to include the interpretation of inputs and to provide diverse outputs ranging from videos-to-voice formats. Research continues to address challenges in contemporary medicine that have prompted the development of LLMs with multimodal capabilities. Artifacts of GenAI provide both educators and learners in medicine and health sciences with innovative opportunities for teaching and learning [22].

COVID-19

The COVID-19 pandemic transformed the final academic year of approximately 21,000 graduating medical students in the USA during the 2020–2021 academic year [32]. This disruption caused the reorganization of rotations to occur in an online format to protect medical students, conserve personal protective equipment, and limit the spread of the coronavirus. Deficits in performance of medical procedures that may have existed prior to the pandemic have worsened during the educational changes prompted by COVID-19. This suggests a level of difficulty in developing core clinical skills with distance learning modalities.

The pandemic has posed several challenges in medical and surgical education. For example, shortage of personal protective equipment, suspension of clinical clerkships, and reduction in elective surgical cases are challenges that have significantly affected medical and surgical education [33]. Additionally, medical students have received decreased exposure to certain medical and surgical specialties, which has reduced the students' examination performance, confidence, and abilities as future healthcare professionals [34]. Restrictions as a result of the COVID-19 pandemic have forced healthcare systems to reimagine their work structures, educational programming, and delivery of patient care [35]. Despite the restrictions, the pandemic has sparked the active engagement for transformative approaches in critical introspection around future work. The pandemic has thus spotlighted cultural norms and social practices, forcing healthcare professionals to consider these concepts through a holistic and critical lens [34–35].

Significant loss of income was also experienced by hospitals and physician practices due to the COVID-19 pandemic. Healthcare spending was reduced by approximately 18% in the first quarter of 2020, with the most significant decline experienced in the surgical and pediatric clinics and practices. This decline includes offices cutting pay, furloughing, and laying off medical staff due to cancellations of elective procedures [36]. Additionally, medical education-related funding was limited by institutions. Adaptations to medical education during the COVID-19 pandemic initially centered around distancing and limiting travel to prevent the spread of the coronavirus. The recommendations included maintaining social distancing of greater than 6 feet, limiting the number of people present in workspaces, monitoring symptoms and signs, limiting personal or business travel, altering service structures to allow residents to work from home, and providing didactics via virtual platforms [36–37]. Digital approaches to healthcare education and delivery played a major role as an invaluable and reliable resource to overcome restrictions imposed during the COVID-19 pandemic [38]. This allowed for effective, accessible, and consumer-friendly care for several patients and families.

Education-Centered Medical Home

Education-centered medical home (ECMH) is a longitudinal education model, or clerkship, that integrates medical students as consistent members of a primary care team throughout the entirety of their medical school training [39]. Longitudinal clerkships in undergraduate medical education aim to provide ECMH experiences early in medical training [40]. Clerkships provide continuity of care between medical students, patients, and preceptors. This enables advantages in primary care education, such as the opportunity to learn about chronic care in an authentic setting and to participate in managing the presenting concerns of patients over time. Thus, the ECMH model achieves effective care delivery by emphasizing continuity as part of its mission [39]. Primary care physicians (PCPs) are considered the first point of contact for patients in accessing resources through the medical system [40]. Thus, it is important for PCPs to serve as an active gatekeeper, or quarterback, in appropriately managing presenting concerns while also referring patients to other specialists.

Innovative Ideas in Health Equity/Cultural Humility

Patient Safety

Ensuring patient safety is central to the practice of medicine. Traditionally one of the primary ways physicians, especially surgeons, address patient safety is through morbidity and mortality (M&M) conferences [41]. M&M conferences involve the discussion of cases with adverse events among peers and faculty, where attendees ask questions to promote learning opportunities so future adverse events in similar patient presentations can be avoided. M&M conferences have been a staple in surgical training programs since 1983, when the ACGME mandated their inclusion for residency training [41]. However, there is evidence that this traditional method of discussing patient safety leads to underreporting of complications, which in turn limits patient safety and educational opportunities [41].

It is estimated that 80% of all injuries are preventable, with certain types of errors relating to diagnosis, prescription, and medication administration causing the most adverse effects for patients [42]. Due to the high percentage of preventable error, there is a strong emphasis on curricula that focuses on patient safety in all training levels for medical professionals [42]. A comprehensive bibliometric analysis of nearly 600 papers identified five main areas of focus in patient safety education research: quality improvement of patient safety teaching and learning, patient safety teaching content, specialized teaching in patient safety, integrating patient safety and clinical teaching, and patient safety teaching assessment content [42]. This analysis showed that although substantial research exists on patient safety, gaps remain in implementing patient safety education particularly in medical schools and hospitals [42].

Improving integration of patient safety education is an important task to raise the level of patient care that is provided. There needs to be an effective way for medical trainees to appropriately identify and learn from adverse events during patient care so future events can be minimized. Faculty development, longitudinal research, and greater attention to cultural perspectives are a few ways in which patient safety education can be enhanced to ensure effective implementation [43].

Health Equity

Research revealed that priority and marginalized communities may have limited access or may not have equal access to the underlying technologies of digital health technologies (DHTs) [6]. Such studies emphasize the need for cultural considerations in health messaging and technologies. One scoping review identified 42 frameworks and 243 concepts related to digital health equity, underscoring both the complexity of the field and the need for consolidated definitions and frameworks [44]. Currently, there does not appear to be a standardized framework to model digital health equity, making consolidation and integration of existing frameworks an essential goal.

Once a cohesive framework is developed, its implementation may be relatively straightforward. One example is the Global Health Education for Equity, Anti-Racism, and Decolonization (GHEARD) curriculum, an open-access modular program designed to integrate equity, anti-racism, and decolonization into graduate medical education [45]. Pilot testing for this curriculum showed that it was effective in delivering its content and implementation was feasible [45]. Health equity in medical education is an important component for teaching the next generation of physicians. This is of high priority as currently, without health equity education, there are many marginalized populations that are facing systemic inequities in the field of medicine [46].

Another model is the Health Equity Implementation Framework (HEIF) which is a structured way for educators to assess and address equity when implementing evidence-based practices [47]. Within this model, three main domains of focus are emphasized: (1) the clinical encounter, (2) the societal context, and (3) culturally relevant factors [47]. This framework is one of the many options to provide equitable care. From the available research, integration of these frameworks and curricula appears relatively simple, and therefore, the first step is to develop a standardized curriculum that provides holistic education on systemic inequities and culturally competent care for patients of all backgrounds. For example, one study found that delivering 11 sessions to teach pediatric residents about how climate change impacts human health was successful in increasing understanding among the study population [48]. Additionally, even a single lecture can make a difference, as evidenced by a study that analyzed medical student reflections after one lecture on racial issues in psychiatry. A total of 108 third-year medical students were studied and students reported that the lecture enhanced their understanding of racism's role in psychiatry, its connection to social determinants of health, and its influence on clinical care [49].

Cultural Humility

Cultural humility is an essential component in medical education as it values a comprehensive approach and teaches medical professionals to communicate and work with patients who may have different cultural beliefs than their own [50]. Spiritual care is often not provided in the medical setting by physicians even though it is valued by patients [51]. Training residents to approach spirituality with cultural humility helps normalize spiritual care as part of comprehensive medical practice. This training does not have to be extensive and even one brief well-designed training for residents has been shown to highlight the value of integrating spiritual care into practice [51]. One particular longitudinal study of 120 preclinical medical students found that an art observation course maintained empathy levels, improved cultural self-efficacy, and increased tolerance for ambiguity [52]. These results suggest that integrating humanities into medical education fosters resilience, cultural sensitivity, and adaptability while supporting professional identity formation [52].

Therefore, integrating cultural humility is possible at any level of medical training, with a variety of approaches available for incorporating this knowledge into traditional medical school or residency curricula. Integrating cultural humility and related humanities earlier in medical education could help to foster the development of clinically competent and culturally aware physicians who are equipped to serve patients from diverse backgrounds. Cultural diversity education should be broadened to include lived experiences and systemic inequities to decolonize medical knowledge [53]. Emphasis should be placed on cultural humility, critical consciousness, and global perspectives [53]. Curricula should include historical, cultural, and experiential learning, as this would help increase empathy, self-reflection, and bias recognition among medical professionals [54]. Experiential learning method frameworks such as simulation-based training (SBT) and unconscious bias training (UBT) can offer practical strategies for improving competence around diversity issues [54]. One example in which programs could incorporate this type of education is by providing funding to pay members of the community to come into training clinics and be "patient actors" for training during scheduled simulation center days. Furthermore, multimodal approaches that are supported by institutional policies are necessary to ensure long-lasting, meaningful impacts on medical education [54]. These approaches ensure a more comprehensive education that incorporates viewpoints from diverse cultures.

Medical Decision-Making and Delivery of Optimized Care

An integral component of CDM is the conversation between the healthcare professional and the patient on the patient's medical history. Thus, CDM is intertwined with the concept of CR. Large language models (LLMs) have been shown to enhance CDM training for medical students through LLM-generated feedback that resulted in significant improvements in medical history gathering [11].

The implementation of LLMs into clinic workflows helps automate patient registration, billing, scheduling, and documentation [31]. This allows for more time for patient-centered activities. A pilot workshop aimed to evaluate two new low-cost surgical simulation models in a lower middle-income country [55]. Both simulators were ranked as "good" or outstanding" by the majority of workshop attendees and, thus, valued for their low-cost design and immersive design elements.

Innovative Ideas in Medical Specialties and Subspecialties

Telehealth

Despite some of the challenges posed in implementing telemedicine services, telemedicine has become a great alternative approach to access to healthcare for those in rural and remote areas of middle- and low-income countries. Telemedicine services can lower medical costs in comparison to specialized in-person care by 31% with its ability to provide a higher volume of consultations [56]. Healthcare is increasingly reliant on digital solutions such as telehealth, virtual health education, and patient portals. Thus, the utilization of digital health calls for the continuing need to develop unified conceptualizations of digital health equity that capture its complexity. Digital health equity, then, aims to provide communities with the information technology capacity that is needed for full participation in the economy with the highest level of health for all people [44]. An example of digital health equity is the approach of human-centered design (HCD). HCD generates empathetic and ethnographic-oriented insights and ideas for solutions to address complex medical problems [57]. HCDs are thought to complement other strategies within healthcare delivery, including patient-oriented research, quality improvement, and implementation science.

International studies highlighted the acceptance of telemedicine as a valuable tool in medical education. A study evaluating the impact of a pilot online learning platform (OLP) and standardized coaching program on the quality of medical student clinical skills found significant increases in recruitment and retention rates [58]. Both the OLP and standardized coaching program were well received, deemed feasible, and demonstrated efficacy in improving clinical skills using telemedicine. Virtual consults as part of telemedicine are often utilized for safe and effective patient care as well as for resident education [33]. Telemedicine also allows for medical students to perform structured video-based encounters with live patients who present to the emergency department (ED) to help aid in triaging. Ongoing, regulatory changes are essential in supporting safe and wide adoption of telehealth approaches. Thus, involving relevant stakeholders in addressing any current and potential future challenges, including logistical, technological, and financial barriers, is recommended for the success of the utilization of telemedicine [38].

Program initiatives and telemedicine curricula helped broaden the scope and accessibility of advance care planning (ACP) discussions, ensuring that healthcare remained aligned with patient values and goals. Studies have shown that ACP discussions can occur remotely, with tailored approaches to individual needs [59]. ACP can help foster better communication and understanding between healthcare professionals and patients, which ultimately can lead to more coordinated and compassionate care. However, there continues to be a need for ACP to be routine, adaptable, and patient-centered, and that future innovations be made to help facilitate those goals.

Telemedicine has played an important role in health and medicine education by providing insight into real-world scenarios while training appropriate medical skills. Despite telemedicine becoming integrated into medical curricula in the early 2000s, the teaching of telemedicine to medical students was still limited [60]. Training healthcare professionals in telemedicine requires a form of interactive and immersive teaching method. The use of telemedicine in both medical education and clinical delivery has substantially increased as a result of the removal from in-person clinical duties. However, the experiences with telemedicine have continued post-pandemic [61]. This suggests that the continued value of telemedicine is an integral part of the formal education of medical students and residents.

Telehealth in Psychological Services

To meet the needs of constantly growing mental health concerns, mental health providers have had to provide clinical services in novel ways. As a result of the COVID-19 pandemic, access to and training of psychological services has become increasingly difficult for both clients and providers. The use of telepsychology services pre-pandemic to post-pandemic has increased significantly, from about 7% to 85%, respectively [62]. A study surveying responses from psychology training directors, predoctoral internship trainees, and postdoctoral fellowship trainees at pediatric sites supported the changes in telepsychology training that was provided during the COVID-19 pandemic [62]. One major example of a resource that was a big undertaking to increase access to psychological services during the pandemic was PSYPACT. This resource is an interstate compact that aims at advancing the interjurisdictional practice of psychology by facilitating the practice of telepsychology across state boundaries. Given the ongoing need for telepsychology services to optimize access to psychological care, there continues to be a growing need for formal training in best practices for the utilization of telepsychology and telesupervision.

A study surveying predoctoral psychology interns and multidisciplinary staff members of an inpatient psychiatry unit highlighted short-term strategies to adapt clinical settings in delivering mental health services [63]. Modifications include redesigning existing virtual training models, utilization of video technology via iPads for simultaneous in-person rounds and virtual observations, and continued track-specific training that is held remotely. A continuing goal is to guide supervisors and trainees in adapting their psychology training programs to meet the evolving demands of telehealth services.

A big innovation that was not included in this book was psychology's role in GME. The ACGME put out new requirements for the inclusion of behavioral and mental health training for medical residents this year. The ACGME requirements involve four major rotations with a duration of 4 weeks for each rotation, including Adolescent Medicine, "mental health training," Developmental and Behavioral Pediatrics (DBP), and outpatient experience with no fewer than two subspecialties in the first 24 months of residency. Given that these new requirements include little-to-no details of what the rotations entail, there is currently no existing literature on the topic of behavioral and mental health training, and additional research and program development on this topic is needed.

Surgical Innovations

Efficient collaborative technological tools have been reported in a variety of specialties, such as surgery [33]. There is a continued demand for improved simulation training for surgical trainees and providers. The development of medical and surgical training centers can be expensive and time-consuming [55]. Low-cost simulation training models are valuable options to improve the level of competency training. Surgical simulation training allows for the objective, real-time feedback and assessment of learners' performance in a safe and standardized environment.

Lifestyle Medicine

Lifestyle medicine (LM) has gained attraction in promoting health among the general population. LM focuses on addressing six key areas of health: nutrition, physical activity, stress management, sleep health, social connection, and the avoidance of risky substances [64]. The integration of LM helps shift the medical paradigm toward holistic patient care, preparing future healthcare professionals for twenty-first century medical practice.

Integrating nutrition into medical curricula is crucial in increasing both medical educators' and students' level of competency in discussing and counseling patients on the topic of lifestyle medicine [65]. To be most effective in implementing lifestyle or nutrition medicine, education must be delivered as early as undergraduate medical curricula. It is important to incorporate a multidisciplinary approach in lifestyle or nutrition education to better understand the roles of each healthcare professional for a patient's nutritional care. Nutrition education should be embedded in a sociocultural framework to enhance patient-centered care and improve long-term health outcomes. Despite its growing evidence, LM is not widely practiced, particularly due to lack of provider knowledge and training on its adoption [66]. An online continuing medical education (CME) course centered around LM can help improve LM knowledge, confidence, attitudes, and practice.

Advantages of and Considerations for Innovation

Innovations in medical education strive to aim for better learning achievements for future and current healthcare professionals. Innovations in medical education provide the opportunity to enhance competency-based education, promote technological innovations, improve curricular and evaluation innovations, and emphasize emerging innovations [67]. New and emerging innovative ideas come with several advantages. Innovations have grown in acceptability across students, educators, and other professionals, increasing its frequency of use. Innovations hold a strong emphasis on active and collaborative learning, immersion and interaction with contents, and construction of experiences. Innovations often favor personalized, global education and the access to and self-management of learning, influencing the level of life-long learning. Innovations also facilitate the connection between formal and informal learning in safe environments between the student and patient care. Innovations can come in a multi-platform format and can enhance productivity, in which the platforms are used until one's level of competency is reached. Innovations also allow for real-time information, which results in greater satisfaction, enjoyable learning, and a stronger sense of motivation.

While there are several advantages to innovations in medical education and training, there are several components to consider with the utilization of such innovations [67]. The time and cost of such materials and the equipment acquisition can hinder the utilization of innovative technologies. Available resources, such as institutional support, may also be limited. As new technologies continue to quickly develop and evolve, their quality can be variable. As the field of healthcare has been around for many generations, a generational barrier may exist as healthcare professionals attempt to learn and stay up to date with the latest developments. Additionally, there may be some level of preoccupied ideas about or resistance to innovative changes. The complex concepts of generative AI and LLMs can be poorly understood and, thus, naturally introduces skepticism into its adoption [31].

Technological advancements are anticipated to continue growing and its challenges require ongoing attention [60]. Such challenges include the need for improved accessibility to relevant technologies as well as improved internet connectivity. Ethical challenges may arise, such as ensuring consent, confidentiality, and ownership of the material use. Institutional support, such as mentorship opportunities and user-friendly interfaces, is crucial in building confidence and competence for users of technological advancements. A new generation of online resources, such as SketchyMedical and Picmonic using visual learning mnemonics, has emerged to help with study preparations [68]. This new generation emphasizes the pedagogical innovations that evolves traditional study approaches. Librarians have been at the forefront of open access, educational resources, and courseware movements for universities and medical training institutions.

Efforts have been made through the American Medical Association (AMA) Innovation Grant Program to promote innovations in content areas including health systems science, competency-based medical education, and emerging technology [69]. Fifteen different proposals for innovations were funded in 2018, resulting in several published articles and presentations at national conferences. The next steps of the grant program involve examining the long-term outcomes of the completed innovation projects, the professional development of the grantees, and the dissemination of the innovations.

References

1. Tokuç B, Varol G. Medical education in the era of advancing technology. Balkan Med J. 2023;40(6):395–9. https://doi.org/10.4274/balkanmedj.galenos.2023.2023-7-79.
2. Rohani N, Gal K, Gallagher M, Manataki A. Providing insights into health data science education through artificial intelligence. BMC Med Educ. 2024;24(1):564. https://doi.org/10.1186/s12909-024-05555-3.
3. Thibault LP, Bourque CJ, Luu TM, Huot C, Cardinal G, Carriere B, Dupont-Thibodeau A, Moussa A. Residents as research subjects: balancing resident education and contribution to advancing educational innovations. J Grad Med Educ. 2022;14(2):191–200. https://doi.org/10.4300/JGME-D-21-00530.1.
4. Singaram VS, Pillay R, Mbobnda Kapche EL. Exploring the role of digital technology for feedback exchange in clinical training: a scoping review. Syst Rev. 2024;13(1):298. https://doi.org/10.1186/s13643-024-02705-y.
5. Tolentino R, Baradaran A, Gore G, Pluye P, Abbasgholizadeh-Rehimi S. Curriculum frameworks and educational programs in AI for medical students, residents, and practicing physicians: scoping review. JMIR Med Educ. 2024;10:e54793. https://doi.org/10.2196/54793.
6. Burns K, Bloom S, Gilbert C, Merner B, Kalla M, Sheri S, Villanueva C, Matenga Ikihele A, Nazer L, Sarmiento RF, Stevens L, Blow N, Chapman W. Centering digital health equity during technology innovation: protocol for a comprehensive scoping review of evidence-based tools and approaches. JMIR Res Protoc. 2024;13:e53855. https://doi.org/10.2196/53855.

7. Altintas L, Sahiner M. Transforming medical education: the impact of innovations in technology and medical devices. Expert Rev Med Devices. 2024;21(9):797–809. https://doi.org/10.1080/17434440.2024.2400153.
8. Mistry D, Brock CA, Lindsey T. The present and future of virtual reality in medical education: a narrative review. Cureus. 2023;15(12):e51124. https://doi.org/10.7759/cureus.51124.
9. Dhar P, Rocks T, Samarasinghe RM, Garth S, Smith C. Augmented reality in medical education: students' experiences and learning outcomes. Med Educ Online. 2021;26(1):1953953. https://doi.org/10.1080/10872981.2021.1953953.
10. Herrera-Aliaga E, Estrada LD. Trends and innovations of simulation of twenty first century medical education. Front Public Health. 2022;10:619769. https://doi.org/10.3380/fpubh.2022.619769.
11. Brügge E, Ricchizzi S, Arenbeck M, Keller MN, Schur L, Stummer W, Holling M, Lu MH, Darici D. Large language models improve clinical decision making of medical students through patient simulation and structured feedback: a randomized controlled trial. BMC Med Educ. 2024;24(1):1391. https://doi.org/10.1186/s12909-024-06399-7.
12. Challa KT, Sayed A, Acharya Y. Modern techniques of teaching and learning in medical education: a descriptive literature review. MedEdPublish. 2021;10:18. https://doi.org/10.15694/mep.2021.000018.1.
13. Garvin RD, Carney PA. Residency education redesign: the interplay of innovation and standardization. Fam Med. 2021;53(7):611–7. https://doi.org/10.22454/FamMed.2021.862031.
14. Khong ML, Tanner JA. Surface and deep learning: a blended learning approach in preclinical years of medical school. BMC Med Educ. 2024;24(1):1029. https://doi.org/10.1186/s12909-024-05963-5.
15. Groenier M, Spijkerboer K, Venix L, Bannink L, Yperlaan S, Eyck Q, van Manen JG, Miedema HAT. Evaluation of the impact of technical physicians on improving individual patient care with technology. BMC Med Educ. 2023;23(1):181. https://doi.org/10.1186/s12909-023-04137-z.
16. Archana S, Nilakantam SR, Hathur B, Dayananda M. The need and art of establishing skill and simulation centers to strengthen skill-based medical education: learning insights and experience. Ann Afr Med. 2021;20(4):247–54. https://doi.org/10.4103/aam.aam_53_20.
17. Velásquez ST, Ferguson D, Lemke KC, Bland L, Ajtai R, Amezaga B, Cleveland J, Ford LA, Lopez E, Richardson W, Saenz D, Zorek JA. Interprofessional communication in medical stimulation: findings from a scoping review and implications for academic medicine. BMC Med Educ. 2022;22(1):204. https://doi.org/10.1186/s12909-022-03226-9.
18. Elendu C, Amaechi DC, Okatta AU, Amaechi EC, Elendu TC, Ezeh CP, Elendu ID. The impact of simulation-based training in medical education: a review. Medicine (Baltimore). 2024;103(27):e38813. https://doi.org/10.1097/MD.0000000000038813.
19. Borg A, Georg C, Jobs B, Huss V, Waldenlind K, Ruiz M, Edelbring S, Skantze G, Parodis I. Virtual patient simulations using social robotics combined with large language models for clinical reasoning training in medical education: mixed methods study. J Med Internet Res. 2025;27:e63312. https://doi.org/10.2196/63312.
20. Guraya SY. Transforming simulation in healthcare to enhance interprofessional collaboration leveraging big data analytics and artificial intelligence. BMC Med Educ. 2024;24(1):941. https://doi.org/10.1186/s12909-024-05916.
21. Scott AE, Campbell KK, Carey J, Velez L, Ambardekar A, Scott DJ. Understanding ACGME standards for simulation: a document analysis of institutional and program requirements. J Grad Med Educ. 2024;16(6):691–700. https://doi.org/10.4300/JGME-D-24-00127.1.
22. Tran M, Balasooriya C, Jonnagaddala J, Leung GK, Mahbookbani N, Ramani S, Rhee J, Schuwirth L, Najafzadeh-Tabrizi NS, Semmler C, Wong ZS. Situating governance and regulatory concerns for generative artificial intelligence and large language models in medical education. NPJ Digit Med. 2025;8(1):315. https://doi.org/10.1038/s41746-025-01721-z.
23. Harrison JH, Gilbertson JR, Hanna MG, Olson NH, Seheult JN, Sorace JM, Stram MN. Introduction to artificial intelligence and machine learning for pathology. Arch Pathol Lab Med. 2021;145(10):1228–54. https://doi.org/10.5858/arpa.2020-0541-CP.

24. Almansour M, Soliman M, Aldekhyyel R, Binkheder S, Temsah MH, Malki KH. An academic viewpoint (2025) on the integration of generative artificial intelligence in medical education: transforming learning and practices. Cureus. 2025;17(3):e81145. https://doi.org/10.7759/cureus.81145.
25. Abid A, Murugan A, Banerjee I, Purkayastha S, Trivedi H, Gichoya J. AI education for fourth-year medical students: two-year experience of a web-based, self-guided curriculum and mixed methods study. JMIR Med Educ. 2024;10:e46500. https://doi.org/10.2196/46500.
26. Botha NN, Segbedzi CE, Dumahasi VK, Maneen S, Kodom RV, Tsedze IS, et al. Artificial intelligence in healthcare: a scoping review of perceived threats to patient rights and safety. Arch Public Health. 2024;82(1):188. https://doi.org/10.1186/s13690-024-01414-1.
27. Hallquist E, Gupta I, Montalbano M, Loukas M. Applications of artificial intelligence in medical education: a systematic review. Cureus. 2025;17(3):e79878. https://doi.org/10.7759/cureus.79878.
28. Kolachalama VB. Machine learning and pre-medical education. Artif Intell Med. 2022;129:102313. https://doi.org/10.1016/j.artmed.2022.102313.
29. Ehrmann D, Harish V, Morgado F, Rosella L, Johnson A, Mema B, Mazwi M. Ignorance isn't bliss: we must close the machine learning knowledge gap in pediatric critical care. Front Pediatr. 2022;10:864755. https://doi.org/10.3389/fped.2022.864755.
30. Mooney SD. Technology platforms and approaches for building and evaluating machine learning methods in healthcare. J Appl Lab Med. 2023;8(1):194–202. https://doi.org/10.1093/jalm/jfac113.
31. Kunze KN, Nwachukwu BU, Cote MP, Ramkumar PN. Large language models applied to health care tasks may improve clinical efficiency, value of care rendered, research, and medical education. Arthroscopy. 2025;41(3):547–56. https://doi.org/10.1016/j.arthro.2024.12.010.
32. Guldner G, Wells J, Ayutyanont N, Iyengar R, Sprenger S, Siegel JT, et al. COVID-19 related disruptions to medical education and perceived clinical capability of new resident physicians: a nationwide study of over 1200 first-year residents. Med Educ Online. 2023;28(1):2143307. https://doi.org/10.1080/10872981.2022.2143307.
33. Dedeilia A, Sotiropoulos MG, Hanrahan JG, Janga D, Dedeilias P, Sideris M. Medical and surgical education challenges and innovations in the COVID-19 era: a systematic review. In Vivo. 2020;34(3 Suppl):1603–11. https://doi.org/10.21873/invivo.11950.
34. Wilcha RJ. Effectiveness of virtual medical teaching during the COVID-19 crisis: systematic review. JMIR Med Educ. 2020;6(2):e20963. https://doi.org/10.2196/20963.
35. Burm S, Luong V, LaDonna K, Bogie B, Cowley L, Klasen JM, MacLeod A. From struggle to opportunity: reimagining medical education in a pandemic era. Perspect Med Educ. 2022;11(2):115–20. https://doi.org/10.1007/s40037-022-00702-2.
36. Kaul V, Gallo de Moraes A, Khateeb D, Greenstein Y, Winter G, Chae J, Stewart NH, Qadir N, Dangayach NS. Medical education during the COVID-19 pandemic. Chest. 2021;159(5):1949–60. https://doi.org/10.1016/j.chest.2020.12.026.
37. Ho PA, Girgis C, Rustad JK, Noordsy D, Stern TA. Advancing medical education through innovations in teaching during the COVID-19 pandemic. Prim Care Companion CNS Disord. 2021;23(1):20nr02847. https://doi.org/10.4088/PCC.20nr02847.
38. Badawy SM, Radovic A. Digital approaches to remote pediatric health care delivery during the COVID-19 pandemic: existing evidence and a call for further research. JMIR Pediatr Parent. 2020;3(1):e20049. https://doi.org/10.2196/20049.
39. Mesa AS, Tschoe M. Comparison of quality metrics in an education-centered medical home with local and national benchmarks. Med Educ Online. 2022;27(1):2073806. https://doi.org/10.1080/10872981.2022.2073806.
40. Henschen BL, Shaunfield S, Golden BP, Gard LA, Bierman J, Evans DB, Wayne DB, Ryan ER, Yang M, Cameron KA. From passive gatekeeper to quarterback: evolving perceptions of primary care among medical students in longitudinal outpatient clerkships. J Gen Intern Med. 2022;37(3):608–14. https://doi.org/10.1007/s11606-021-06914-2.

41. Johnson CR, Noorzad A, Pujari A, Paiement G, Lin C. There is an app for that: mobile technology improves complication reporting and resident perception of their role in patient safety. JB JS Open Access. 2021;6(1):e20.00077. https://doi.org/10.2106/JBJS.OA.20.00077.
42. Zhou L, Sun Y, Wang J, Huang H, Luo J, Zhao Q, Xiao M. Trends in patient safety education research for healthcare professional students over the past two decades: a bibliometric and content analysis. Med Educ Online. 2024;29(1):2358610. https://doi.org/10.1080/10872981.2024.2358610.
43. Aldardeir N, Abdullah QK, Jones L. Patient safety education in undergraduate medical education through a global lens: a scoping review. BMC Med Educ. 2025;25(1):544. https://doi.org/10.1186/s12909-025-07159.
44. Kim KK, Backonja U. Digital health equity frameworks and key concepts: a scoping review. J Am Med Inform Assoc. 2025;32(5):932–44. https://doi.org/10.1093/jamia/ocaf017.
45. Rule ARL, Haq HA, Barnes A, Bowen D, Chiume-Kayuni M, Cameron W, Fanny SA, Groothuis E, Hodge B, Howard C, Hudspeth JC, Langford S, McHenry MS, Opara IN, Kamath-Rayne BD, Suchdev PS, Tam RP, Taylor F, Musiime V. GHERD: an open-access modular curriculum to incorporate equity, anti-racism, and decolonization training into global health education. J Grad Med Educ. 2025;17(1):28–37. https://doi.org/10.4300/JGME-D-24-00264.1.
46. Bakunda L, Crooks R, Johnson N, Osei-Tutu K, Bharwani A, Gye E, Okoro D, Hinz H, Nearing S, Peer L, Kassam A, Smyth P, Chu P, Ruzycki S, Joneja M, Rabi D, Barnabe C, Roach P. Redefining professionalism to improve health equity in competency based medical education (CBME): a qualitative study. MedEdPublish. 2024;14:237. https://doi.org/10.12688/mep.20489.1.
47. Ramadurai D, Shea JA. Leveraging the health equity implementation framework to foster an equity focus in medical education. Adv Health Sci Educ Theory Pract. 2024;29(3):1047–58. https://doi.org/10.1007/s10459-023-10277-0.
48. Marwah H, Thapar I, McShane M, Silva GS, Goodhall H, Lewis N, Bottone PD, Hussain F. A longitudinal pediatric residency climate justice curriculum. J Grad Med Educ. 2024;16(6 Suppl):115–9. https://doi.org/10.4300/JGME-D-24-00058.1.
49. Pickerl P, Sorrell T, Blue M, Patterson K, Sheth N, Givens S. Racial issues in psychiatry: a thematic analysis of an initial health equity educational activity for medical students. BMC Med Ethics. 2025;26(1):53. https://doi.org/10.1186/s12910-025-01215-3.
50. Jones AC, Bertsch KN, Williams D, Channell MK. The tensegrity curriculum: a comprehensive curricular structure supporting cultural humility in undergraduate medical education. Adv Med Educ Pract. 2024;15:381–92. https://doi.org/10.2147/AMEP.S442569.
51. Drumright B, Sacro Y, Nussbaum A. Enriching spiritual care in medical residents through cultural humility and courage. MedEdPORTAL. 2024;20:11423. https://doi.org/10.15766/mep_2374-8265.11423.
52. Srinivasan S, Rachoin JS, Gentile M, Hunter K, Cerceo E. Empathy and cultural competence remains stable for medical students: do the humanities have an effect? BMC Med Educ. 2024;24(1):1301. https://doi.org/10.1186/s12909-204-06040-7.
53. Zanting A, Frambach JM, Meershoek A, Krumeich A. Exploring the implicit meanings of 'cultural diversity': a critical conceptual analysis of commonly used approaches in medical education. Adv Health Sci Educ Theory Pract. 2025;30(3):859–77. https://doi.org/10.1007/s10459-024-10371-x.
54. Linde P, Hallal H, Charkina P, Adams A, Frank J, Wegen S, Fan J, Nadjiri L, Zima H, Stosch C, Baues C. Diversity competence in medical education: short-term effectiveness of an interprofessional diversity-specific undergraduate learning. BMC Med Educ. 2025;25(1):226. https://doi.org/10.1186/s12909-025-06824-5.
55. Irfanullah EA, Chandra A, Solaiman RH, Siems C, Chethan S, Belani K, Harmon J. Simulation training in a lower middle-income country: supporting a new center and developing low-cost models for critical skill acquisition. Cureus. 2023;15(6):e40950. https://doi.org/10.7759/cureus.40950.

56. Alnasser Y, Proaño A, Loock C, Chuo J, Gilman RH. Telemedicine and pediatric care in rural and remote areas of middle-and-low-income countries: narrative review. J Epidemiol Glob Health. 2024;14(3):779–86. https://doi.org/10.1007/s44197-024-00214-8.
57. Levander XA, VanDerSchaaf H, Barragan VG, Choxi H, Hoffman A, Morgan E, Wong E, Wusirika R, Cheng A. The role of human-centered design in healthcare innovation: a digital health equity case study. J Gen Intern Med. 2024;39(4):690–5. https://doi.org/10.1007/s11606-023-08500-0.
58. Greengold J, Spahic H, Serwint J, Dlhosh S, Barouch L, Gattamorta K, Pahwa A, Hughes H. Novel educational strategies to improve the telemedicine clinical skills of medical students. Prim Health Care Res Dev. 2025;26:e10. https://doi.org/10.1017/S1463423625000040.
59. Mayers T, Sakamoto A, Inokuchi R, Hanari K, Ring HZ, Tamiya N. Situation, education, innovation, and recommendation: a large-scale systematic review of advance care planning in the age of COVID-19. Healthcare. 2024;12(6):667. https://doi.org/10.3390/healthcare12060667.
60. Ogundiya O, Rahman TJ, Valnarov-Boulter I, Young TM. Looking back on digital medical education over the last 25 years and looking to the future: narrative review. J Med Internet Res. 2024;26:e60312. https://doi.org/10.2196/60312.
61. Henschen BL, Jasti H, Kisielewski M, Pincavage AT, Levine D. Teaching telemedicine in the COVID-19 era: a national survey of internal medicine clerkship directors. J Gen Intern Med. 2021;36(11):3497–502. https://doi.org/10.1007/s11606-021-07061-4.
62. Frye WS, Feldman M, Katzenstein J, Gardner L. Modified training experiences for psychology interns and fellows during COVID-19: use of telepsychology and telesupervision by child and adolescent training programs. J Clin Psychol Med Settings. 2022;29(4):840–8. https://doi.org/10.1007/s10880-021-09839-4.
63. Stein MB, O'Keefe S, Mace R, Foley JD, White AE, Ruchensky JR, Curtiss J, Moran E, Evans C, Beck S. Psychology internship training amidst COVID-19: balancing training opportunities, patient care, and risk of exposure. J Clin Psychol Med Settings. 2023;30(1):61–71. https://doi.org/10.1007/s10880-022-09890-9.
64. Bansal S, Shubrook JH. Pioneering the future: incorporating lifestyle medicine tools in osteopathic medical education. J Osteopath Med. 2025. https://doi.org/10.1515/jom-2024-0121.
65. Xie JY, Abramovich N, Burridge J, Jaffee A, Broadley I. Nutrition education in core medical curricula: a call to action from tomorrow's doctors. Future Healthc J. 2021;8(1):19–21. https://doi.org/10.7861/fhj.2020-0207.
66. Ames ML, Staffier KL, Kees A, Freeman K, Shetty P, Gittelsohn J, Karlsen MC. Online lifestyle medicine continuing medical education (CME) course completion predicts increases in clinician knowledge, confidence, and practice of lifestyle medicine. Am J Lifestyle Med. 2024:15598276241279523. https://doi.org/10.1177/15598276241279523.
67. Lifshitz-Guinzberg A, Abreu-Hernández LF, Sepúlveda-Vildósola AC, Urrutia-Aguilar ME, Córdova-Villalobos JA, López-Bárcena J, Sánchez-Mendiola M. Pros and cons of innovations in medical education. Gac Med Mex. 2021;157(3):325–34. https://doi.org/10.24875/GMM.M21000568.
68. O'Hanlan R, Laynor G. Responding to a new generation of proprietary study resources in medical education. J Med Libr Assoc. 2019;107(2):251–7. https://doi.org/10.5195/jmla.2019.619.
69. Santen SA, Van Rite E, Hammoud M, Lomis KD, Elliott VS, Heckman K, Andrews JS, Ayala SB, Richardson J. Supporting medical education innovation: evaluation of a grants initiative. Acad Med. 2023;98(10):1159–63. https://doi.org/10.1097/ACM.0000000000005279.

New and Innovative Ideas in Medical Education

Definitions and Introduction to Medical Innovation

Peter T. Le and Cheryl A. Dickson

Definition of Medical Innovation

Medical innovation encompasses a broad definition of products, processes, ideas, technologies, and systems that improve health care through modalities such as patient satisfaction, efficiency, and accessibility [1]. Medical innovations often overlap with other disciplinary fields such as artificial intelligence, biotechnology, and business. For now, we will look at 3 focuses of medical innovation: clinical, technological, and entrepreneurial innovation.

Clinical innovation refers to changes in the interactions between clinicians and their patients [2]. This can be through changes in patient care methodology (e.g., guidelines), implementations of multidisciplinary teams, or even federal programs that influence hospital and physicians' decisions. Ultimately, these changes hope to improve patients' quality of life, patient satisfaction, and even survival.

Technological innovation, on the other hand, is the incorporation of new technologies or significant improvements of existing ones, leading to advancements in the products and services provided by the healthcare sector [3]. This includes both hardware and software components that have led to better patient outcomes and allowed the delivery of health care to be more efficient. Technological innovation has become one of the most exciting medical evolutions in the past decade. With the incorporation of AI, new processors, and hardware technology, many specialties

P. T. Le
Western Michigan University Homer Stryker M.D. School of Medicine, Kalamazoo, MI, USA
e-mail: peter.le@wmed.edu

C. A. Dickson (✉)
Department of Pediatric and Adolescent Medicine, Western Michigan University Homer Stryker M.D. School of Medicine, Kalamazoo, MI, USA
e-mail: cheryl.dickson@wmed.edu

S. S. Chahin et al. (eds.), *Innovation in Medical Education and Clinical Practice*, https://doi.org/10.1007/978-3-032-19116-8_2

like Ophthalmology and Radiology have become rapidly evolving fields that require physicians to be up to date with the newest gadgets [4, 5].

At its core definition, entrepreneurial innovation` refers to implementing new ideas, processes, or products through a business scope that ultimately creates unique value while also providing a competitive advantage. Although medicine should not be viewed as a business chasing profit, many ideas from a business model have proven fruitful in patient innovation [6]. Many of our surgical centers run in a procedural fashion (much like a business), and optimizing surgical procedures without compromising patient care allows for more patients to be operated on, decreases physician work hours and burnout, and can reduce the overall strain on the healthcare system [7, 8]. This is because proper optimization can reduce waiting times for patients who may need life-changing surgery, will allow physicians to operate on more patients in a shorter amount of time, and should ultimately lead to reduced overtime hours needed by the surgical staff.

Framework of Medical Innovation

Medical innovation is a unique, complex process that requires multidisciplinary input to transform creative ideas into tangible improvements in patient care. While the pathway from concept to clinical adoption will differ for each case of innovation, most medical innovations follow a general framework consisting of different stages of production. Having a general understanding of this framework is important for healthcare professionals, inventors, and policymakers who may be involved in medical innovation in the future.

1. Idea Brainstorming
    - Every medical innovation starts with an idea. Many come from novel solutions inspired by clinical challenges, unmet consumer needs, or advancements in scientific knowledge or technology. These may arise from frontline healthcare workers noticing gaps in patient care (diagnosis and treatment), researchers discovering new biological mechanisms, or technological upgrades and breakthroughs. At this stage, innovators need to clearly define what the problem is, propose innovations to address the problem, and research how their intervention has the potential to impact patient care, safety, or efficiency.
    - Once the idea has been generated and refined, innovators will pitch their ideas to investors or collaborations that can provide resources such as funding, expertise, or infrastructure. Oftentimes, this required crafting a compelling proposition, conducting market research, and early data supporting their idea. Many innovators find their investors and collaborators through pitch meetings, innovation competitions, or connections with venture capital firms or academic hospitals.

2. Prototype Development

    - Once enough support has been secured, innovators will develop their first prototypes. These will be early working models that demonstrate the core function of the innovation; however, it is expected that there will be pitfalls, glitches, and errors. Prototypes serve several purposes that include identifying design flaws, determining the feasibility of implementation, and gauging user experience. For medical devices, this may include building the hardware and testing whether certain materials meet quality control measures. For drugs, it may involve synthesizing candidate molecules and determining their biosafety. For digital health tools, it may include beta testing software versions and looking for possible security flaws within the software architecture.
    - This phase can become quite repetitive and is often where most innovations get stuck. Because of the complexity of most medical innovations, most feedback loops involve an interdisciplinary team involving engineers, clinicians, regulation experts, patients, and potentially government policymakers. Testing may also try simulating real-life scenarios through lab environments, animal models, or even standardized clinical encounters. An iterative feedback loop is important as this allows the prototype to evolve from a simple concept with multiple flaws to a reliable, manufacturable, and scalable product that meets the needs of the market. Once the product has matured, intellectual property protection (trademarks) and cost modeling are formulated.

3. Clinical Trials and Evaluation

    - Medical innovations are unique in the fact that they are intended for human use and that any errors have serious consequences. Hence, clinical trials have become the cornerstone of validating these medical inventions as they are structured studies that assess the safety, efficacy, dosing, and side effects in large samples meant to simulate the intended patient population. Generally, trials progress through different phases [9]:

        - Phase 1—Small patient groups testing for the safety of the innovation or dosage of the drug.
        - Phase 2—Medium-sized patient groups that evaluate the efficacy of the innovation of the possible side effects of the drug.
        - Phase 3—Large, randomized controlled trials that confirm statistical effectiveness and monitor the severity of adverse drug reactions.

    With clinical trials, data must be rigorously collected and analyzed to determine the meaningful clinical benefit that the innovation offers. These benefits are then compared to the risks associated with the innovation, and analysis is used to determine if the pros outweigh the cons. If it is determined that the pros do not outweigh the cons, then innovators revert back to the Prototype Development Phase, where they take the new information and make necessary modifications in their design or protocol. On the other hand, if the pros outweigh the cons, then the product is almost ready to be introduced into the market and must undergo regulatory approval.

4. Regulations and Approval

    - Given the substantial impact on human health and also the potential breach of patient privacy, medical innovators must comply with strict regulations set by federal agencies. Agencies like the FDA in the United States or the EMA in Europe help oversee the approval process for medical products. This includes reviewing the data from clinical trials, investigating manufacturing practices, analyzing product blueprints, and confirming post-market surveillance plans. Examples of these procedures include new drug applications (NDAs) for medications, and premarket approval (PMA) or clearance (501(k)) for medical devices.
    - Regulatory compliance is important as it protects patients, ensuring that the products are up to safety and quality standards. This also provides a framework to monitor adverse events in case something goes wrong once the product enters the market. Regulation approval can prove to be quite tedious as this requires detailed documentation, more extensive testing, and constant communication with regulatory authorities. Furthermore, innovators must also align with laws safeguarding patient data and ethics, such as HIPAA.

5. The Idea Is Introduced to the Market

    - Once approval is granted by regulatory agencies, the innovation is able to enter the market. Despite the tedious testing done through clinical trials and the agency regulations, the product is usually gradually adopted into the market. Implementation of the product usually occurs in well-funded areas. This includes well-resourced academic medical centers or clinics located in urban areas. This allows clinicians who are usually apt to implement innovation and are experts in the field of interest to assess and incorporate these new technologies in their practice. These clinicians become the "early adopters" who play a critical role in validating the real-world benefits, identifying additional challenges in workflow integration, and generating additional evidence for the manufacturer. These clinicians also influence other healthcare providers as their recommendations bring credit to the validity of the product.
    - In addition to marketing toward these early adopters, training programs, user support systems, and feedback are vital at this stage of production. Therefore, manufacturers work closely with healthcare providers to collect post-market data, which will allow them to further refine the product and create user guidelines. Once final changes are made, conversations with insurance companies begin, which focus on insurance reimbursement and cost-effective analysis based on broader accessibility.

6. Widespread Accessibility and Standardization
    - If there is a successful introduction to the market, the innovation will shift its focus to providing wider accessibility. This includes optimization in the manufacturing process, reductions in production costs, and increased clinical acceptance in community hospitals, outpatient centers, and low-resource settings. At this point, professional societies and guidelines committees start incorporating the innovation into clinical protocols, leading to more standardization of the product.
    - Furthermore, educational initiatives are made to target a broader audience. This includes physicians outside of academic hospitals and other clinicians, such as nurses. This builds competence and confidence when using the innovation to treat patients. With time, the innovation transforms from a new technology to the norm for the standard of care. Although, at this point, innovators can consider their product "finalized," many continue to have open feedback and post-market surveillance to ensure a high standard of quality, safety, and efficacy, and also to make iterative improvements for the next-generation versions of their product.

Drivers of Medical Innovation

Medical innovation is propelled by a combination of factors that motivate inventors, funders, policymakers, and clinicians to develop new solutions aimed at improving patient outcomes, improving healthcare delivery, and improving healthcare efficacy. Oftentimes, these drivers overlap or intertwine with one another, creating a dynamic ecosystem that drives creativity and accelerates the implementation of new ideas into clinical practice. Below are key drivers that shape the landscape of current medical innovation.

Unmet Clinical Needs

- The basis of any medical innovation attempts to solve problems that current medical knowledge, technologies, or current practices cannot adequately address. These unmet clinical needs may arise from new diseases, limitations with current treatments, or disparities in healthcare access and quality. For example, common chronic diseases such as diabetes, heart failure, and neurodegenerative diseases present ongoing challenges in patients due to their untreatable natures and patient variability. Innovations in medicine, such as glucose monitors, cardiac pacemakers, and personalized medications, have emerged directly as a response to prevent worsening of the disease course or even prevent disease onset [10–12].

- Input from frontline physicians is often the earliest ideas of innovation, which are due to their first-line position to identify unmet needs through their day-to-day patient interactions. Their input is vital as it highlights real-world gaps in diagnosis, therapy, or care coordination. Moreover, they act as a bridge for patient communication and feedback. An example of their importance can be seen through traditional insulin delivery methods. Due to poor patient adherence with insulin injections, physician input helped with the development of insulin pumps and smart pens, which ultimately improved the effectiveness of insulin [13].
- Furthermore, physicians are able to provide input related to patient safety. For instance, due to their oversight in the hospital, physicians have identified causes of hospital-acquired infections and medication errors. With their first-hand experience, they have helped develop innovations in infection control protocols, barcode medication systems, and clinical decision algorithms. Having physicians play the role of recognizing and articulating these essential needs through first-hand experiences is essential for gaining support for innovation.

Technological Advances

- Technological evolution has served as both a catalyst and driver of medical innovation. Evolutions in fields such as molecular biology, information technology, and artificial intelligence offer new tools, platforms, and scientific knowledge that expand the current clinical information available for healthcare providers and patients. A notable example of this is the innovation of next-generation sequencing technologies that have changed the way the medical field views genomics. Technologies like this allow clinicians to rapidly decode a patient's DNA in an affordable manner, which opens up the field of precision medicine [14, 15].
- Artificial Intelligence and machine learning algorithms have transformed medical imaging by improving the accuracy of medical diagnosis, and can also act as an assistant when interpreting X-rays, MRIs, and pathology slides, reducing medical errors [16–18].
- Nanotechnology has enabled targeted drug delivery systems that improve drug effectiveness while reducing adverse side effects seen in typical liposomal chemotherapy agents [19, 20].
- New breakthroughs in material sciences have created new biocompatible implants that mimic human physiology, leading to new venues of innovation in regenerative medicine.
- One thing to note with these examples is that most of the technological innovation occurs outside of the healthcare sector (telecommunications, engineering, consumer electronics). However, many innovators are able to adapt these

advancements into medicine, which opens new avenues for innovation. For example, the creation of miniature sensors and compact batteries has influenced the development of handheld monitors and implantable technologies.

Economic Incentives

- Like many other fields, financial motivation is one of the most influential factors that drive innovation. In market-driven healthcare systems, companies and investors look for innovations that offer a competitive advantage that is also profitable. Therefore, it should be no surprise that patents and intellectual property rights play a role in driving innovation, as they protect investments and also bring market exclusivity.
- Furthermore, due to the potential for profits in market shares and revenues, particularly in areas where there is lack of a solution and innovation can replace the existing standard of care, funding from venture capital and private equity funding can provide motivation for innovation. A recent example of this came with the biotech boom over the last two decades. Due to the success in gene therapies and novel drug delivery systems, significant investments have been made into healthcare companies focusing on these innovations.
- Besides investment from the public market, governments and non-profit organizations can also provide resources through grants, subsidies, and prize funds. Government programs are also providing payment models that reward value-based care, which further incentivize innovations that improve outcomes while reducing costs. Examples of this include remote patient monitoring, preventive health technologies, and antibiotic stewardship programs.
- Although, for the majority of the time, economic incentives improve patient outcomes, they can sometimes misalign with public health priorities. This can lead to challenges such as high drug prices or minimal research in diseases that are extremely rare. More effort needs to be placed in addressing this issue through policy interventions, as there should be a balance between innovation incentives and equitable healthcare access.

Regulation and Policy Shifts

- Government policies and regulations can play a role in driving medical innovation as they set safety and efficacy standards, protect patient rights, and control access to patient health records. The FDA can influence the pace and direction of innovation through approval or rejection of pathways with guidance documents.

For example, the FDA's Breakthrough Therapy designation (an expedited approval mechanism) has accelerated access to promising drugs for serious diseases [21].
- The FDA oversees policies that promote data interoperability and privacy protection, which can be another driver where digital health innovations can evolve and adapt.

Patient Advocacy and Empowerment

- Patient feedback is extremely valuable when it comes to accessing health care. Therefore, it is vital that they become active partners and drivers of innovation. Due to the technological evolution, patients now have greater access to medical information and digital health tools. Empowered with their greater access to medical information, patient advocacy groups have influenced research priorities, regulatory decisions, and clinical trials.
- Advocacy organizations can raise funds to support research for a specific disease, lobby for accelerated approvals, and collaborate with innovators to ensure that patient needs are met. Due to the rise in patient-reported outcomes and personal health data, innovations have shifted to prioritize precision medicine. Moreover, patient empowerment has fostered a team-based approach where decision-making and creation of health technologies not only include the "traditional" innovators, but also the consumers.

Global Health Changes

- Global health crises and long-term demographic changes can exert pressure on healthcare systems to rapidly innovate on a worldwide scale. A prime example of this is with COVID-19, which triggered unprecedented collaboration between different countries, scientists, world leaders, and biotech companies to rapidly develop a vaccine, create new diagnostic guidelines, and expand telecommunications [22].
- Due to healthcare advancements, the average life expectancy has increased to about 78.4 years [23]. As a result, the aging population in many countries has placed an increased demand for chronic disease management, long-term care technologies, and age-friendly healthcare delivery models. Moreover, the rising burdens of non-communicable diseases in resource-limited countries motivate the development of inexpensive and scalable technologies specifically for these populations.

- Due to the growing health disparities, addressing health inequalities also inspires innovation through mobile clinics, digital platforms, and task-shifting strategies that extend care to the underserved population. Global organizations such as the World Health Organization call for universal health coverage and help drive policy change through funding, further supporting innovations that improve affordability and accessibility.

Examples of Medical Innovation

Because the three focuses of medical innovation we discussed above are so broad, it should be no surprise that many examples we see in medicine today can encompass more than one field of innovation. Here, we will briefly discuss historical examples of medical innovation in the past.

Therapeutic Drugs

- The first antibiotic (penicillin) was discovered by Dr. Alexander Fleming in 1928 [24]. As science became more advanced and different spectrums of antibiotics were being formulated, treatments of infectious diseases became revolutionized, saving many lives and extending the average life expectancy of a human. As the use of antibiotics became widespread, biotech companies became more efficient at formulating them, causing the price of antibiotics to become more accessible to the general population. For example, penicillin prices when first formulated hovered around $20 per dose; currently, it hovers around $0.40 per dose (not accounting for inflation) [25].
- A notable example of clinical innovation seen in the context of therapeutic drugs is how our healthcare system views the use of antibiotics. Particularly, as more research uncovers the mechanisms of certain antibiotics and how bacterial strains respond to these drugs, the topic of antibiotic resistance has become a large concern, with the CDC labeling it as an urgent global public health threat [26]. Antibiotic resistance becomes problematic since it places a larger burden on our healthcare system and takes the lives of millions of people worldwide. Fortunately, programs like the antibiotic stewardship program have coordinated an effort to optimize antibiotic use in hospitals by improving antibiotic use monitoring, following up-to-date evidence-based guidelines that suggest narrow-spectrum antibiotics, and implementing a multidisciplinary team made up of physicians, pharmacists, nurses, and infection control specialists [27]. Ultimately, efforts like these reduce resistance, side effects, and healthcare-associated infections, with papers even showing reduced Clostridium difficile infections and improved patient outcomes [28].

- One recent innovation that many of us have witnessed come to light is the invention of the first mRNA vaccine genetically modified to encode the spike protein of SARS-CoV-2 [29]. This reflects the leaps in technological evolution, as researchers were able to create a paradigm shift in how we view vaccines, because, unlike traditional vaccines, mRNA vaccines allow for a more rapid and targeted immune response. Furthermore, due to rapid mutations of the viruses, researchers are now able to fine-tune the vaccine based on its evolving genomic data [30]. With the case of COVID-19, we see why technological innovation is important in society, as COVID-19 vaccines were developed within 10 months of genome publication, created vaccines that are safer for patients, as no actual viral pathogens are exposed to patients, and opened up new doors for genomic modification for patient-specific therapies.

Medical Devices and Wearables

- In 1816, René Laennec created what many considered to be the first modern medical device, the stethoscope [31]. This allowed physicians to better assess a patient's health by amplifying sounds, leading to better diagnosis of cardiovascular, pulmonary, and gastrointestinal abnormalities. Although it's been over 200 years since the invention of the stethoscope, no major invention has replaced it or drastically changed the way it has been used in the medical field. This is quite evident as it is the main tool that many medical students and doctors carry with them when visiting patients. However, there have been innovations that have optimized how a stethoscope is used.
  - Physicians used to manually measure blood pressure by inflating blood pressure cuffs and using the stethoscope to listen to the first Korokoff sound (systolic pressure) and the last sound (diastolic pressure). Because of this, there was the possibility of human error as different noise environments may have affected when physicians heard a change in sound, and readings of the barometers could be inconsistent between providers. In 1976, Dinamap produced the first commercially available automatic blood pressure monitor. This helped remove user error, optimized how quickly blood pressure could be measured, and made it more accessible (in both clinical but also personal use at home settings) [32].
  - In the future, a Digital Stethoscope (like the Eko Core) may become the mainstream stethoscope used among the medical community. These are particularly beneficial as they can use technology to filter out background noise and amplify specific sounds, improving the clarity of auscultation [33]. Furthermore, these stethoscopes can transmit sounds wirelessly, possibly allowing for remote consultations and monitoring, which would be extremely beneficial for patients in remote areas or those with mobility restrictions. Furthermore, many companies are starting to integrate AI algorithms to

analyze these sounds and assist in diagnosis, which helps clinicians determine potential issues earlier on in the disease course.

- As society shifts from treating symptoms to treating the underlying cause of disease, a higher focus is being placed on preventive medicine. The effectiveness of preventive medicine places a large emphasis on patient involvement in their care. Giving patients control over their health has become a trend of many technological companies (especially ones that aren't traditionally involved in the healthcare sector), like Apple, Google, Samsung, etc. These companies have made handheld devices (like watches) that can track vitals such as heart rate, blood pressure, respiratory rate, blood oxygenation, wrist temperature, sleep duration, and even possibly ECGs [34]. Furthermore, the apps these companies have made can present this information in real time to patients in an easy-to-understand manner and provide suggestions for their lifestyle. These tech companies have also seemed to gamify health, allowing you to set daily goals and to compete with friends and family based on the number of steps taken per day, calories burned, minutes exercising, etc. Overall, since the introduction of consumer-focused handheld devices, many doctors are recommending this technology to patients as it gives them more autonomy over their health and allows them to be more engaged in healthy habits.
- Point-of-care ultrasound (POCUS) represents one of the most transformative medical device innovations of the twenty-first century. Traditional ultrasounds are bulky; however, innovation has miniaturized this technology while also implementing cloud computing and wireless capabilities, causing ultrasound devices to become more portable, affordable, and user-friendly while providing similar accuracy [35]. Modern handheld devices like Butterfly Network and GE's Vscan are starting to integrate AI-assisted interpretation tools, which have shown promise in assisting users in image interpretation [36]. Ultimately, these improvements allow clinicians to share live imaging with specialists remotely, which can make medical training more accessible and provide better quality of care in low-resource settings [37].

Medical Equipment

- Innovations in medical hardware have also been used to change the way we diagnose and treat patients. In the 1970s, Dr. Damadian published a groundbreaking paper in Science about the use of magnetic resonance imaging (MRI) in cancer detection [38]. Keep in mind that before medicine, MRIs had industrial applications in the material sciences field. Nowadays, MRIs have become an integral part of diagnosis in many major hospitals, allowing physicians to rapidly diagnose emergent soft tissue diseases that may require immediate resolution. Moreover, MRIs have become a routine part of cancer screenings, allowing physicians to diagnose and control cancer before it becomes metastatic. With these innovations in hardware, diagnostic tools like X-ray machines, CT scanners, MRI machines, ultrasounds, PET scanners, etc. have created the field of radiology and are used every day, allowing us to diagnose patients with higher accuracy and before symptoms become severe.

- Over the past two decades, one of the most transformative advances in surgical care was the creation of the Da Vinci Surgical System. The Da Vinci is a marvel of engineering that combines the interdisciplinarity of surgical work and robotic precision. This has redefined the possibilities of minimally invasive surgery since the Da Vinci System provides benefits for both patients and surgeons. With patients, due to its tools' small footprint and robotic precision, smaller incisions are made, leading to less scarring, which has been shown to reduce the risk of infection and pain/discomfort. This has also led to quicker recovery times and fewer post-surgery complications, particularly those involving nerve-sparing techniques [39]. For surgeons, programs in the Da Vinci Surgical System can filter out tremors, provide greater ranges of motion with instruments, magnify the surgical field with better depth perception and resolution, and can also improve access to difficult-to-reach anatomical spaces [40]. Funny enough, it also provides surgeons with better comfort as they can operate from a seated console, which has been shown to reduce physical strain and fatigue, especially in long, complex procedures.

Digital Health

- In the 1960s, hospitals began experimenting with storing patient information electronically to improve record-keeping. Although inconvenient due to limitations in computing and database technology, it slowly started being incorporated at larger hospitals. The early 2000s marked the turning point for policy-driven adoption of Electronic Health Records (EHRs) as the United States introduced the HITECH Act of 2009, which offered financial incentives for adopting and using certified Electronic Medical Records (EMRs). Since then, EMRs have become the norm for patient documentation and provide benefits for providers as they organize patient data in a predictable manner and allow for interoperability and real-time data sharing across healthcare systems [41].
- Since the 1870s, when the telephone was first invented, it has slowly become incorporated in medical communication. In the 1960s, NASA developed telemedicine capabilities that allowed physicians to monitor astronauts' health in space [42]. Since the early twentieth century, telemedicine has been mainly used for remote medical advice in rural and military settings. However, there was a surge in telemedicine during the COVID-19 pandemic when public health restrictions prevented traditional doctor visits. Since then, COVID-19 has accelerated the adoption of telemedicine, with options of video consultations and remote patient monitoring provided by most clinics [43].

Stakeholders Involved in the Innovation Ecosystem

The medical innovation ecosystem comprises a dynamic, multifaceted network of individuals, organizations, and institutions that all play a collective role in guiding an innovation from its concept to clinical adoption. Innovations rarely happen with just a single individual or team. In fact, it requires collaboration between diverse stakeholders, each bringing unique perspectives, expertise, and resources when developing a concept. Understanding the roles and motivations of certain stakeholders is critical for anyone who is interested in bringing a new medical idea to the market.

Clinicians

- Physicians, nurses, physician assistants, and other healthcare providers are considered to the frontline in medical treatment. They are also often the first to identify unmet needs based on their direct interactions with patients. Not only can they act as a messenger for patients' needs, but they also bring technical knowledge about disease presentation, workflow dynamics, and real-world metrics of current treatments. Their unique position as direct providers with their scientific background makes them essential contributors when it comes to assessing innovative ideas, providing prototype feedback, and adopting new innovations.
- In innovation, clinicians can play the role of
  - Inventors—Develop tools and protocols to solve problems based on issues they see in their daily practice.
  - Advisors—Offer counseling to innovators who lack clinical experience and are trying to break into the healthcare sector.
  - Gatekeepers—Determine if innovations are feasible to implement into their practice, and are early adopters of new ideas.
  - Leaders—Advocate innovations toward their colleagues, accelerating the adoption of the innovation to become the norm in health care.

Patients

- In the recent decade, patients have increasingly become more and more involved in the innovation process. Given the emphasis on health in our society, patients are no longer passive recipients of care but instead are active participants in changing healthcare solutions. They provide essential feedback on the feasibility of services, accessibility of innovations, and impacts on their quality of life. It is important to involve patients when creating healthcare solutions, as it is ultimately their lives that are going to be impacted.

- In innovation, patients can play the role of
  - Feedback providers—Provide feedback based on their anecdotal experiences, which can help guide product modifications and influence priorities set by innovators.
  - Clinical Trial Subjects—Participate in clinical trials to help with testing for the safety and efficacy of new inventions.
  - Advocates—Voice public opinion on policies or the needs of the public, which can facilitate faster access to new therapies and medications.
  - Co-inventors—Kickstart development of tools and protocols based on problems they witness in their lived experiences.

Researchers

- Researchers play a foundational role in understanding the biology that makes medical innovation possible. Many work within academic universities, government-sponsored laboratories, or privately sponsored research companies. Research that contributes to innovation can span from basic research in biochemical pathways to translation research that transitions from animal research into human clinical trials to applied research that focuses on refining technologies that are currently being used.
- In innovation, research can play the role of
  - Integrators—Researchers often partner with clinicians and industry workers to move concepts from bench work to clinical experiences.
  - Corroborator—Due to their scientific background, researchers can statistically analyze and generate evidence that supports an innovation's safety, efficiency, and cost-effectiveness.
  - Inventor—Given that many researchers are at the forefront of scientific discovery, it is no surprise that any breakthrough findings place researchers as one of the forefront drivers of innovation.

Entrepreneurs

- Entrepreneurs act as the backbone for innovative concepts. They allow products to be scalable and sustainable. Specifically, they provide resources and focus on the business management processes needed to commercialize medical technologies.

- In innovation, entrepreneurs can play the role of
  - Startups—Entrepreneurs can pitch their new products to the market, leading to increased funds, employment recruitment, and public name recognition.
  - Fundraisers—Entrepreneurs can navigate fundraising means of venture capital, public markets, and government grants.

One thing to note is that many biotechnology entrepreneurs consider themselves "clinical-entrepreneurs" who combine medical expertise with business, ensuring that their solutions are both clinically relevant and business-driven. This is because it is harmful to label medical inventions as solely for-profit endeavors.

Industry (Pharmaceuticals, Medical Technology, Diagnostics)

- Established Medical Industry Companies are critical innovations to pass production for global distribution. Their experience with previous innovations quickens the process of integrating an idea into day-to-day practice.
- In innovation, industry giants contribute
  - Manufacturing capacity with experience in quality control systems.
  - Distribution networks that can reach global markets.
  - Regulation expertise for processes that require government approval.
  - Marketing and sales infrastructure.

Given the dominance that certain Biotech companies have on the market share of medical innovation (Johnson & Johnson, Roche, Novartis, Merck, AbbVie, etc.), most innovations that have exited their early stages of development are acquired by these companies, leading to an optimized implementation of innovation into large-scale markets.

Regulators (FDA, EMA, etc.)

- Regulatory agencies prioritize public health and do so by ensuring that new medical products meet rigorous standards before entering the market. They can also influence guidelines for manufacturing, labeling, marketing, and post-marketing surveillance.
- In medical innovation, regulators play the role of
  - Authenticators—Regulators evaluate evidence from preclinical and clinical studies and ensure that results are accurate and can do minimal harm when the product is brought to the market.
  - Gatekeepers—Regulators can approve or reject new drugs, devices, and diagnostics based on their efficacy and adverse effects.
  - Managers—Regulators can establish compliance frameworks that allow for ongoing monitoring and feedback.

Investors

- Investors play the most indirect role in innovation. They provide the financial resources needed to move an idea from its concept to commercialization. Given the high-cost environment of medical innovation, investors are not just financiers, but are strategic partners who can influence timelines and market strategies, as many want to see a return on their investment.

Limitations of Innovation

While there is no doubt that medical innovation has changed modern medicine, the journey from concept to clinical adoption has limitations that have led many innovators to abandon their projects. Although most limitations can be sourced from technical problems, they can also emerge from economic hardships, human behavior, regulatory frameworks, and societal views.

- Funding and investment hurdles
  - With the rigorous standards that medical products must follow, medical innovation can be an expensive task. Expenses can include the high cost of labor, skilled personnel, regulatory submissions, and large-scale clinical trials. Hence, there is increased pressure to invest in "high-profit" innovations, which can lead to less focus on less marketable products such as rural health solutions or rare diseases.
- Ethical and legal concerns
  - New technological advancements operate in areas where ethical regulations are not fully established. For example, AI-driven tools require large datasets to train their computer algorithms. However, this opens up the possibility of security breaches and unauthorized data being accessed without consent. Another example where ethics are placed in murky waters is through genomic editing. Technologies of CRISPR allow for human gene editing, but there is a political divide on whether CRISPR is being used for disease prevention or human enhancement [44].
- Regulatory complexity
  - Regulatory agencies aim to protect patients and put less priority on the speed of innovation. Therefore, entrepreneurs run into the challenge of long approval timelines, which can stall lifesaving therapies or allow competitors to catch up. Furthermore, given the climate of shifting to digital health, many innovators need to redesign their products to appease expectations created by regulatory agencies. Moreover, given that regulatory agencies cover a geographic area, products are only approved in one region and require approval from multiple agencies before being implemented globally, further limiting the spread of the product.

- Integration into clinical practice
  - Unfortunately, innovation doesn't end at FDA approval. It must also be implemented in the real world. This requires training and slow workflow integration, particularly with new medical hardware like surgical robots or AI imaging systems. This further deepens the required resources needed for medical implementation. Moreover, given that most of health care is transitioning to digital health platforms, EHRs struggle to integrate new concepts seamlessly, creating additional work for clinicians. These barriers cause many innovations to be underutilized despite their proven clinical benefits.
- Equity and accessibility
  - New products and services are often unevenly distributed, with high-resource areas receiving new technologies first. This leads to a lack of accessibility in rural areas and low-income countries. Since feedback plays a vital role in further development of products, having a lack of input from these communities further contributes to the health disparities present in our society.
- Resistance to change
  - Although medical culture values evidence, it also emphasizes stability. The saying "if it ain't broke, don't fix it" is quite common in the physician community as they prefer more familiar, proven methods over untested ones. Furthermore, with technological advancements, younger clinicians are more apt to embrace new technology changes, while older clinicians are slower to transition, given the learning curve. Large healthcare systems also follow this trend as they are more reluctant to overhaul protocols due to costly transitions and invest in unproven architectures. Without visible champions and trusted peers, adoption can lag for years or even decades.
- Public trust
  - Trust is at the core of healthcare adoption. Unfortunately, in the past, there has been abuse of patient trust (like the Tuskegee Syphilis Study) that has left communities hesitant to participate in medical research [45, 46]. This is especially prominent in marginalized communities, which has led to research data that is inaccurate and more skewed toward better-resourced communities [47].

Case Study: Theranos—A Cautionary Tale

- One recent example of public mistrust in health care came through the story of Theranos, a Silicon Valley startup that promised to revolutionize blood testing with finger-prick devices. Having raised over $700 million from investors and collaborating with high-profile partners like Walgreens and the Cleveland Clinic, the company's prototypes had misled the public. The company made claims that were not scientifically plausible, given the current technological developments. Due to pressured regulatory oversight, whistleblowers, and investigative journalism, it was revealed that Theranos had misled investors, patients, and clinicians [48]. Through this case, it becomes clear that innovation without rigorous regulations, transparency, and effective communication not only harms patient outcomes but can also contribute to hesitancy in investing in future innovations.

Innovation and Its Implementation into Medical Education

Environments where curiosity meets education act as breeding grounds for medical innovation [49]. As health care rapidly evolves with the introduction of artificial intelligence and focuses on precision medicine, medical education must not only keep up with the pace of evolution, but also should be a leader for change. Future physicians need to be comfortable with rapidly adapting environments. Therefore, innovation must be one of the core competencies in medical training. Traditionally, the medical school curriculum consisted of classroom/textbook learning that contained right answers with little room for risk-taking or problem-solving, which often led students to feel unprepared for clinical practice [50]. However, medical school curricula have slowly adopted a more creative approach with emphasis on case-based learning, partnerships with other interdisciplinaries (pharmacy, engineering, business), and early adoption of medical education technologies like VR Anatomy programs [51]. By hosting events with fields outside of health care, students get early exposure to team-based work, as many physicians will be collaborating with engineers, computer scientists, public health specialists, etc.

Finally, most medical students become future physicians who will directly enter the workforce. Without a doubt, they are likely to encounter problems that require solutions, discover new diseases, and gain access to new technologies. By teaching medical students the current framework of innovation, we are not just training physicians to learn how to adapt; we are also empowering them to shape the future medical landscape.

References

1. Kosiol J, Silvester T, Cooper H, Alford S, Fraser L. Revolutionising health and social care: innovative solutions for a brighter tomorrow—a systematic review of the literature. BMC Health Serv Res. 2024;24(1):809. Available from: https://bmchealthservres.biomedcentral.com/articles/10.1186/s12913-024-11099-5.
2. Wiersma M, Kerridge I, Lipworth W. Clinical innovation ethics frameworks: a systematic narrative review. Health Policy. 2023;129:104706.
3. Avelar AFM, dos Santos LM. Technological innovation in health: back to origins. Rev Bras Enferm. 2021;74(suppl 5):e74suppl501.

4. Mack HG. Technology driving advances in ophthalmology. Aust J Gen Pract. 2019;48(8):501. Available from: https://pubmed.ncbi.nlm.nih.gov/31422586/.
5. Heggie JCP. Technical developments in radiology in Australasia dating from 1977. Australas Phys Eng Sci Med. 2007;30(3):160–77. Available from: https://pubmed.ncbi.nlm.nih.gov/18044300/.
6. Bloch C, Bak MS, Glud SZ. Enhancing health innovation and entrepreneurship through an entrepreneurial fellowship program. Ann Biomed Eng. 2025;53(7):1703. Available from: https://pmc.ncbi.nlm.nih.gov/articles/PMC12185631/.
7. Rothstein DH, Raval MV. Operating room efficiency. Semin Pediatr Surg. 2018;27(2):79–85. Available from: https://www.sciencedirect.com/science/article/pii/S1055858618300040.
8. Harders M, Malangoni MA, Weight S, Sidhu T. Improving operating room efficiency through process redesign. Surgery. 2006;140(4):509–16.
9. Umscheid CA, Margolis DJ, Grossman CE. Key concepts of clinical trials: a narrative review. Postgrad Med. 2011;123(5):194–204. Available from: https://www.ncbi.nlm.nih.gov/pmc/articles/PMC3272827/.
10. Lee EY, Cha SA, Yun JS, Lim SY, Lee JH, Ahn YB, et al. Efficacy of personalized diabetes self-care using an electronic medical record–integrated mobile app in patients with type 2 diabetes: 6-month randomized controlled trial. J Med Internet Res. 2022;24(7):e37430.
11. Seidu S, Kunutsor SK, Ajjan RA, Choudhary P. Efficacy and safety of continuous glucose monitoring and intermittently scanned continuous glucose monitoring in patients with type 2 diabetes: a systematic review and meta-analysis of interventional evidence. Diabetes Care. 2023;47(1):169–79. Available from: https://diabetesjournals.org/care/article-abstract/47/1/169/154009/Efficacy-and-Safety-of-Continuous-Glucose?redirectedFrom=fulltext.
12. Ngo L, Nour D, Denman RA, Walters TE, Haqqani HM, Woodman RJ, et al. Safety and efficacy of leadless pacemakers: a systematic review and meta-analysis. J Am Heart Assoc Cardiovasc Cerebrovasc Dis. 2021;10(13):e019212. Available from: https://www.ncbi.nlm.nih.gov/pmc/articles/PMC8403316/.
13. Karges B, Schwandt A, Heidtmann B, Kordonouri O, Binder E, Schierloh U, et al. Association of insulin pump therapy vs insulin injection therapy with severe hypoglycemia, ketoacidosis, and glycemic control among children, adolescents, and young adults with type 1 diabetes. JAMA. 2017;318(14):1358–66. Available from: https://pmc.ncbi.nlm.nih.gov/articles/PMC5818842/.
14. Slatko BE, Gardner AF, Ausubel FM. Overview of next-generation sequencing technologies. Curr Protoc Mol Biol. 2018;122(1):e59. Available from: https://www.ncbi.nlm.nih.gov/pmc/articles/PMC6020069/.
15. Hu T, Chitnis N, Monos D, Dinh A. Next-generation sequencing technologies: an overview. Hum Immunol. 2021;82(11):801–11. Available from: https://www.sciencedirect.com/science/article/abs/pii/S0198885921000628.
16. Wu BM, Moeckel G. Application of digital pathology and machine learning in the liver, kidney and lung diseases. J Pathol Inf. 2023;14:100184.
17. Zhou SK, Greenspan H, Davatzikos C, Duncan JS, van Ginneken B, Madabhushi A, et al. A review of deep learning in medical imaging: imaging traits, technology trends, case studies with Progress highlights, and future promises. Proc IEEE. 2021;109(5):1–19. Available from: https://arxiv.org/pdf/2008.09104.pdf.
18. Roest C, Fransen SJ, Kwee TC, Yakar D. Comparative performance of deep learning and radiologists for the diagnosis and localization of clinically significant prostate cancer at MRI: a systematic review. Life. 2022;12(10):1490.
19. Rommasi F, Esfandiari N. Liposomal Nanomedicine: applications for drug delivery in cancer therapy. Nanoscale Res Lett. 2021;16(1):95.
20. Yao Y, Zhou Y, Liu L, Xu Y, Chen Q, Wang Y, et al. Nanoparticle-based drug delivery in cancer therapy and its role in overcoming drug resistance. Front Mol Biosci. 2020;7:193. Available from: https://www.ncbi.nlm.nih.gov/pmc/articles/PMC7468194/.

21. Herink MC, Irwin AN, Zumach GM. FDA breakthrough therapy designation: evaluating the quality of the evidence behind the drug approvals. Pharmacotherapy. 2018;38(9):967–80.
22. Druedahl LC, Minssen T, Nicholson PW. Collaboration in times of crisis: a study on COVID-19 vaccine R&D partnerships. Vaccine. 2021;39(42):6291–5. Available from: https://www.ncbi.nlm.nih.gov/pmc/articles/PMC8410639/
23. Schneider L. US life expectancy is rebounding. JAMA. 2025;334(10):849.
24. Fleming A. On the antibacterial action of cultures of a penicillium, with special reference to their use in the isolation of *B. influenzæ*. Br J Exp Pathol. 1929;10(3):226–36. Available from: https://pmc.ncbi.nlm.nih.gov/articles/PMC2048009/
25. USDA. Penicillin: opening the era of antibiotics: USDA ARS [Internet]. Usda.gov; 2018. Available from: https://www.ars.usda.gov/midwest-area/peoria-il/national-center-for-agricultural-utilization-research/docs/penicillin-opening-the-era-of-antibiotics/.
26. CDC. In: CDC, editor. Antimicrobial resistance facts and stats [Internet]. Antimicrobial resistance; 2024. Available from: https://www.cdc.gov/antimicrobial-resistance/data-research/facts-stats/index.html.
27. Dyar OJ, Huttner B, Schouten J, Pulcini C. What is antimicrobial stewardship? Clin Microbiol Infect. 2017;23(11):793–8. Available from: https://www.clinicalmicrobiologyandinfection.com/article/S1198-743X(17)30489-5/fulltext.
28. Baur D, Gladstone BP, Burkert F, Carrara E, Foschi F, Döbele S, et al. Effect of antibiotic stewardship on the incidence of infection and colonisation with antibiotic-resistant bacteria and Clostridium difficile infection: a systematic review and meta-analysis. Lancet Infect Dis. 2017;17(9):990–1001. Available from: https://www.sciencedirect.com/science/article/pii/S1473309917303250?via%3Dihub
29. Lamb YN. BNT162b2 mRNA COVID-19 vaccine: first approval. Drugs. 2021;81(4):1–7. Available from: https://www.ncbi.nlm.nih.gov/pmc/articles/PMC7938284/.
30. Fang E, Liu X, Li M, Zhang Z, Song L, Zhu B, et al. Advances in COVID-19 mRNA vaccine development. Signal Transduct Target Ther. 2022;7(94):94. Available from: https://www.ncbi.nlm.nih.gov/pmc/articles/PMC8940982/.
31. Roguin A. Rene theophile hyacinthe laennec (1781–1826): the man behind the stethoscope. Clin Med Res. 2006;4(3):230–5. Available from: https://pmc.ncbi.nlm.nih.gov/articles/PMC1570491/.
32. Juraschek SP, Ishak A, Mukamal KJ, Cohen ML, Beach JL. Impact of clinic-based blood pressure approaches on blood pressure measurement. Am J Hypertens. 2020;33(1):26–30. Available from: https://pubmed.ncbi.nlm.nih.gov/31350541/
33. Silverman B, Balk M. Digital stethoscope—improved auscultation at the bedside. Am J Cardiol. 2019;123(6):984–5.
34. Isakadze N, Martin SS. How useful is the smartwatch ECG? Trends Cardiovasc Med. 2020;30(7):442–8. Available from: https://www.sciencedirect.com/science/article/pii/S1050173819301495.
35. Gibbons RC, Jaeger DJ, Berger M, Magee M, Shaffer C, Costantino TG. Diagnostic accuracy of a handheld ultrasound vs a cart-based model: a randomized clinical trial. West J Emergency Medicine. 2024;25(2):268–74.
36. Papadopoulou SL, Sachpekidis V, Kantartzi V, Styliadis I, Nihoyannopoulos P. Clinical validation of an artificial intelligence-assisted algorithm for automated quantification of left ventricular ejection fraction in real time by a novel handheld ultrasound device. Eur Heart J Digital Health. 2022;3(1):29–37.
37. Dana E, Nour M, Kpa'Hanba GA, Khan JS. Point-of-care ultrasound (PoCUS) and its potential to advance patient care in low-resource settings and conflict zones. Disaster Med Public Health Prep. 2023;17:e417.
38. Damadian R. Tumor detection by nuclear magnetic resonance. Science. 1971;171(3976):1151–3. Available from: https://science.sciencemag.org/content/171/3976/1151.

39. Morris B. Robotic surgery: applications, limitations, and impact on surgical education. MedGenMed: Medscape Gen Med. 2005;7(3):72. Available from: https://pubmed.ncbi.nlm.nih.gov/16369298/.
40. Rivero-Moreno Y, Echevarria S, Vidal-Valderrama C, Pianetti L, Cordova-Guilarte J, Navarro-Gonzalez J, et al. Robotic surgery: a comprehensive review of the literature and current trends. Cureus. 2023;15(7):e42370. Available from: https://www.cureus.com/articles/166890-robotic-surgery-a-comprehensive-review-of-the-literature-and-current-trends#.
41. Adler-Milstein J, Jha AK. HITECH Act drove large gains in hospital electronic health record adoption. Health Aff. 2017;36(8):1416–22. Available from: https://www.healthaffairs.org/doi/10.1377/hlthaff.2016.1651.
42. Doarn CR. Development of telemedicine and NASA'S contribution. Aerosp Med Hum Perform. 2015;86(5):504–5.
43. Nittari G, Savva D, Tomassoni D, Tayebati SK, Amenta F. Telemedicine in the COVID-19 era: a narrative review based on current evidence. Int J Environ Res Public Health. 2022;19(9):5101.
44. Brokowski C, Adli M. CRISPR ethics: moral considerations for applications of a powerful tool. J Mol Biol. 2019;431(1):88–101. Available from: https://www.sciencedirect.com/science/article/pii/S0022283618305862.
45. Brandt AM. Racism and research: the case of the Tuskegee Syphilis Study. Hast Cent Rep. 1978;8(6):21–9. Available from: https://pubmed.ncbi.nlm.nih.gov/721302/.
46. Katz RV, Lee Green B, Kressin NR, Kegeles SS, Wang MQ, James SA, et al. The legacy of the Tuskegee Syphilis Study: assessing its impact on willingness to participate in biomedical studies. J Health Care Poor Underserved. 2008;19(4):1168–80. Available from: https://www.ncbi.nlm.nih.gov/pmc/articles/PMC2702151/.
47. Corbie-Smith G. The continuing legacy of the Tuskegee Syphilis Study: considerations for clinical investigation. Am J Med Sci. 1999;317(1):5–8.
48. Lackner KJ, Plebani M. The Theranos saga and the consequences. Clin Chem Lab Med. 2018;56(9):1395–6.
49. Koh DLK. Creativity and innovation in medical education: it's time to let the trees grow freely. Ann Acad Med Singap. 2013;42(11):557–8. Available from: https://pubmed.ncbi.nlm.nih.gov/24356650/.
50. Kadmon M, Ten Cate O, Harendza S, Berberat PO. Postgraduate Medical Education – an increasingly important focus of study and innovation. GMS J Med Educ. 2017;34(5):Doc70. Available from: https://www.ncbi.nlm.nih.gov/pmc/articles/PMC5704613/.
51. Altintas L, Sahiner M. Transforming medical education: the impact of innovations in technology and medical devices. Expert Rev Med Devices. 2024;21(9):797–809. Available from: https://pubmed.ncbi.nlm.nih.gov/39235206/.

Use of Simulation Centers in Medical Education

Kalista Tapas, Jonathan Greve, Sydney Slepian, Berrin Ergun-Longmire, and Gerrit J. Bouma

Introduction

Simulation in health care refers to the replication of real-life clinical scenarios, such as cardiac arrest or trauma resuscitation, in a controlled, safe environment. Simulation can exist in various forms including part-task trainers, computer-based systems, simulated patients and environments, and integrated simulators. All these components can be incorporated into a central location as seen in simulation centers. Simulation centers have evolved into the gold standard training environment for young medical professionals.

Simulation centers serve as a centralized hub where diverse modalities, procedural training, standardized patients, and immersive team-based exercises are integrated into an organized educational experience. Simulation centers are designed to provide training for medical students and healthcare providers in a manner that improves both the educational experience and the safety of patients [1].

Kalista Tapas, Jonathan Greve and Sydney Slepian contributed equally with all other contributors.

K. Tapas · J. Greve · S. Slepian
Western Michigan University Homer Stryker M.D. School of Medicine, Kalamazoo, MI, USA

B. Ergun-Longmire
Department of Pediatrics and Adolescent Medicine, Division of Pediatric Endocrinology, Western Michigan University Homer Stryker M.D. School of Medicine, Kalamazoo, MI, USA

G. J. Bouma (✉)
Department of Biomedical Sciences, Western Michigan University Homer Stryker M.D. School of Medicine, Kalamazoo, MI, USA
e-mail: gerrit.bouma@wmed.edu

S. S. Chahin et al. (eds.), *Innovation in Medical Education and Clinical Practice*, https://doi.org/10.1007/978-3-032-19116-8_3

In this chapter, first we'll provide a historical perspective on the origins and development of simulation in health care, its standardization and accreditation, and an example of a modern-day simulation center. Then, we'll discuss the implementation of simulation into undergraduate and postgraduate medical education curriculum and student perspectives; and finalize it with an overview of the advantages and disadvantages of implementation and application of simulation and simulation centers in healthcare training.

The History of Healthcare Simulation

Simulation and its use in professional training today have its origins in the aviation industry. Flight simulation has been routinely used since the 1930s, creating a controlled environment for amateur pilots to encounter dangerous scenarios [2]. This pioneering approach to simulation laid the groundwork for simulation's entrance into the healthcare landscape to address the need for clinical skills practice in a safe environment. The type of simulation that first enabled learners to build hands-on skills in health care was procedural simulation and can be traced back as early as the 1700s. French midwife, Angelique Marguerite Le Boursier du Coudray (1712–1790), was recruited by King Louis XV to educate rural midwives with the overall goal of improving health outcomes in pregnancy and reduce infant mortality rates [3]. She developed the first obstetric manikin ("The Machine") which was a life-size manikin that included human pelvic bones, dye liquids for amniotic fluid and blood, mechanical straps for the birthing canal, and a neonate attached via a fabric umbilical cord, which allowed rural midwives to simulate the birthing process and movement of baby's head through the birthing canal.

The development of the first commercialized manikin to teach resuscitation techniques was in 1960, when Norwegian toymaker Asmund Lærdal created *Resusci Anne*. *Resusci Anne* was a task trainer manikin designed to teach mouth-to-mouth ventilation and led to mass production of the device enabling widespread use across the United States in the twentieth century. The introduction of *Resusci Anne* was a major contribution to simulation in healthcare education and marked a turning point in the simulation movement [4].

Shortly after the introduction of the *Resusci Anne* manikin, standardized patients were introduced into the simulation landscape. Soon after, neurologist Dr. Howard Barrows pioneered the use of "simulated patients" by hiring a paraplegic woman to help evaluate third-year medical students' ability to assess neurological signs in 1963. This marked the first documented use of a simulated patient [4]. At first this approach was met with skepticism, yet the concept gained traction as it was modified and adapted. It was Geoff Norman at McMaster University who later coined the term *standardized patient* to highlight their reliability and consistency in both clinical teaching and assessment. Standardized patients are real people trained to provide an authentic and medically relevant patient encounter. With real people acting as patients, clinical reasoning and communication skills were transformed into a "real-life" experience.

The role of the standardized patients increased, becoming not just a way to practice communication and clinical skills but also a method of assessment and evaluation for undergraduate medical students. In 1975, the University of Dundee introduced the Objective Structured Clinical Examination (OSCE). The OSCE quickly became the gold standard for assessing students' clinical skills and it was adopted by the United States in 2004 [4]. Currently, the OSCE standardized patient encounters are routinely used to assess student's clinical skills and the effectiveness of curricula.

Medical simulation continued to evolve with the introduction of immersive, high-technology simulations. In the 1990s, advanced simulations became part of Crisis Resource Management training. One of the earliest high-tech simulators developed and used was *Sim One* at the University of Southern California for anesthesiology training. This electronic manikin could blink, move its pupils, simulate pulse, breathe, sleep, cough, and vomit providing a remarkably lifelike experience [2, 4]. By the 1980s, software systems like Sleeper, BodySim, and Anesthesia Simulator-Recorder expanded the reach of simulation in fields like cardiology and anesthesia. Today, simulation has entered the digital frontier with virtual reality tools, including head-mounted displays and vestibular sensors, offering even more immersive learning opportunities [2]. Along with the various types of simulation, the idea of having a centralized location to incorporate a variety of simulation experiences gained interest resulting in development of simulation centers.

Modern-Day Simulation Centers

As simulation-based medical education (SBME) continues to expand, institutions are increasingly pursuing formal accreditation as a means to validate the quality and effectiveness of their simulation programs. Accreditation not only enhances the credibility and prestige of a simulation center but also promotes consistency by establishing minimum standards and defining best practices for this evolving educational modality [5]. In 2004 the Society for Simulation in health care (SSH) was established. Today the SSH remains the largest accrediting body of simulation centers in the United States, with more than 290 programs earning the distinction of SSH accreditation [6]. The SSH works to serve members by fostering education, professional development, and the advancement of research and innovation, and SSH core accreditation lists 7 core standards that are fundamental to the fulfillment of the accreditation [6]. Each core standard has a subset of 2–4 criteria that the program must provide documentation to meet requirements for accreditation. A summary of the 7 core standards are as follows:

1. *Mission and governance*: They address the intent and function of the program, documenting the governing structure and strategic planning of the organization.

2. *Program management*: It ensures the organization has appropriate financial resources to support mission and vision. It provides the program's current financial status and day-to-day operations.
3. *Resource management*: It maintains that the organization has the ability to obtain and support equipment and relevant technologies. It provides accreditation with inventory list, facility description, and past 24 months of simulation activity and learner contact hours.
4. *Human resources*: It ensures the program is directed by qualified individuals and provides job descriptions for simulation program staff.
5. *Program improvement*: It describes the use of a quality management system and documentation processes instituted to address concerns and complaints.
6. *Ethics*: It commits to and describes ethical standards the program abides by.
7. *Expanding the field*: It provides a list of activities that contribute to knowledge in simulation community and how the program has potential to contribute to knowledge with or about simulation.

In addition to credentialing of simulation centers, the SSH established the Certified Healthcare Simulation Educator (CHSE) and the Certified Healthcare Simulation Operations Specialist (CHSOS) certifications. As of 2025, the SSH has certified 3122 and 719 individuals for the CHSE and CHSOS certifications respectively [6]. The credentialing promotes professional development and continued education while providing a method of standardization for staff members within the simulation center. Before discussing the use and implementation of SBME, an example and overview are provided next of a top-tier, regional, and SSH reaccredited medical simulation center in academia, Western Michigan University Homer Stryker M.D. School of Medicine (WMed).

Western Michigan University Homer Stryker M.D. School of Medicine (WMed)

Located in Kalamazoo, Michigan, the WMed Upjohn M.D. Campus is a prime example of a successful simulation center accredited by the SSH. This center is the largest regional academic simulation center in Southwest Michigan, with over 24,000 square feet. The educational spaces include a 13-bed virtual hospital including an operating room and three debriefing rooms, a 12-room ambulatory clinic, and two large control rooms. Additionally, the center encompasses two procedure labs, two classrooms, a standardized patient staging suite, an ultrasonography suite, and a virtual endoscopic surgery room. It's unique in its integration in both undergraduate medical and residency education, with over 14,000 learners logging over 67,000 h of training in 2022–2023 [7].

Undergraduate and graduate learners utilize the spaces for role-playing, tabletop exercises, partial task trainers, computerized simulations, and manikin-based simulations. Learners interact with low-to-high fidelity manikins, standardized patients,

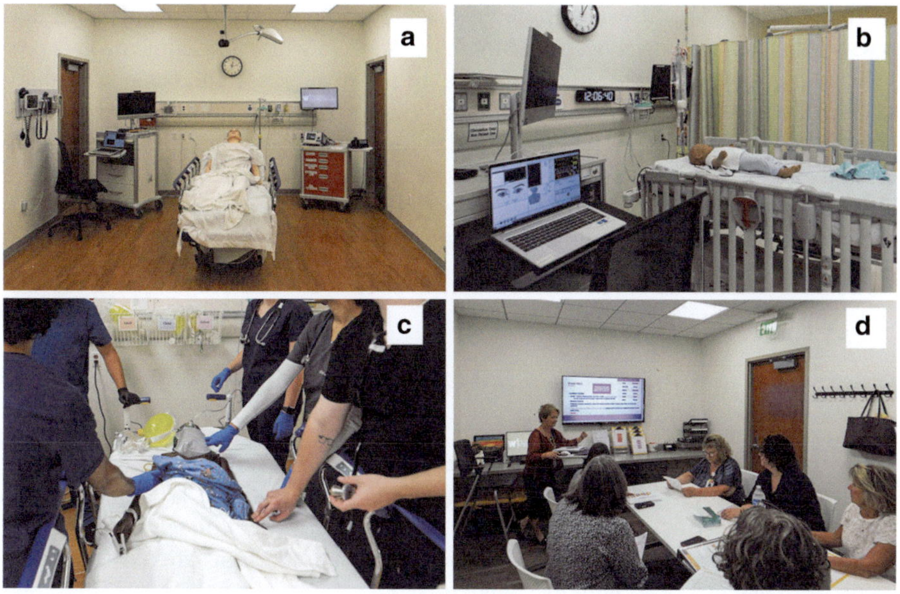

Fig. 1 (**a**) WMed Virtual hospital room with standard setup and high-fidelity manikin. (**b**) Neonatal intensive care unit (NICU) room with high-fidelity manikin, including a view of the control computer used by staff to adjust vital signs during simulation. (**c**) Medical students interacting with a pediatric manikin during a medical first responder training course. (**d**) Standardized patients receiving a pre-brief for an Objective Structured Clinical Examination (OSCE) patient encounter

hybrid simulators, and virtual reality devices. The medical school's undergraduate curriculum alone includes more than 100 h of simulation-based learning, providing dedicated learning spaces and opportunities for interprofessional collaboration with directed feedback in a patient-safe environment. Examples of various simulation environments are shown in Fig. 1.

In the next section, we'll discuss practical implementation of simulation centers in both undergraduate and graduate medical education and highlight how these facilities are integrated into curricula to support skill development, clinical reasoning, and interprofessional collaboration.

Implementation of Simulation Centers within Medical Education

Having a medical simulation center on-site at medical schools and hospitals allows simulation sessions to be more accessible to learners, easier integration into curriculum programs, and continued practice throughout the medical school curriculum. Simulation may be implemented throughout the entirety of medical training, within pre-clinical and clinical years of medical school and postgraduate residencies, fellowship, and continuing education. Simulation centers within pre-clinical years provide students a centralized space for learning physical exams and basic procedural skills including CPR, securing airways, applying tourniquets, suturing, and endotracheal tube placements. Within the clinical and postgraduate years, the centers allow students and health professionals to practice a range of technical skills from basic procedures to complex surgeries before performing them on real patients, as well as sharpening interpersonal skills with patients, their families, and with other medical providers.

Simulation in Undergraduate Medical Education

While undergraduate medical students may learn skills effectively using high-fidelity manikins in simulations, simulation centers are unique as they offer the opportunity to interact with standardized patients in a variety of settings. Medical procedural and interpersonal skills are more realistic and translational to clinical medicine when practiced with the standardized patients compared to manikins, and standardized patients help improve students' overall clinical competence, communication skills, and diagnostic accuracy [8].

The role of simulation and standardized patients has become vital to the education of medical professionals. All Liaison Committee on Medical Education (LCME) accredited medical schools and several physician assistant programs require OSCEs, which are timed interactions with the standardized patients. Students are given a prompt to follow where they must elicit the patient's chief complaint, history, and pertinent physical exam findings, and then devise a written assessment and plan for the patient. These examinations are held at certain time points within the medical curriculum and serve to give medical students opportunities to practice interactions with simulated patients, hands-on physical exam skills on real people, and time management skills in controlled settings. Additionally, mock OSCEs allow for debriefing and feedback by standardized patients and medical educators for the medical students to recognize strengths and deficits to perform more effectively on their summative OSCEs, and ultimately when interacting with patients in the clinical and hospital settings.

Simulation in Postgraduate Medical Education

Simulation centers are not only important within the context of undergraduate medical education but are also vital for acquisition of more advanced competencies during residencies and clinical settings. Simulation-based learning has been shown to lead to improved clinical outcomes as clinicians are less likely to make errors and more likely to have more timely and accurate diagnoses [8]. Furthermore, the ability to repeat hands-on and communication techniques within simulations has demonstrated improved adherence to protocol and guidelines in procedures and emergency scenarios. For example, second year residents with simulation-based training adhered to American Heart Association standards 68% of the time compared to their counterparts without simulation training who adhered to the guidelines 44% of the time [9]. Furthermore, credentialing for some procedures such as carotid stenting requires competency of the procedure in a simulation [10, 11]. Providers can simulate procedures such as laparoscopy, endoscopy, lumbar punctures, placing central lines, and numerous other techniques to learn how to best approach them, receive feedback, and correct errors before performing them on patients in the hospital or clinic.

In addition to acquisition and mastering of more practical skills through simulation, simulation centers allow for residents and clinicians to practice communication skills with patients and within the medical team which they operate. Internal medicine residents felt significantly more confident in their ability to give patients discharge instructions and use the electronic medical record (EMR) discharge navigator after performing simulations of patient discharge interactions with standardized patients and receiving feedback from nurses and medical assistants [12]. Furthermore, for these postgraduate physicians, simulation of ethically challenging scenarios and conversations such as end-of-life care, delivering bad news, and navigating care in a mass casualty event allow these providers to identify strengths and areas for growth [10]. Additionally, performing simulations with students or providers from other disciplines creates an environment where roles can be established and protocols strengthened to optimize team communication and performance. In this way, usage of simulation centers within postgraduate medical education is helpful to learn and sharpen hands-on and communication skills, practice complex procedures, and improve outcomes for patients.

Debriefing in Simulation

One crucial component of simulation-based training for learners is debriefing the simulated scenarios after their performance. Simulation centers are unique as most are equipped with audio and visual equipment to record and play back simulations for students that encourages them to critically analyze their actions, share perspectives, and consolidate learning [13, 14]. There are many ways to provide feedback based on the simulation being performed and aim of the instructor and learner. For example, asking the learner how they believed they performed and any gaps they identified allows them to have an active role in identifying their mistakes and taking the necessary steps to mitigate and improve them. More direct feedback from instructor to learner allows for quick corrections during procedures but may not be preferred in a team-based environment. A discussion-based model gives the opportunity for all team members to participate in mutual and collective feedback to recognize gaps in team performance. This method can be helpful within interdisciplinary settings to better establish roles for the various levels of providers such as students, nurses, techs, and physicians [15].

Debriefing sessions allow time for active reflection, constructive feedback, and advice on how to improve gaps in skills and/or knowledge immediately following simulations and have been shown to significantly improve learning and improve clinical outcomes [8]. Structured reflection is a foundational element in adult learning theory and plays a critical role in promoting deeper understanding and knowledge retention [16]. Effective debriefings have been shown to enhance team performance by up to 25% and are adaptable across various organizational contexts [14]. Simulation centers often offer distraction-free environments that replicate clinical settings while minimizing interruptions, thereby promoting and facilitating meaningful debriefings and emotional processing [17, 18]. In addition to fostering cognitive growth, simulation has also been shown to reduce anxiety and significantly improve learner confidence, particularly in high-stakes or unfamiliar clinical scenarios [19]. Through repeated exposure and deliberate practice, students gain not only competence but also a greater sense of preparedness for real-world encounters. While the success of debriefing depends heavily on the quality of facilitation, it remains an indispensable element of the simulation learning cycle.

Student and Patient Perspectives on Simulation

Overall, students, faculty, and patients indicate that simulation-based training is beneficial to their medical experiences. For example, students at WMed who participate in simulation trainings like those provided through simulation centers generally value and look positively upon the experiences as they can practice and improve communication skills and hands-on procedures within controlled, risk-free environments (Fig. 2).

Simulation training was vital for many programs during the COVID-19 pandemic, as hospital practice for students was limited due to shutdowns. In the beginning of their experience in the clinical setting, students often lack confidence with patient care skills due to lack of practice, which may manifest as increased anxiety and stress. This increased anxiety and stress can then negatively impact performance, which further reduces confidence for the student. Medical students with more medical experience and opportunities to interact with patients are more likely to demonstrate confidence within the clinical setting. In fact, students repeatedly exposed to simulation scenarios within their education have significantly lower anxiety and higher confidence and exhibit higher psychological stability and increased competency following the simulations [19]. In addition, students not only boost their confidence and skillsets through simulation, but simulation-based training has been found to have a significant role in the professional identity formation for students. In one study, 90% of students who participated in their clinically relevant simulation-based orientation to medical school agreed that it helped them

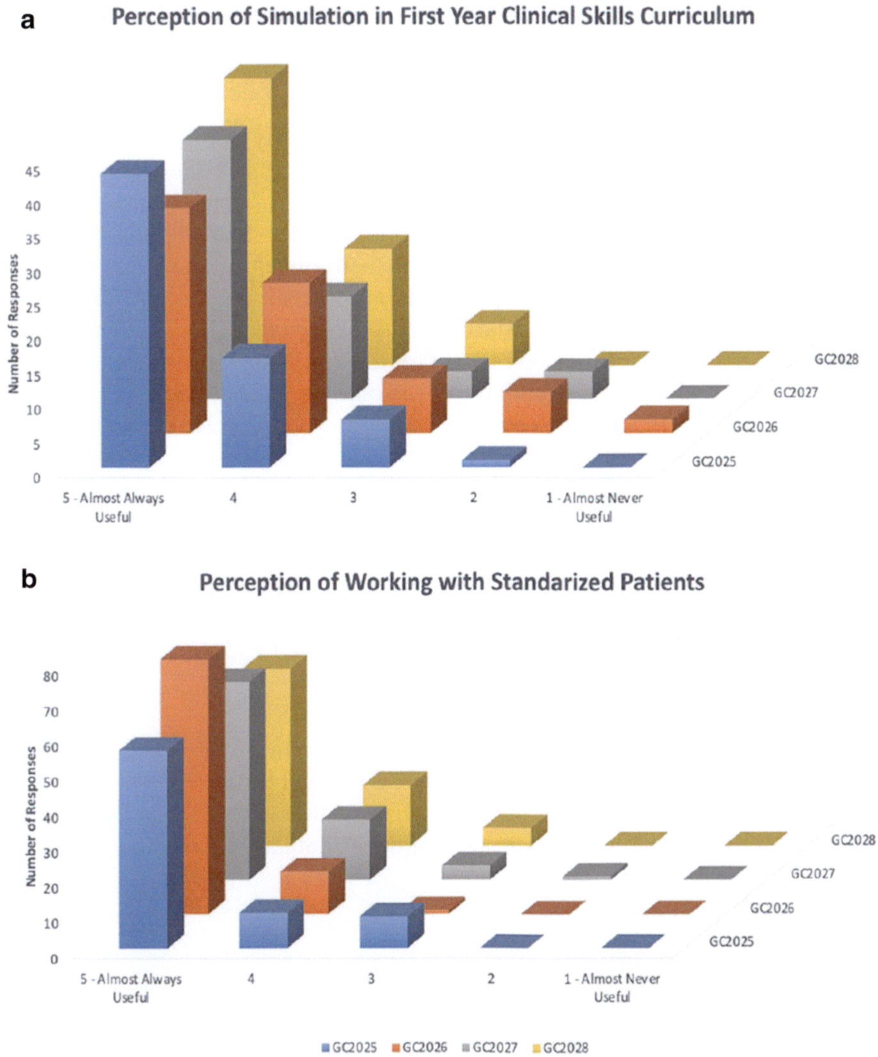

Fig. 2 Perceptions of simulation in the first-year clinical skills curriculum (**a**) and combined across four medical school graduating classes (GC2025–GC2028) (**b**). Responses were measured on a 5-point Likert scale (1 = almost never useful, 5 = almost always useful). Most students rated simulation as highly useful, with the majority selecting 4 or 5 across all classes

transition to their role as a medical student and make them feel like a physician by acting in their role [20].

Patients themselves also support simulation-based training as it improves the preparedness and competency of their providers, and see simulation-based training as a vital way to reduce medical errors as providers have the opportunity to recognize these errors within simulations, reflect, and correct rather than performing them in the clinical setting when patient safety and health are at risk [8]. Therefore, training within simulation centers not only boosts confidence among students and providers, but performing and mastering simulations helps to put patients at ease and decreases errors to improve outcomes.

In summary, students and patients alike look favorably upon simulation-based learning, with students appreciating the opportunity to gain confidence in a controlled environment and receive constructive feedback before interacting with patients, and patients having more trust in their providers knowing that they have developed hands-on and communication skills before their interactions. However, developing, running, and maintaining simulation centers is not an easy feat considering the high cost of equipment, staffing, and maintenance, but the centers have shown to have notable return on investment for their programs with decreased medical errors, surgery times, and overall improved outcomes for patients.

Benefits and Challenges of Developing and Maintaining a Simulation Center

Most medical schools contain some form of simulation-based education with their requirements [21]. The natural progression of this trend has led to an increasing prevalence of simulation centers to provide the necessary resources and personnel to facilitate this form of education. The benefits of such resources are well documented, and its future possibilities are considerable. There also are many challenges associated with implementing and operating SBME and especially when developing a dedicated simulation center. The following section will focus and summarize benefits and challenges inherent to the utilization of simulation in medical education.

Benefits and Advantages

The ability of SBME to enhance technical and procedural skills, and essential non-technical competencies such as communication, leadership, and decision-making, has made it an invaluable component of modern medical training. SBME also plays a critical role in advancing interprofessional education by fostering collaboration and improving team dynamics. As a dynamic and evolving modality, SBME has several significant benefits and advantages for continued advancement of medical education.

Performance in Technical Skills

SBME has some of its earliest and most notable applications in teaching cardiopulmonary resuscitation (CPR), a skill in which simulation training has demonstrably improved both educational outcomes and patient survival [22, 23]. Since then, SBME has expanded well beyond resuscitation training and is now widely used to teach a broad range of procedural and technical skills [22]. A substantial body of literature supports the effectiveness of SBME in facilitating both acquisition and long-term retention of technical competencies, with many studies suggesting that simulation training is superior to traditional didactic methods alone [24]. Furthermore, as simulation has become more popular and technology has improved, it has been applied beyond fundamental medical skills and into residency programs and specific procedural specialties. Overall, some of the most compelling evidence for the implementation of simulation centers to enhance medical education is from the benefit in learning technical skills [25].

Performance in Non-technical (Soft) Skills

SBME also provides a critical framework for developing non-technical or soft skills such as communication, leadership, and teamwork, competencies that are all essential for safe, high-quality health care. These skills are often more difficult to teach and assess through traditional didactic methods. However, SBME, through structured debriefing and experiential learning, allows learners to effectively practice these skills in a controlled environment. As optimal medical treatment becomes increasingly complex, learners must not only understand clinical protocols and procedures, but also demonstrate appropriate behaviors under pressure, including collaboration, clear communication, and delegation of tasks. SBME has proven to be a valuable novel modality in teaching these skills [26].

The transition of health care from individual expertise to team-based systems underscores the importance of these competencies. SBME prepares learners for real-world scenarios by creating opportunities to engage in dynamic team-based interactions that mirror the fast-paced, interdependent nature of modern healthcare systems. Evidence supports that SBME improves essential Accreditation Council for Graduate Medical Education (ACGME) core competencies, particularly interpersonal and communication skills, professionalism, and systems-based practice [27]. Furthermore, simulation promotes critical skills like situational awareness and decision-making under uncertainty [28, 29]. By immersing learners in lifelike scenarios, SBME enhances their ability to anticipate challenges, adapt under pressure, and function effectively as part of a cohesive unit, fostering not only individual growth but also system-level readiness.

Clinical Outcomes

An important question that remains is whether SBME training translates into tangible improvements in clinical practice and patient outcomes. Despite the widespread adoption of SBME, only about 5% of medical education studies report on patient outcomes, reflecting a persistent gap in the literature that connects educational interventions with real-world clinical impact [30]. However, there is evidence suggesting that SBME contributes meaningfully to clinical outcomes. A meta-analysis found that SBME, especially when used for procedural training, yields a small to moderate benefit in patient-related outcomes, indicating that skills acquired in simulation are successfully transferred to clinical environments and impact patient care [30]. Furthermore, SBME not only improves the technical proficiency of learners but also enhances interventional success rates, reduces patient discomfort, and decreases the frequency of procedural errors, all of which contribute to better patient experiences and outcomes [31]. In addition, simulation has also been associated with reductions in healthcare costs by minimizing complications and avoiding unnecessary interventions.

Safety

A key strength of clinical application of SBME lies in its potential to enhance patient safety. Studies indicate that simulation-based training improves the recognition and management of emergent clinical conditions, leading to quicker and more effective interventions [32–34]. These improvements are especially critical in acute care settings, where rapid decision-making can significantly alter a patient's clinical trajectory. Simulation has also been used successfully to train teams for crisis resource management and high-risk procedures, further supporting a systems-level improvement in care delivery [33, 34]. Notably, there is emerging data that suggests simulation can contribute to reduced morbidity and mortality. For example, decreased neonatal mortality following implementation of a simulation-based resuscitation curriculum was reported, offering compelling evidence that SBME can have life-saving implications [35]. Moreover, an 84.5% reduction in catheter-related blood stream infections following the implementation of a simulation-based training regimen on central line insertion has been reported [36]. Although further high-quality, outcome-focused studies are warranted, these findings highlight the translational potential of simulation beyond the classroom and provide evidence that SBME is a powerful educational modality with the capacity to meaningfully enhance patient outcomes and improve the quality and safety of healthcare delivery.

While SBME has shown clear advantages in developing non-technical skills such as leadership, communication, and teamwork, these competencies have not yet been definitively linked to improvements in patient outcomes. Although improved non-technical skills likely contribute to safer and more efficient care delivery, a direct causal relationship between non-technical skills acquisition through simulation and specific clinical metrics remains to be established [37].

Beyond refining individual and team performance, SBME also serves a critical role in identifying latent safety threats within clinical systems, risks that may otherwise go unnoticed until they contribute to patient harm. Simulation centers, therefore, not only provide skills training but also function as dynamic platforms for safety surveillance, quality improvement, and culture change within healthcare organizations [1, 38].

Ethics

An often-underappreciated advantage of SBME lies in its ethical implications. The traditional model of clinical training "see one, do one, teach one" places medical trainees in a position where they must eventually perform procedures on real patients despite having minimal to no hands-on experience [39]. This approach inherently risks patient safety by potentially subjecting individuals to care from inexperienced providers. Furthermore, it creates an ethical tension where experienced physicians may feel compelled to entrust procedures to trainees to facilitate learning, even when the trainee's skill level may not guarantee the same standard of care. Given that the overarching goal in health care is to provide the safest and most effective care possible, this tension highlights a conflict between educational needs and patient well-being.

Simulation offers a resolution to this dilemma. By allowing learners to develop technical, cognitive, and teamwork skills in a controlled, consequence-free environment, SBME enables trainees to gain competence before ever interacting with patients [40]. This shift from patient-based to simulation-based initial learning not only enhances skill acquisition and retention but also minimizes the ethical burden of learning through patient exposure. Indeed, simulation has been shown to improve both provider performance and patient outcomes, reinforcing its role as not just a pedagogical or andragogical tool, but an ethical imperative in modern medical education.

The benefits of SBME are extensive and well supported by the literature. SBME has been shown to enhance both technical proficiency and non-technical. Importantly, there is growing evidence that simulation training translates into improved clinical performance and patient safety while also addressing ethical concerns.

Challenges and Disadvantages

Despite the numerous benefits of SBME and its growing role in the future of healthcare training, its implementation is not without significant challenges and costs. One of the most prominent barriers is the financial burden associated with acquiring and maintaining the necessary equipment, infrastructure, and personnel. In addition to logistical and financial challenges, integrating SBME into existing medical curricula presents its own complexities. While SBME has demonstrated considerable promise, it cannot fully substitute for real-world clinical experience, and its ultimate capacity to prepare learners for practice is still being evaluated.

Costs

One of the most fundamental and immediate challenges in SBME is securing adequate space and infrastructure. Although SBME can be integrated flexibly across a range of settings, the increasing demand for high-fidelity simulation has prompted construction of dedicated simulation centers. The development of such centers is not only financially challenging but also logistically complex. The design and planning process involves an interdisciplinary team that includes simulation educators, information technology professionals, architects, faculty, and institutional administrators each contributing to the cost and complexity of the project [40]. These logistical considerations span architectural planning, integration of audio-visual and networking systems, and decisions around layout and accessibility. Once a facility is established, additional operational decisions must be made including how simulation spaces will be utilized, how to ensure flexibility for multiple disciplines, how much equipment and storage are necessary, and how frequently the space will be in use [41].

Once a SBME program has secured a physical space or virtual platform, one of the most significant and ongoing operational costs is staffing [40]. The personnel requirements of simulation centers vary widely depending on factors such as the scope of the curriculum, complexity of the simulations, and institutional goals. However, many centers across the United States function with fewer than six full-time staff members, reflecting both budgetary limitations and variable institutional support [42]. Simulation centers require a multidisciplinary team that may include simulation technicians, standardized patients, instructional designers, program managers, and faculty educators. Each of these roles demands specialized and years of on-the-job training and competencies, which introduces further financial burdens in the form of onboarding, continuing education, and skills maintenance. Additionally, typical organizational expenses, such as those related to staff turnover, recruitment, and human resource management, can add to the financial strain. Finally, although there is growing consensus of its benefits, simulation training fellowships have not yet been recognized by ACGME [43, 44]. In conclusion, the challenge of maintaining a skilled and sustainable workforce remains a universal and costly aspect of SBME operations.

Another major financial hurdle in SBME lies in the acquisition and upkeep of simulation equipment and consumable materials. Core simulation assets, such as manikins, vary dramatically in cost, ranging from several hundred dollars for low-fidelity models to well over $100,000 for high-fidelity simulators [45]. Beyond manikins, many commonly used items, such as central line kits, airway management tools, and IV training supplies, are designed to be disposable, contributing to an ongoing consumable expense. Additionally, specialized medical equipment like ultrasound machines, laparoscopic instruments, and other procedure-specific devices carry high initial costs and require regular servicing, warranties, and sometimes even staff training for proper use and upkeep [41]. These cumulative expenses quickly strain simulation center budgets, particularly when scaled to support an expanding curriculum. However, there are several cost-mitigation strategies. These include sourcing expired, but still usable hospital materials for training purposes, reusing supplies when safe and feasible, and incorporating low-fidelity models to meet specific educational objectives without incurring unnecessary cost [45, 46].

Beyond the expense and sophistication of high-fidelity simulators, even basic simulation programs face challenges in integrating technology into their operations [47]. Many simulation centers rely on audio-visual recording systems for debriefing, while others incorporate virtual reality platforms or augmented reality tools to enhance immersive learning experiences. The acquisition, maintenance, and updating of such technologies can significantly increase both the financial and logistical burdens of SBME [48]. Moreover, as new technologies rapidly evolve, institutions may struggle to remain current without incurring unsustainable costs.

However, although there are several costs associated with simulation centers, there is also great evidence for return on investment on their creation. Additional necessary operating room (OR) time necessary to train 15 residents on laparoscopic entero-enterostomies cost the program over $45,000/year. Practicing these procedures in a simulated environment prior to entering the OR can help better prepare the surgical residents for the OR environment which can ultimately cut down on costs for programs long-term [27]. However, there are potential ways simulation centers could generate revenue to off-set some of the costs by offering CME courses, fee-for service, photoshoots for medical equipment brochures, donations, and hosting conferences.

Development of a Simulation Curriculum

While cost remains one of the most prominent barriers to implementing SBME, an equally complex challenge lies in effectively integrating SBME into existing medical curricula [49]. Simulation, though increasingly recognized for its educational value, still represents a relatively novel instructional modality compared to traditional didactic and clinical teaching methods. As such, many institutions are still navigating how best to incorporate simulation into the broader fabric of medical education. While frameworks such as Kern's six-step approach to curriculum development offer a structured pathway for designing educational programs, their successful application to simulation requires faculty expertise in both curriculum design and simulation pedagogy [50, 51]. Moreover, simulation lacks a universally standardized integration model, compelling institutions to independently determine essential components such as learning objectives, syllabi, assessment rubrics, faculty roles, and curricular time allocation. This individualized approach demands extensive coordination between clinical educators, simulation specialists, curriculum committees, and administrative leaders. Without established norms for integration, programs face the risk of underutilizing simulation or misaligning it with broader educational outcomes. Despite SBME's demonstrated effectiveness, its curricular integration remains a complex and resource-intensive endeavor, one that continues to evolve without a consistent, evidence-based standard across institutions.

Realism of Simulation

A persistent challenge in SBME is determining the appropriate degree of realism needed to optimize learning outcomes. Simulation modalities are commonly classified as low- or high-fidelity based on how closely they replicate clinical scenarios [52]. While high-fidelity equipment, such as responsive manikins, advanced software, and immersive virtual reality, can create a more lifelike experience, these resources are often expensive and resource-intensive to maintain, limiting their accessibility across institutions. Despite growing interest in high-fidelity tools, and some indication that it can improve clinical outcomes [53, 54], the literature does not consistently support a proportional improvement in educational or clinical outcomes compared to low-fidelity alternatives [55]. This ambiguity leaves institutions facing the challenge of aligning simulation fidelity with educational value rather than technological sophistication. Therefore, the true effectiveness of SBME lies perhaps not in the realism of the equipment itself, but in the thoughtful integration of simulation into a well-structured curriculum that prioritizes active learning, feedback, and repetition.

Overconfidence with SBME

A potential limitation of SBME that warrants consideration is the development of overconfidence. While high-fidelity simulation offers realistic and practical training opportunities, there is concern that such experiences may inadvertently foster inflated self-assessment and increased risk-taking behavior among learners. For example, medical students trained with high-fidelity simulators were more likely to overrate their performance compared to peers trained with low-fidelity simulators, despite no differences in knowledge assessments or practical outcomes between the groups [56]. Although overconfidence and its risks have been well-documented in medicine, the extent to which SBME may contribute to this phenomenon remains unclear. Nevertheless, one of the very strengths of SBME, its ability to bolster learners' confidence, may carry the unintended consequence of fostering overconfidence if not carefully addressed.

Conclusion and Future Direction

SBME is increasingly recognized as a powerful teaching modality for improving clinical competencies, patient safety, and clinical outcomes. For this reason, there is a growing global consensus, reflected in accreditation standards, that the use of SBME and its proper and deliberate development is not just beneficial, but an ethical imperative.

Healthcare simulation offers more than just technical training. It provides opportunities for skill practice, retention, and accuracy, while also fostering interprofessional development and teamwork. Research shows that simulation enhances team functioning, reduces medical errors, and improves the overall quality of care. Furthermore, simulation serves a greater mission which is to elevate the performance of healthcare providers, teams, and systems in order to positively impact the health of patients, communities, and societies. Achieving this vision will require a unified effort among policymakers, educators, and health systems to integrate and advance simulation-based education globally.

However, SBME implementation is not without obstacles. The financial burden of developing simulation centers, acquiring and maintaining equipment, and managing the curricular, logistical, and personnel demands remains substantial. While the future of SBME is undoubtedly promising, its full impact on medical education continues to be explored.

Author Contribution Kalista Tapas, Jonathan Greve, and Sydney Slepian, all M2 students, collected all the information and wrote the chapter (equal contribution). The chapter has been edited and formatted by me. It has been reviewed by Dr. Neil Highes, Assistant Dean for simulation at WMed, and final edits and review by Dr. Longmire.

References

1. Hunt EA, Nelson KL, Shilkofski NA. Simulation in medicine: addressing patient safety and improving the interface between healthcare providers and medical technology. Biomed Instrum Technol. 2006;40(5):399–404. https://doi.org/10.2345/i0899-8205-40-5-399.1.
2. Singh H, Kalani M, Acosta-Torres S, El Ahmadieh TY, Loya J, Ganju A. History of simulation in medicine: from Resusci Annie to the Ann Myers Medical Center. Neurosurgery. 2013;73(Suppl 1):9–14. https://doi.org/10.1227/NEU.0000000000000093.
3. Jandu GK, Khan A. Angelique Marguerite Le Boursier du Coudray (1712–1790)—pioneer of simulation. J Med Biogr. 2021;29(2):121–2. https://doi.org/10.1177/09677720211002204.
4. Chiniara G, Crelinsten L. A brief history of clinical simulation: how did we get here? In: Chiniara G, editor. Clinical simulation. 2nd ed. London: Elsevier; 2019. p. 3–16. https://doi.org/10.1016/B978-0-12-815657-5.00001-2.
5. Khan M, Sasso RA. Obtaining medical simulation center accreditation. In: StatPearls [Internet]. Treasure Island: StatPearls Publishing; 2022. [cited 2025 Oct 6]. Available from: https://www.ncbi.nlm.nih.gov/books/NBK554424/.
6. Society for Simulation in Healthcare. Home [Internet]. Society for Simulation in Healthcare; 2025. [cited 2025 Aug 12]. Available from: https://www.ssih.org.

7. Western Michigan University Homer Stryker M.D. School of Medicine. Simulation center [Internet]. Western Michigan University; 2026. [cited 2025 Aug 12]. Available from: https://wmed.edu/simulationcenter.
8. Elendu CB, Amaechi DC, Okatta AU, Amaechi EC, Elendu TC, Ezeh CP, Elendu ID. The impact of simulation-based training in medical education: a review. Medicine (Baltimore). 2024;103(27):e38813.
9. Wayne DB, Didwania A, Feinglass J, Fudala MJ, Barsuk JH, McGaghie WC. Simulation-based education improves quality of care during cardiac arrest team responses at an academic teaching hospital. Chest. 2008;133(1):56–61.
10. Ogden PE, Sokolovskaya G, Howell M, et al. Clinical simulation: importance to the internal medicine educational mission. Am J Med. 2007;120(9):820–4.
11. Gallagher AG, Cates CU. Approval of virtual reality training for carotid stenting: what this means for procedural-based medicine. JAMA. 2004;292(24):3024–6.
12. Sizemore J, Bailey A, Sankineni S, et al. Training to transition: using simulation-based training to improve resident physician confidence in hospital discharges. MededPortal. 2023;19:11348. https://doi.org/10.15766/mep_2374-8265.11348.
13. Eppich W, Cheng A. Promoting Excellence and Reflective Learning in Simulation (PEARLS): development and rationale for a blended approach to health care simulation debriefing. Simul Healthc. 2015;10(2):106–15.
14. Allen JA, Reiter-Palmon R, Crowe J, Scott C. Debriefs: teams learning from doing in context. Am Psychol. 2018;73(4):504.
15. Schertzer K, Patti L. In situ debriefing in medical simulation. In: StatPearls. Treasure Island: StatPearls Publishing; 2022.
16. Schaepkens SP, Veen M, de la Croix A. Is reflection like soap? A critical narrative umbrella review of approaches to reflection in medical education research. Adv Health Sci Educ Theory Pract. 2022;27(2):537–51. https://doi.org/10.1007/s10459-021-10082-7.
17. Mirza MB, Sulaiman A, Hashmi S, Zaki S, Rehman R, Akbar R. Use of simulation based technology in pre-clinical years improves confidence and satisfaction among medical students. J Pak Med Assoc. 2021;71(4):1296–302.
18. Ahmad M, Page M, Goodsman D. What is simulation-based medical education (SBME) debriefing in prehospital medicine? A qualitative, ethnographic study exploring SBME debriefing in prehospital medical education. BMC Med Educ. 2023;23(1):625. https://doi.org/10.1186/s12909-023-04592-8.
19. Yu JH, Chang HJ, Kim SS, et al. Effects of high-fidelity simulation education on medical students' anxiety and confidence. PLoS One. 2021;16(5):e0251078.
20. Feldman M, Edwards C, Wong A, Randolph J, Woleben C, Nguyen A, Grossman C. The role for simulation in professional identity formation in medical students. Simul Healthc. 2022;17(1):e8–e13.
21. Campbell KK, Wong KE, Kerchberger AM, Lysikowski J, Scott DJ, Sulistio MS. Simulation-based education in US undergraduate medical education. Simul Healthc. 2023;18(6):359–66. https://doi.org/10.1097/SIH.0000000000000705.
22. Bradley P. The history of simulation in medical education and possible future directions. Med Educ. 2006;40(3):254–62.
23. Mundell WC, Kennedy CC, Szostek JH, Cook DA. Simulation technology for resuscitation training: a systematic review and meta-analysis. Resuscitation. 2013;84(9):1174–83.
24. McGaghie WC, Issenberg SB, Cohen ER, Barsuk JH, Wayne DB. Does simulation-based medical education with deliberate practice yield better results than traditional clinical education? A meta-analytic comparative review of the evidence. Acad Med. 2011;86(6):706–11. https://doi.org/10.1097/ACM.0b013e318217e119.
25. Irfanullah EA, Chandra A, Solaiman RH, Siems C, Chethan S, Belani K, et al. Simulation training in a lower middle-income country: supporting a new center and developing low-cost models for critical skill acquisition. Cureus. 2023;15(6):e40950.

26. Hammond KM, Morgan CJ. Development of interprofessional healthcare teamwork skills: mapping students' process of learning. J Interprof Care. 2022;36(4):589–98.
27. Kothari LG, Shah K, Barach P. Simulation based medical education in graduate medical education training and assessment programs. Prog Pediatr Cardiol. 2017;44:33–42.
28. Tseng LP, Hou TH, Huang LP, Ou YK. Effectiveness of applying clinical simulation scenarios and integrating information technology in medical-surgical nursing and critical nursing courses. BMC Nurs. 2021;20(1):229.
29. Chow KM, Ahmat R, Leung AW, Chan CW. Is high-fidelity simulation-based training in emergency nursing effective in enhancing clinical decision-making skills? A mixed methods study. Nurse Educ Pract. 2023;69:103610. https://doi.org/10.1016/j.nepr.2023.103610.
30. Zendejas B, Brydges R, Wang AT, Cook DA. Patient outcomes in simulation-based medical education: a systematic review. J Gen Intern Med. 2013;28(8):1078–89.
31. Griswold-Theodorson S, Ponnuru S, Dong C, Szyld D, Reed T, McGaghie WC. Beyond the simulation laboratory. Acad Med. 2015;90(11):1553–60. https://doi.org/10.1097/ACM.0000000000000938.
32. Park O, Jeon M, Kim M, Kim B, Jeong H. The effects of a simulation-based patient safety education program on compliance with patient safety, perception of patient safety culture, and educational satisfaction of operating room nurses. Healthcare. 2023;11(21):2824. https://doi.org/10.3390/healthcare11212824.
33. Schaad S. Simulation-based training: malignant hyperthermia: patient safety first. AORN J. 2017;106(2):158–61. https://doi.org/10.1016/j.aorn.2017.06.008.
34. Lewis KA, Ricks TN, Rowin A, Ndlovu C, Goldstein L, McElvogue C. Does simulation training for acute care nurses improve patient safety outcomes: a systematic review to inform evidence-based practice. Worldviews Evid-Based Nurs. 2019;16(5):389.
35. Goldshtein D, Krensky C, Doshi S, Perelman VS. In situ simulation and its effects on patient outcomes: a systematic review. BMJ Simul Technol Enhanc Learn. 2020;6(1):3. https://doi.org/10.1136/bmjstel-2018-000387.
36. Barsuk JH, Cohen ER, Feinglass J, McGaghie WC, Wayne DB. Use of simulation-based education to reduce catheter-related bloodstream infections. Arch Intern Med. 2009;169(15):1420–3. https://doi.org/10.1001/archinternmed.2009.215.
37. Gjeraa K, Møller TP, Østergaard D. Efficacy of simulation-based trauma team training of non-technical skills. A systematic review. Acta Anaesthesiol Scand. 2014;58(7):775–87.
38. Geis GL, Pio B, Pendergrass TL, Moyer MR, Patterson MD. Simulation to assess the safety of new healthcare teams and new facilities. Simul Healthc. 2011;6(3):125–33.
39. Schmidt E, Goldhaber-Fiebert SN, Ho LA, McDonald KM. Simulation exercises as a patient safety strategy: a systematic review. Ann Intern Med. 2013;158(5 Pt 2):426–32.
40. Senvisky JM, McKenna RT, Okuda Y. Financing and funding a simulation center. In: StatPearls [Internet]. Treasure Island: StatPearls Publishing; 2023. [cited 2025 Oct 6]. Available from: https://www.ncbi.nlm.nih.gov/books/NBK568786/.
41. Eliadis M, Verkuyl M. Balancing the budget in the simulation Centre. Clin Simul Nurs. 2019;37:14–7.
42. Tranel GE, Johanneck MD, Thompson RJ, Campbell KK. Results of a nationwide descriptive survey on simulation center operations. Clin Simul Nurs. 2021;53:32–41.
43. Natal B, Szyld D, Pasichow S, Bismilla Z, Pirie J, Cheng A, International Simulation Fellowship Training Investigators. Simulation fellowship programs: an international survey of program directors. Acad Med. 2017;92(8):1204–11. https://doi.org/10.1097/ACM.0000000000001668. PMID: 28379935.
44. Kotal ER, Sivertson RM, Wolfe SP, Lammers RL, Overton DT. A survey of simulation fellowship programs. J Emerg Med. 2015;48(3):351–5. https://doi.org/10.1016/j.jemermed.2014.10.004. PMID: 25456774.
45. Kumar EJ, Parameswari A, Manickam A, Purva M. Establishment of a simulation Centre: challenges and solutions. Indian J Anaesth. 2024;68(1):45–51.

46. Gable B, Ballas D, Ahmed RA. Enhancing simulation education using expired materials. BMJ Simul Technol Enhanc Learn. 2020;6(3):129–31.
47. Zendejas B, Wang AT, Brydges R, Hamstra SJ, Cook DA. Cost: the missing outcome in simulation-based medical education research: a systematic review. Surgery. 2013;153(2):160–76.
48. Gupta S, Wilcocks K, Matava C, Wiegelmann J, Kaustov L, Alam F. Creating a successful virtual reality-based medical simulation environment: tutorial. JMIR Med Educ. 2023;9:e41090.
49. Sawaya RD, Mrad S, Rajha E, Saleh R, Rice J. Simulation-based curriculum development: lessons learnt in Global Health education. BMC Med Educ. 2021;21(1):33. https://doi.org/10.1186/s12909-020-02430-9.
50. Khamis NN, Satava RM, Alnassar SA, Kern DE. A stepwise model for simulation-based curriculum development for clinical skills, a modification of the six-step approach. Surg Endosc. 2016;30(1):279–87. https://doi.org/10.1007/s00464-015-4206-x.
51. Motola I, Devine LA, Chung HS, Sullivan JE, Issenberg SB. Simulation in healthcare education: a best evidence practical guide. AMEE Guide No. 82. Med Teach. 2013;35(10):e1511–30.
52. Al-Elq A. Simulation-based medical teaching and learning. J Fam Community Med. 2010;17(1):35–40.
53. Zeng Q, Wang K, Liu WX, Zeng JZ, Li XL, Zhang QF, Ren SQ, Xu WM. Efficacy of high-fidelity simulation in advanced life support training: a systematic review and meta-analysis of randomized controlled trials. BMC Med Educ. 2023;23(1):664. https://doi.org/10.1186/s12909-023-04654-x.
54. Cheng A, Lockey A, Bhanji F, Lin Y, Hunt EA, Lang E. The use of high-fidelity manikins for advanced life support training—a systematic review and meta-analysis. Resuscitation. 2015;93:142–9. https://doi.org/10.1016/j.resuscitation.2015.04.004.
55. Norman G, Dore K, Grierson L. The minimal relationship between simulation fidelity and transfer of learning. Med Educ. 2012;46(7):636–47.
56. Massoth C, Röder H, Ohlenburg H, Hessler M, Zarbock A, Pöpping DM, Wenk M. High-fidelity is not superior to low-fidelity simulation but leads to overconfidence in medical students. BMC Med Educ. 2019;19(1):29. https://doi.org/10.1186/s12909-019-1464-7.

Innovations in the Preclinical Curriculum: Third-Party Resources and Modern Strategies in Medical Education

Sarah Zalubas, John Paul Arslanian, Alexander Lindsay, and Kelsey Temprine Grellinger

Introduction

The Flexner Report and the Preclinical Curriculum

Over a century ago, the Carnegie Foundation for the Advancement of Teaching invited Abraham Flexner to evaluate the state of medical education in the United States and Canada. From 1908 to 1909, Flexner toured all 155 medical schools in the United States and Canada. He found medical education in the early twentieth century to be lacking in quality, taking issue with the commercial identity of medical schools and the unstandardized curriculum across different medical schools [1].

As a result, the Flexner Report in 1910 set modern standards for medical education in the United States. Among other directives, this report urged the linkage between medical schools and research universities, emphasizing basic science training for medical students. Correspondingly, the Flexner Report established the standard for 2 years of basic laboratory science education succeeded by 2 years of clinical training for all medical students.

Sarah Zalubas, John Paul Arslanian and Alexander Lindsay contributed equally with all other contributors.

S. Zalubas · J. P. Arslanian · A. Lindsay
Western Michigan University Homer Stryker M.D. School of Medicine, Kalamazoo, MI, USA

K. T. Grellinger (✉)
Department of Biomedical Sciences, Western Michigan University Homer Stryker M.D. School of Medicine, Kalamazoo, MI, USA
e-mail: kelsey.grellinger@wmed.edu

S. S. Chahin et al. (eds.), *Innovation in Medical Education and Clinical Practice*, https://doi.org/10.1007/978-3-032-19116-8_4

In modern times, while some schools have shortened the length of the preclinical curriculum, the arrangement of preclinical instruction prior to clinical application still comprises the fundamental structure of the 4 years of medical school that we recognize today [2].

The COVID-19 Pandemic and the Shift to Virtual Learning

In Flexner's time during the early twentieth century, preclinical education consisted of lectures to students in the classroom and the laboratory. These preclinical medical students learned solely from their instructors in person, a model that has become less prominent today due to technological advances and a recent global event that changed the mode of education forever.

In March 2020, the COVID-19 pandemic and associated stay-at-home orders sent all students out of the classroom. In the years leading up to the pandemic, many medical schools had begun to offer their students the option to view their preclinical lectures virtually, but the pandemic hastened the transition for the masses. With no opportunity for in-person lectures, the medical education community was forced to determine how effective instruction could be delivered to students in an alternative fashion.

Today, several years after the COVID-19 pandemic, medical students have returned to the classroom, but it looks quite different. With the requirement for in-person attendance at every lecture no longer in play at many medical schools, lecture halls are much emptier. Many medical students choose to livestream the lectures from the comfort of their own homes or watch uploaded recordings at a later time.

Medical Student Learning Today

Perhaps even more significant than virtual lectures is the use of "third-party" online resources to enhance medical student learning. Medical education resources from companies outside of the purview of medical schools have come to light as a form of "parallel curriculum" to supplement, and, in some cases replace, institution-specific lectures [3]. These third-party resources occupy several niches in the medical education curriculum, specializing in high-yield review and alternative ways of presenting information. The advantage to many of these resources is that they draw from modern learning theories rooted in cognitive psychology. In other words, they use what psychology researchers have learned about the process of learning in the last 100 years to help modern medical students learn, synthesize, and apply information that has traditionally been presented as a lecture in the classroom.

Some resources offer practice questions in the style of USMLE Step 1 questions to prepare students to think in the way that will be required of them to pass the exam. Others provide shortened lecture videos that cover the highest yield topics, maximizing efficiency in reviewing material. Even more resources take advantage of psychology concepts such as the memory palace and spaced repetition, which have been demonstrated to be effective in improving long-term recall [4, 5]. These third-party resources are not bound by the traditional instructor-student relationship and therefore have the potential to offer innovative advantages.

Of course, a discussion about the modern tools of medical student learning would be incomplete without the mention of artificial intelligence tools that are quickly changing the educational landscape. ChatGPT is a popular tool among medical students used for writing, quickly summarizing material, and more. However, while AI tools deliver tempting advantages, they also bring to the forefront the dangers and ethical questions associated with all these novel tools [6].

Since Flexner's time, medical student education has changed in innovative ways as our understanding of education and technology has advanced. This chapter will discuss common resources used by today's medical students, explore how they are used, and analyze why students must be careful when using them.

Third-Party Lecture Videos

What are Third-Party Lecture Videos?

As technology continues to improve, the modalities in which medical students consume information are continuously changing. For example, third-party companies separate from specific medical schools are now creating medical education lecture videos designed to cover high-yield topics. The development of these third-party video resources by companies such as Boards and Beyond, Pathoma, and Bootcamp has led to a significant shift from the traditional style of classroom-based learning to a student self-teaching approach through the use of asynchronous, third-party lecture videos [7]. In fact, nearly 70% of medical students state that they use third-party online videos weekly for their medical education [7]. The magnitude of this trend indicates that further discussion is necessary on the impact of these videos on medical education.

Strengths

There are numerous reasons that medical students choose to use third-party lecture videos. Some students elect to use these videos as supplements to the lectures given by faculty, while other students choose to solely rely on these videos for their learning. Students often claim that institution-specific lectures contain extraneous information that is not covered on exams or not clinically relevant, leading to frustration due to their busy schedules [8]. This has discouraged many students from solely engaging with institution-specific lectures as they have identified that third-party videos tend to present high-yield details in a concise manner, ultimately enhancing the efficiency of studying [8]. The medical students that treat third-party lecture videos as supplemental content to institution-specific lectures value the ability to hear similar information from multiple different sources and instructors [7]. This method empowers students to use these succinct videos to cement content knowledge by filling in the gaps of knowledge that they had after engaging with institution-specific lectures.

In addition to providing students alternative descriptions of important concepts, third-party lecture resources typically provide several ways for students to interact with the content. Medical students have stated their appreciation for opportunities to interact with content as they feel it better allows them to direct their learning [7]. This feeling of autonomy over one's learning has been shown to be critically important to the learning process. Adult learners have improved performance and satisfaction as a result of self-directed learning. By providing options such as short videos, practice questions, and flashcards, these third-party lecture resources empower students to take control of their medical education [7].

Weaknesses

While self-directed learning has been demonstrated to have a positive impact on medical student learning, there is evidence suggesting that using video resources may not be as effective as alternative studying methods. This stems from the consumption of lecture videos being a passive form of studying. A study conducted at the University of Arkansas for Medical Sciences College of Medicine found that there was an improvement in USMLE Step 1 scores associated with active study strategies, but no such improvement was identified with passive study strategies [9]. Therefore, the rate of consumption of lecture videos should be closely monitored to ensure productive preparation for licensure exams. An additional limitation of the shift from traditional classroom-style learning to online, third-party learning involves the disconnect that is formed between students and institutional faculty [8]. The lack of human interaction results in isolation from classmates as well as the inability of institutional faculty to identify areas in which they could address the personal academic needs of each student.

Conclusion

Third-party lecture videos are commonly used by medical students as their concise descriptions of high-yield information enable students to be self-directed learners by helping to efficiently fill in their gaps of knowledge. The utilization of these videos in this manner has been demonstrated to have positive impacts on medical student performance. However, medical students should not over-rely on learning through online lecture videos due to the inefficiency of this passive learning style. Thus, these tools can be maximized when used alongside active learning strategies, whether provided by the institution or by third-party sources. By understanding the specific ways in which these tools can improve and hinder learning, medical students can be well-equipped self-directed learners through thoughtfully formulating their study schedules.

Question Banks

What are Question Banks?

Question banks are some of the most popular tools used by medical students throughout their education. Some medical schools provide faculty-generated question banks to help students prepare for exams, but the most popular resources are from third parties like UWorld and ScholarRX. These tools are typically formatted with a clinical vignette followed by multiple-choice questions with explanations presented after the answers are submitted. On average, students complete approximately 2666 practice questions in preparation for the USMLE Step 1 exam, accounting for up to 50% of their total study time [10].

Learning Theory

The effectiveness of question banks is supported by three major learning theories: the testing effect, gamification, and cognitive load theory. The testing effect refers to the observation that repeated testing of learned material enhances long-term memory by promoting active recall and providing immediate feedback [11]. This repeated testing is a core feature of question banks and forces students to engage with the material before advancing. Furthermore, engaging with material in a low-stakes environment allows students to benefit from the testing effect prior to high-stakes exams that have a much higher consequence of failure. After a session, many platforms provide feedback on performance relative to other users. This combination of immediate feedback and peer-score comparisons introduces a form of gamification. Gamification refers to the use of game-like elements such as scoring, competition, and progress tracking in non-game contexts, and it can enhance motivation and engagement [10].

Cognitive load theory suggests that individuals have limited working memory and that learning can be hindered by three types of cognitive load: intrinsic, extraneous, and germane. Intrinsic load reflects the inherent difficulty of a concept; thus, harder topics require more mental effort. Extraneous load includes non-essential distractions that reduce learning efficiency, such as background noise or poorly designed learning material. Germane load is the cognitive effort used to encode information into long-term memory [12]. Many question banks are built around carefully constructed vignettes and focused topic coverage, which minimizes extraneous load and frees up working memory to process new information, helping to encode information into long-term memory [13]. Additionally, they help reduce intrinsic load by breaking down complex subjects into smaller, more manageable parts [13].

Strengths

The success of question banks is demonstrated by their strong correlation with USMLE Step 1 scores (prior to the exam becoming pass/fail in 2022). In fact, studies found a dose-response relationship: the more practice questions completed, the higher the expected score [9]. This suggests that the emphasis students place on question banks is well-founded, and that beginning earlier in medical school may be advantageous for maximizing question volume. Students should be informed that using practice questions as a review tool, rather than a primary method of learning, is associated with better exam performance [13]. The widespread use of question banks is grounded in both theory and evidence, indicating that they can be an efficient way to spend a medical student's time.

Weaknesses

Medical students often have limited time, and many question banks do not align perfectly with their school's curriculum [11]. As a result, students may end up learning content that is not immediately relevant, or waste time discerning which questions apply to their current coursework. Additionally, students tend to not check the veracity of the information presented through question banks. Given the rapidly evolving nature of medical education, it is critical to evaluate content against individual curricula and the expectations of licensing exams.

The gamified nature of question banks may also encourage unproductive behaviors. For instance, some students select easier questions when given the option in order to maintain high scores. Moreover, students often report using question banks because of extrinsic motivations, like anxiety or fatigue [10]. While having an easy-access study tool can be beneficial for short bursts of last-minute review, relying on it in the long term may contribute to burnout, a common issue among medical students.

Conclusion

Practice questions have been a cornerstone of medical student study strategies for decades. This method is supported by both robust theoretical frameworks and experimental data, but its drawbacks must also be acknowledged. Students should be mindful of how gamification can distort learning habits and ensure that their study efforts align with their school's curriculum and licensure requirements. By recognizing question banks as both powerful educational tools and potential sources of inefficiency, students can develop study strategies that support both academic success and long-term well-being.

Anki

What is Anki?

Anki is a digital flashcard-based learning tool utilized by many medical students. The program uses spaced repetition to optimize learning and support the retention of vast amounts of information.

Learning Theory

The theoretical underpinnings supporting the use of Anki are grounded in the spacing effect, which states that practice via repetition spread out over time tends to produce stronger and longer lasting memories than learning information all at once. Additionally, spaced repetition has been shown to increase the generalizability of learned information [14]. Since medical school curricula tend to refer back to previously learned topics, it is highly advantageous to utilize programs that are efficient at retaining knowledge and adaptable for future application.

Strengths

The unique strength of Anki is its blend of flexibility and customizability with the consistency it demands. There are several ways that users can build their spaced-repetition algorithm. Upon seeing and completing each flashcard, users have the option to select "again," "hard," "good," or "easy" based on the perceived difficulty of that card. The harder the card is, the sooner the user will see it again. The length of time between when a card is seen each time varies depending on how many times the user has seen the card previously and the previous inputs the user gave regarding its difficulty.

Flashcards can be made in different ways, which further increases the flexibility of Anki in supporting medical education [15]. The most popular card type used among students is the "cloze deletion" style. In this card style, a pre-written sentence will appear with one or more missing words. For visual learning, images can be pasted into cards and through the "image occlusion" card type, areas of the image can be blocked. This is especially useful for anatomy-focused events where images of labeled structures and diagrams can be pasted with the labels blocked until the card is completed.

Flashcards can be made individually and shared with others. Using decks made by other students is a common practice at many medical schools and is increasingly popular among certain residency programs [15]. While exact figures vary, over half of medical students likely use Anki regularly [5, 16]. Usage patterns vary, but most students use Anki to reinforce learning after a lecture has been completed [16].

The use of Anki is optimized when students adhere to the daily regimen of cards due. Among Anki users, students who adopted its use earlier in the curriculum and used it consistently tended to score higher on preclinical exams than those who adopted its use later and used it sporadically [17]. Furthermore, students who use Anki consistently tend to avoid "cramming" before exams and, in some cases, even decrease their overall study time [17], likely reflecting greater exam preparedness. Additionally, students who create their own flashcards may achieve greater improvements in exam performance than those who rely on premade decks [18]. This suggests that students who create and review their own flashcards may derive the greatest gains in exam performance. There is also some evidence that using Anki is correlated with better sleep quality among preclinical medical students [19], which could be a result of the reduced cramming and more structured daily routines.

Academic performance is highly correlated to engagement with Anki as a study tool. Anki users tend to score higher on the Comprehensive Basic Science Examination (CBSE), a test used by medical schools to gauge readiness for USMLE Step 1. Moreover, there is a dose-response relationship between self-reported dependency on Anki as the primary study tool and higher CBSE scores [5]. Prior to the USMLE Step 1 transition to pass/fail scoring, Anki use was linked to significantly higher exam scores. The Anki program has internal metrics like card retrievability and true retention percentage, but it is important to note that there is currently no evidence that exam scores are correlated to these metrics [5]. Students should use these metrics as guides for studying but be cautious in interpreting them as predictive of future exam scores.

Weaknesses

Using the program optimally, meaning everyday use, can be challenging. Medical school students are exceptionally busy with many different activities to balance. Finding the time to complete several hundred cards per day is daunting and missing a day means those uncompleted cards move to the next day, which can be demoralizing. One of the biggest challenges in using Anki is translating lecture material into high-quality flashcards. Many medical schools use exams written by institution-specific faculty, which can necessitate a more personalized set of flashcards than what is available on the Internet. Finally, much like SketchyMedical, Anki can promote the memorization of facts, rather than promoting a deeper understanding of the content. It is critical to be aware of this while studying to ensure both the learning of new information and the integration of facts into a wider understanding of the content.

Conclusion

Anki is one of the most potent digital learning tools available to undergraduate medical students. The use of spaced repetition with optimized flashcard intervals makes it possible to retain the massive amount of information that medical students are expected to learn. While it may represent a large time commitment each day and missing a day can lead to a daunting pile-up of flashcards, the strong correlation with CBSE test scores demonstrates the large payoff in its use for students in the preclinical phase of their curriculum. When used appropriately, Anki is a powerful tool in the medical student's arsenal.

SketchyMedical

What is SketchyMedical?

With the vast amount of content retention required throughout medical school, medical students often rely on the use of memory aids such as pictures and acronyms to properly develop and maintain their understanding of complex concepts. SketchyMedical provides over 1400 narrated sketches covering a wide variety of important medical topics (Fig. 1). Within SketchyMedical, there are sections dedicated to specific subjects like microbiology, pathophysiology, pharmacology, and more [21]. Through the use of recurring symbols, concept grouping, and narration, SketchyMedical's sketches help students remember the most important components of each diagnosis or medication.

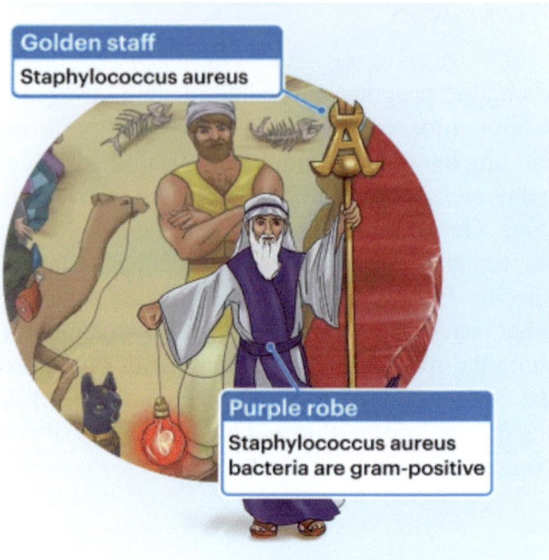
Golden staff
Staphylococcus aureus
Purple robe
Staphylococcus aureus
bacteria are gram-positive

Fig. 1 An example image and description of a recurring symbol in SketchyMedical [20]

Learning Theory

SketchyMedical empowers each student to expand and maximize their personal memory palace, a mnemonic technique that utilizes the underlying principles of the Method of Loci. The Method of Loci is a popular memory activation technique that maximizes the brain's ability to efficiently store spatial data and its capacity to visually recall information [21]. Traditionally, the Method of Loci has involved visualized navigation through an imagined environment. Within this imaginary environment, items to be remembered are located along the route to associate a spatial location to each item for enhanced recall [22]. Individuals who use the Method of Loci have substantially improved memory recall relative to individuals who do not use any specific memory technique [22]. The advancement of technology has empowered companies such as SketchyMedical to take advantage of this method through the creation of virtual environments with recurrent items or symbols placed around the sketch. These newly designed virtual environments have been shown to provide similar improvements in memory recall as the traditional Method of Loci.

In support of the utilization of spatial learning strategies for formation and retention of concepts, it has been demonstrated that "world-renowned outstanding memories" are not a result of increased intellectual abilities of those individuals but rather based upon their use of a spatial learning strategy. In fact, individuals who used spatial learning techniques have an increase in brain activity in the right hippocampus, an area critically important in the formation and development of long-term memory [23]. This increase in hippocampal involvement is crucial to creating a memory trace that can be retrieved at later instances, which is vital for medical students in their roles as test-takers and future physicians.

Strengths

Anecdotally, medical students have noted many benefits from incorporating cartoon-style resources such as SketchyMedical into their study routines. Students often feel the cartoon nature of the sketches tricks their brain into being more engaged with the content. Furthermore, these students mention that the cartoon-style resources enable them to better memorize large chunks of information, stating visualization of an image is more efficient than rote memorization of facts. Some students even mentioned that they often watch these sketches as a primer to their in-class lectures. They cite the utilization of recurrent symbols and imagery that resemble the long and complex names of various drugs, organisms, and pathophysiological conditions as an effective way to organize their memory palace. By priming their minds, students state they are less likely to get overwhelmed by the vast amount of content that is presented during their standard lectures [7].

SketchyMedical appeals to students with a variety of learning preferences as a result of its multimodal instructional approach. While visual learners are typically drawn to cartoon drawings, there are also narrations for auditory learners. Furthermore, SketchyMedical is designed by medical students [21]. As a result, the resource has been developed to include high-yield concepts in consolidated and sectioned videos. This enables students to pick and choose which topics they would like to learn and helps make SketchyMedical an efficient study tool in preparation for standardized licensing exams such as USMLE and COMLEX [21].

Weaknesses

SketchyMedical, however, does have limitations as a tool in medical education. One area of limitation involves the over-reliance on memorization-based learning rather than on forming a conceptual understanding. In fact, some argue that because of the vast amount of information readily available for students to memorize, they experience a form of information overload which can lead to a reliance on the memorization of facts rather than an actual understanding of the reasoning [24]. While memorization of facts certainly has its place in medical education, there are often complex pathways and clinical situations that require a deeper understanding and the ability to problem-solve that are not effectively learned through the simple recollection of facts.

Conclusion

While not without its drawbacks, SketchyMedical is a commonly used tool that is effective in helping medical students manage the wealth of knowledge that they are required to learn. Through the formation of memory palaces by using the Method of Loci, the recurrent symbols in these sketches have been shown via multiple studies to improve students' ability to form and retrieve memories. Via its consolidated and multimodal approach, SketchyMedical serves as an effective medical education tool for many students.

ChatGPT

What is ChatGPT?

ChatGPT is a large language model (LLM) that has recently grown in popularity among many segments of the workforce and education, including medical students. LLMs are a specific type of artificial intelligence (AI) designed for natural language processing [25]. ChatGPT allows students to type into an online chat box and have a natural-sounding conversation with the software. Given the rapid response times and the complexity of medical topics, students gravitate toward its use.

The use of ChatGPT in medical education is broad and polarizing. Roughly half of medical students report using ChatGPT weekly [6]. The natural language processing feature of ChatGPT makes it easy for students to ask questions and engage in a dialogue while it assesses their understanding. For this reason, many students are more likely to ask ChatGPT a question than to consult a textbook, lecture, or professor [6]. However, while the future is bright for artificial intelligence in medical education, its current state leaves much to be desired, and users must be aware of its strengths and limitations.

Strengths

ChatGPT's uses are broad but generally fall into three categories: writing, understanding complex topics, and generating practice questions [6, 26]. Through these uses, medical students attempt to streamline their education. Students can use ChatGPT to help with low-stakes assignments by refining ideas, finding resources and publications, and editing [26]. This frees up time for other scholarly activities. The same can be said for breaking down complex medical topics. The chatbot feature of ChatGPT gives students a rapid way to find answers to questions that may be difficult to answer using a typical Internet search. Finally, generating practice questions and scenarios is one of the main ways students engage with course material and prepare for exams. ChatGPT gives students a method to generate practice questions for highly specific medical school content. ChatGPT's speed and adaptability offer a swift method for obtaining answers and accelerating previously laborious tasks, thereby significantly enhancing the efficiency of medical education.

Weaknesses

While ChatGPT may be updated frequently, it is not updated continuously. This means that the data fed into ChatGPT to generate dialogue may not reflect the most current medical guidelines [26]. These inaccuracies can be compounded by hallucinations, a phenomenon in which AI models present false information as true [25]. Although observant medical students might occasionally detect AI hallucinations, the awareness of their possibility hinders complete trust in ChatGPT or even lead to students learning incorrect information, particularly during the initial stages of learning a new subject. While ChatGPT can streamline medical education, it is imperative that students and educators be aware of its drawbacks and remain cautious in its use in the classroom.

Conclusion

The use of ChatGPT and other types of AI represents one of the next major steps in advancing the efficacy of medical education. It allows for less time spent on low-stakes tasks and more time spent understanding challenging concepts that will help shape students into great physicians. In its current state, however, information presented by ChatGPT cannot be blindly trusted. Students and educators must approach its use with skepticism and exercise judgment regarding how and when it is appropriate. With thoughtful integration and continued improvement, ChatGPT holds the potential to become an indispensable ally in shaping the next generation of physicians and medical educators.

Dangers and Ethics

Cost and Disparity in Learning Opportunities

One of the considerations at the forefront of most medical students' minds is cost. As of 2024, the average medical student graduates with $234,597 in debt from medical school alone, excluding any potential debt from premedical studies. This debt burden also falls inequitably on minority communities. 91% of Black non-Hispanic medical students carry debt compared to an average of 72% across all other medical students. Possibly due to the prospective debt, the proportion of low-income students starting medical school has been declining since 2017 [27].

The third-party resources discussed earlier in this chapter come at an additional cost beyond medical school tuition. Some of these companies charge over $500 for a one-year subscription to their service (Table 1). A subscription to any of these third-party resources, in addition to debt already accumulated from tuition, living expenses, board exams, and more, results in an even greater financial burden to medical students.

Should some students opt to forego the use of these resources due to financial concerns, there is the potential to create a disparity in learning opportunities between those who can afford to pay for these subscriptions and those who cannot. This difference in learning opportunities could affect a student's chance of passing USMLE Step 1. A failed attempt at USMLE Step 1 greatly decreases a medical student's chance at matching into the residency of their choice [34]. Therefore, the cost of third-party resources could potentially generate a difference in residency match rates and specialty choices between those who can afford to pay for them and those who cannot.

Accuracy Concerns

In addition to the concern of cost, medical students must be careful when considering the accuracy of the material presented by third-party resources. Third-party resources are not vetted by individual schools for their accuracy nor assessed for alignment with institution-specific material [3]. Additionally, as mentioned previously, ChatGPT and other AI tools may suffer from hallucinations, or the presentation of inaccurate information as true [25]. It may be risky, therefore, to adopt external resources as pure replacements for school-specific lectures rather than as supplements. It is possible that future accuracy concerns could be mitigated as the

Table 1 Cost of third-party resources

Third-party resource	Type of resource	Cost for one-year subscription
Boards and Beyond	Third-Party Lecture Videos	$249 [28]
Pathoma	Third-Party Lecture Videos	$99.95 [29]
Bootcamp	Third-Party Lecture Videos Question Bank	$249 [30]
UWorld	Question Bank	$559 [31]
ScholarRx (Rx360+ plan)	Question Bank	$279.30 [32]
Anki	–	Free
Sketchy	–	$449.99 [33]
ChatGPT	Artificial Intelligence	Free

instructor's role transitions from the "sage on the stage" to the "guide on the side" [35] as more instructors embrace third-party resources to deliver content while they help students find, apply, and integrate the information.

Resource Overload and Student Mental Health

Medical students already carry increased levels of depression, anxiety, and stress compared to their non-medical peers. They must juggle intense academic expectations, financial debt, imposter syndrome, and more to stay afloat in the curriculum [36]. The addition of third-party resources to a medical student's plate can result in resource overload, which is the overwhelmed feeling that students experience when inundated by the vast number of resources offered by their school and by third parties [34]. The challenge presented by the overwhelming number of third-party resources is compounded by the learning curve to use them. Given the stress that medical students endure with institution-specific curriculum alone, they must be selective when choosing the third-party resources that they will use and how they will use them.

Conclusions

As the medical education landscape rapidly adjusts alongside technological improvements, one fact remains evident: medical students are committed to learning and retaining information in the most effective and efficient ways possible. As more medical students veer from the traditional pedagogical structure of professor-led lectures at their institution, it is imperative to understand the impact that alternative study tools and strategies can have on their education. Whether through principles of active recall via platforms such as Anki and question banks, memory aids such as those used in SketchyMedical, or targeted ways of getting condensed explanations of high-yield topics such as third-party lecture videos and ChatGPT, these new tools are derived from evidence-based learning techniques.

However, it is necessary to consider the potential for various negative effects of the increased use of these tools, including increased burnout rates, increased financial stress, incorrect use, inaccurate information, and diminished relationships with institutional faculty. Overall, student satisfaction and test scores have demonstrated a role for these tools in the ever-developing field of medical education, but students should be encouraged to be selective on which tools they use to supplement their learning to maximize efficiency while limiting the risks these new tools can present.

References

1. Arky RA. Abe Flexner, where are you? we need you! Trans Am Clin Climatol Assoc [Internet]. 2007 [cited 2025 Jun 22];118:89. Available from: https://pmc.ncbi.nlm.nih.gov/articles/PMC1863593/.
2. Duffy TP. The Flexner report — 100 years later. Yale J Biol Med [Internet]. 2011 [cited 2025 May 25];84(3):269. Available from: https://pmc.ncbi.nlm.nih.gov/articles/PMC3178858/.
3. Verma N, Yui JC, Record JD, Hueppchen NA, Naik RP. The changing landscape of the preclinical medical school curriculum: results from a Nationwide Survey of United States Medical School Curriculum Deans. Am J Med [Internet]. 2024 [cited 2025 Jun 22];137(2):178–184.e2. Available from: https://www.sciencedirect.com/science/article/pii/S000293432300671X.
4. Qureshi A, Rizvi F, Syed A, Shahid A, Manzoor H. The method of loci as a mnemonic device to facilitate learning in endocrinology leads to improvement in student performance as measured by assessments. Adv Physiol Educ [Internet]. 2014 [cited 2025 Jun 22];38(2):140. Available from: https://pmc.ncbi.nlm.nih.gov/articles/PMC4056179/.
5. Gilbert MM, Frommeyer TC, Brittain G V., Stewart NA, Turner TM, Stolfi A, et al. A Cohort Study assessing the impact of Anki as a spaced repetition tool on academic performance in medical school. Med Sci Educ [Internet]. 2023 [cited 2025 Jun 22];33(4):955. Available from: https://pmc.ncbi.nlm.nih.gov/articles/PMC10403443/.
6. Zhang JS, Yoon C, Williams DKA, Pinkas A. Exploring the usage of ChatGPT among medical students in the United States. J Med Educ Curric Dev [Internet]. 2024 [cited 2025 Jun 23];11:23821205241264696. Available from: https://pmc.ncbi.nlm.nih.gov/articles/PMC11292693/.
7. Lawrence ECN, Dine CJ, Kogan JR. Preclerkship medical students' use of third-party learning resources. JAMA Netw Open [Internet]. 2023 [cited 2025 Jun 30];6(12):e2345971. Available from: https://jamanetwork.com/journals/jamanetworkopen/fullarticle/2812522.
8. Kann MR, Huang GW, Pugazenthi S, Kann R, Chen D, Hardi A, et al. Unlocking medical student success: a systematic review and meta-analysis of third-party resources used for medical education and USMLE Board Preparation. Med Sci Educ [Internet]. 2024 [cited 2025 Jul 1];34(6):1603–22. Available from: https://link.springer.com/article/10.1007/s40670-024-02116-7.
9. Clemmons KR, Vuk J, Jarrett DM. Educational videos versus question banks: maximizing medical student performance on the United States medical licensing examination step 1 exam. Cureus. 2023;15:e38110.
10. Fisher J, Leahy D, Lim JJ, Astles E, Salvatore J, Thomson R. Question banks: credit? Or debit? A qualitative exploration of their use among medical students. BMC Med Educ. 2024;24:569.
11. Wynter L, Burgess A, Kalman E, Heron JE, Bleasel J. Medical students: what educational resources are they using? BMC Med Educ. 2019;19:36.
12. Young JQ, Van Merrienboer J, Durning S, Ten Cate O. Cognitive Load Theory: implications for medical education: AMEE guide No. 86. Med Teach. 2014;36:371–84.
13. Sheehy R, Scott D, Davis D, Roffler M, Sweatman T, Nemec E. Medical student use of practice questions in their studies: a qualitative study. BMC Med Educ. 2024;24:1181.
14. Smith CD, Scarf D. Spacing repetitions over long timescales: a review and a reconsolidation explanation. Front Psychol. 2017;8:962.
15. https://www.ama-assn.org/medical-students/usmle-step-1-2/what-anki [Internet]. What is Anki?.
16. Harris DM, Chiang M. An analysis of Anki usage and strategy of first-year medical students in a structure and function course. Cureus. 2022;14:e23530.
17. Mehta A, Brooke N, Puskar A, Woodson MCC, Masi B, Wallon RC, et al. Implementation of spaced repetition by first-year medical students: a retrospective comparison based on summative exam performance. Med Sci Educ. 2023;33:1089–94.

18. Pan SC, Zung I, Imundo MN, Zhang X, Qiu Y. User-generated digital flashcards yield better learning than Premade flashcards. 2022 [cited 2025 Sep 4]; Available from: https://doi.org/10.1037/mac0000083.supp.
19. Wothe JK, Wanberg LJ, Hohle RD, Sakher AA, Bosacker LE, Khan F, et al. Academic and wellness outcomes associated with use of Anki Spaced Repetition software in medical school. J Med Educat Curri Develop. 2023;10:23821205231173290.
20. Sketchy Medical | USMLE/COMLEX Prep Courses & QBank [Internet]. [cited 2025 Sep 4]. Available from: https://www.sketchy.com/explore/medical.
21. The Sketchy Method: Using Visual Memory and Elaborative Encoding to Make Learning Easier [Internet]. [cited 2025 Jun 30]. Available from: https://blog.sketchy.com/visual-memory-and-elaborative-encoding.
22. Legge ELG, Madan CR, Ng ET, Caplan JB. Building a memory palace in minutes: equivalent memory performance using virtual versus conventional environments with the Method of Loci. Acta Psychol (Amst) [Internet]. 2012 [cited 2025 Jun 30];141(3):380–90. Available from: https://www.sciencedirect.com/science/article/pii/S000169181200145X.
23. Maguire EA, Valentine ER, Wilding JM, Kapur N. Routes to remembering: the brains behind superior memory. Nat Neurosci [Internet]. 2003 [cited 2025 Jun 30];6(1):90–5. Available from: https://www.nature.com/articles/nn988.
24. Lujan HL, DiCarlo SE. The Paradox of knowledge: why medical students know more but understand less. Med Sci Educ [Internet]. 2025 [cited 2025 Jul 12];35(3):1761. Available from: https://pmc.ncbi.nlm.nih.gov/articles/PMC12228860/.
25. Tan S, Xin X, Wu D. ChatGPT in medicine: prospects and challenges: a review article. Int J Surg (London, England). 2024;110:3701–6.
26. Ganjavi C, Eppler M, O'Brien D, Ramacciotti LS, Ghauri MS, Anderson I, et al. ChatGPT and large language models (LLMs) awareness and use. A prospective cross-sectional survey of U.S. medical students. PLOS Digital Health. 2024;3:e0000596.
27. Average Medical School Debt [2024]: Student Loan Statistics [Internet]. [cited 2025 Jun 29]. Available from: https://educationdata.org/average-medical-school-debt.
28. Preclinical Online Virtual Curriculum | Boards & Beyond [Internet]. [cited 2025 Jun 29]. Available from: https://www.mheducation.com/highered/digital-products/compass/boards-beyond/products/step-1-preclinical.html.
29. Sign Up | Pathoma [Internet]. [cited 2025 Jun 29]. Available from: https://www.pathoma.com/sign-up.
30. Pricing | Med School Bootcamp [Internet]. [cited 2025 Jun 29]. Available from: https://bootcamp.com/med-school/upgrade.
31. USMLE Step 1 practice questions & exams [Internet]. [cited 2025 Jun 29]. Available from: https://medical.uworld.com/usmle/usmle-step-1/.
32. Pricing | USMLE-Rx [Internet]. [cited 2025 Jun 29]. Available from: https://usmle-rx.com/pricing/.
33. Med School Prep | USMLE Prep Courses | Sketchy [Internet]. [cited 2025 Jun 29]. Available from: https://www.sketchy.com/explore/medical.
34. Mathai R, Patel S, Littman ER, Lo A, Yitzhak B, Hirumi A. Medical students' perceptions and use of formal and informal curriculum resources. Cureus [Internet]. 2024 Jan 17 [cited 2025 Jul 5];16(1):e52454. Available from: https://pmc.ncbi.nlm.nih.gov/articles/PMC10871689/.
35. King A. From sage on the stage to guide on the side. College Teach [Internet]. 1993 [cited 2025 Sep 4];41(1):30. Available from: https://openurl-ebsco-com.wmusom.proxy.liblynxgateway.com/contentitem/doi:10.1080/87567555.1993.9926781?sid=ebsco:plink:crawler&id=ebsco:doi:10.1080/87567555.1993.9926781&crl=c.
36. Nair M, Moss N, Bashir A, Garate D, Thomas D, Fu S, et al. Mental health trends among medical students. Proc (Bayl Univ Med Cent) [Internet]. 2023 [cited 2025 Jul 5];36(3):408. Available from: https://pmc.ncbi.nlm.nih.gov/articles/PMC10120543/.

Artificial Intelligence and Medical Distance Learning and Management

Rami Madani, David M. Richter, and Theotonius J. Gomes

Introduction

Over the past decade, artificial intelligence (AI) has moved from the periphery of technological curiosity to the center of innovation across nearly every industry: medical education is no exception. From adaptive learning platforms that adjust to the needs of individual students, to AI-powered virtual patient simulations and predictive analytics that identify at-risk learners, AI promises to reshape how future physicians are trained and how medical institutions operate. This transformation is occurring against a backdrop of increasing complexity in health care, a growing demand for competency-based education, and a global shift toward distance and hybrid learning models, all of which has been accelerated by the COVID-19 pandemic.

AI's role in medical education extends far beyond replacing traditional teaching tools; it enables entirely new paradigms for learning, assessment, and institutional management. By leveraging algorithms capable of natural language processing, image recognition, and predictive modeling, educators can now provide highly personalized instruction, generate instant feedback, and design immersive simulation environments. At the administrative level, AI facilitates recruitment, optimizes course scheduling, streamlines grading, and assists with holistic student evaluation, which in theory frees faculty to focus on mentorship and higher level educational design. Yet, with these opportunities come challenges. Questions about data privacy,

R. Madani · D. M. Richter
Western Michigan University Homer Stryker M.D. School of Medicine,
Kalamazoo, MI, USA

T. J. Gomes (✉)
Division of Medicine-Pediatrics, Western Michigan University Homer Stryker M.D. School of Medicine, Kalamazoo, MI, USA
e-mail: theotonius.gomes@wmed.edu

S. S. Chahin et al. (eds.), *Innovation in Medical Education and Clinical Practice*, https://doi.org/10.1007/978-3-032-19116-8_5

algorithmic bias, overreliance on automation, and the ethical boundaries of AI in decision-making loom large. As medical education seeks to prepare students not only to acquire knowledge but also to navigate ambiguity, communicate effectively, and exercise clinical judgment, thoughtful integration of AI becomes imperative.

This chapter explores the evolving landscape of AI in medical education and institutional administration. We will examine current applications, from personalized learning tools and AI-powered simulations to administrative support systems, as well as the ethical considerations surrounding their use. In doing so, this chapter aims to provide medical educators, administrators, and policymakers with a comprehensive understanding of how AI can enhance, and responsibly transform the training of the next generation of healthcare professionals.

AI in Medical Education

The integration of AI into medical education marks a paradigm shift from traditional, standardized approaches toward more dynamic, personalized, and competency-driven models of learning. Rather than simply digitizing existing content, AI enables the creation of adaptive platforms, immersive simulations, and intelligent tutoring systems that respond to individual learner needs in real time. Although there are numerous approaches by which AI can enhance medical education, such methods can broadly fit one of three classifications: AI tools that facilitate personalized and active learning, AI-powered simulation, and AI-driven learning support.

Personalization of Learning Using AI

Medical trainees begin their programs with diverse backgrounds—differing in prior knowledge, cultural and linguistic capital, and structural advantages or barriers. As a result, designing curricula that truly meet learners where they are and empower their success presents a significant challenge. However, the emergence of AI has opened the door for enhanced self-regulated learning (SLR), a process by which learners actively set goals, monitor their progress, and strategically regulate their cognition, motivation, and behavior [1]. AI-driven intelligent tutoring systems (ITSs) can help students master complex knowledge domains. MetaTutor, for example, is a hypermedia-based ITS that was originally developed to foster trainees SLR while learning about complex biological topics. This program went beyond traditional e-learning by monitoring behavior in real time (e.g., eye tracking and facial expressions) and deploying animated AI-based virtual tutors—termed pedagogical agents—to guide users through lessons and prompt adoption of adaptive processes essential for medical education. Numerous studies have shown that MetaTutor has improved SLR strategy development and knowledge gains, in addition to providing a framework for analyzing learning processes relevant to medical training [2]. Additionally, perceptual and adaptive learning models (PALMs) have been shown to produce considerable improvements in trainees' pattern recognition skills—tools that are critical to developing in medical education. For example, PALMs have been successfully used to enhance trainees' ECG interpretation [3], transesophageal echocardiography image classification [4], and histopathological identification [5]. Importantly, ITS can be used to augment simulation learning, with a recent randomized controlled trial finding that trainees who received training from a surgical ITS (Virtual Operative Assistant) achieved greater performance in practice tumor resections, as compared to those who received expert instruction [6]. Additional simulation-integrated ITSs, such as Hepius, will be discussed below. Collectively, this demonstrates that AI-driven tutors can be effective tools to personalize knowledge acquisition, accelerate procedural expertise, and scaffold effective learning strategies; however, longitudinal studies are necessary to determine whether AI-guided learning achieves comparable clinical performance.

AI-Enhanced Simulation

AI-powered simulation has been increasingly employed across both undergraduate and graduate medical education, facilitating trainees' acquisition of procedural skills, diagnostic reasoning, and communication skills. In undergraduate medical education (UME), large language model-based digital patients (LLMDPs) have been used to provide students with simulated patients that allow opportunities to practice patient interviews, differential diagnoses, and clinical decision-making. For example, a recent RCT found that students who learned history taking skills via a LLMDP achieved superior outcomes to those who learned by traditional bedside encounters [7]. Furthermore, students using LLMDPs with integrated feedback have shown gains in clinical decision-making abilities [8]. Another LLMDP, Hepius, used natural language processing to simulate authentic patient encounters, offering individualized real-time, targeted feedback and remediation, allowing for individualized tutoring of patient interview and clinical reasoning skills [9]. AI-powered simulations have also shown promise for teaching medical students procedural skills. In addition to the aforementioned Virtual Operative Assistant—which provided automated feedback during a virtual reality tumor resection task—other AI simulation tools have demonstrated potential in UME. For example, the Intelligent Continuous Expertise Monitoring System, which provided students with continuous feedback during surgical simulations, conferred superior performance as compared to students who received in-person instruction [10]. Interestingly, a recent multicenter RCT found that AI-plus-human instruction produced superior results as compared to either alone [11], suggesting hybrid AI-traditional models may prove an effective model for surgical UME. Importantly, students appear to believe AI-powered simulations enhance their education; in a recent study, students reported that a LLMDP (MedSimAI) was beneficial and provided realistic patient history-taking practice [12].

Similarly, in graduate medical education (GME), AI-enhanced simulation has shown promise for improving how procedural skills, clinical reasoning, and communication skills are taught and assessed. For example, VirtaMed—one of the leading surgical simulators—employs AI "feedback assistants" throughout their models; although the specifics are proprietary, it is likely that they employ AI rule-based models to provide enhanced performance tracking. AI is also used throughout their augmented reality platforms to provide real-time instructions and overlays, helping guide hands-on practice of complex technical skills [13]. Such products offer trainees immersive experience to facilitate acquisition of procedural skills that is transferable to the operating room. Additional products are found in Table 1.

Learning Support

Another major avenue for the use of AI in medical education is the augmentation of learning by AI-powered study tools. In our experience, students have increasingly turned to AI platforms to provide an effective and efficient means by which to develop exam-style questions in preparation for exams. For example, Remember Quick extracts information from user-uploaded content (e.g., lecture notes, research papers, and eBooks) to automatically generate individualized quizzes tailored to the user's content; this platform also will produce flashcards for study with AI-optimized spaced repetition to empower optimal retention of information [14]. Though it is not possible to discuss all such resources given the rapid expansion of products within this space, another commonly used product is Quiz Med AI [15]. Though these platforms are becoming increasingly common, subscription fees for third-party study tools pose economic barriers for many students. In response, some schools have begun developing similar platforms for use by their own students. For example, the University of Cincinnati College of Medicine developed an AI tool that would generate USMLE-style questions (along with lengthy explanations) based on lecture content from courses. Their tool has proven effective, with 75%–85% of AI-generated questions meeting USMLE standards. As their AI platform continues to improve in response to feedback, they hope it will become an effective way to lessen the economic barrier that some students face when preparing for examinations [16].

Alternatively, students with auditory learning styles (or who wish to multitask) have experienced success using Google's NotebookLM platform to convert user-uploaded notes into an AI-generated podcast [17]. The AI-generated "hosts" effectively summarize the user's material in a lively discussion reminiscent of established medical education podcasts, such as Behind the Knife—a resource commonly used by surgery residents. Though many alternative products exist

Table 1 Selected products offering AI-enhanced simulation for use in undergraduate medical education (UME) and graduate medical education (GME)

Level	Platform	Modality	Educational application
UME	Shadow Health[a] MedSimAI[b]	Screen-based SPEs	Practice history taking, therapeutic communication, and early clinical reasoning
UME/ GME	PCS Spark[c]	Screen-/ VR-based SPEs	Practice history taking, communication, clinical reasoning, documentation, physical exam, and select procedural skills (e.g., ETT placement, central lines, and arterial lines)
UME/ GME	Oxford Medical Simulation[d]	Screen-/ VR-based SCSs	Single- and multi-user immersive scenarios, allowing practice of history taking, communication, clinical reasoning, and select procedural skills (e.g., venipuncture)
UME/ GME	GigXR[e]	VR-/AR-based anatomy, SPEs, SCSs	Supplement anatomical education, practice history taking, communication, clinical reasoning, and standardized skills (e.g., BLS, ACLS)
UME/ GME	Full Code[f]	Screen-based SCEs	Practice history taking, communication, clinical reasoning, and physical exams. Also offers a tutor mode to help users learn as they progress
GME	FundamentalXR[g]	VR/MR surgical simulation with haptics	Practice procedural skills across numerous surgical subspecialities through single- and multi-user immersive cases. Integrates an insight engine to measure training effectiveness and user progress, in addition to reporting ROI for clinical leaders
GME	VirtaMed[h]	VR surgical simulation with haptics	Practice surgical skills on highly realistic surgical simulators with advanced 3D visualization and AI-driven feedback. Single- and multi-user modes

SPEs simulated patient encounters, *SCSs* simulated clinical scenarios, *VR* virtual reality, *MR* mixed reality, *AR* augmented reality, *BLS* basic life support, *ACLS* advanced cardiac life support, *ROI* return on investment

[a]https://evolve.elsevier.com/studentlife/training/shadow-health/

[b]https://medsimai.com

[c]https://pcs.ai/spark/for-medicine

[d]https://oxfordmedicalsimulation.com

[e]https://gigxr.com

[f]https://fullcodemedical.com/simulator

[g]https://fundamentalxr.com

[h]https://virtamed.com/en

(Table 2), NotebookLM remains distinctive for its dialogue-based review of user-uploaded sources. Some products, such as Coconote, have expanded beyond this, producing multimodal study aids. However, it is important to note that platforms that allow for audio input (e.g., Knowt, StudyFetch) may conflict with certain schools' policies pertaining to audiovisual recording.

Table 2 Selected AI-powered platforms for generating audiovisual study aids based on user-inputted content

Tool	Input type	Output type	Educational application
Google NotebookLM[a]	Text, PDFs	Podcast dialogue	Transforming lecture content into discussion-based audio summaries
Wondercraft AI[b]	Text, PDFs	Narrated podcast	Converting lecture notes into narrated podcasts
NoteGPT[c]	Text	Single-voice narration	Converts spoken version of notes (i.e., uses input as a script, without AI reorganization)
Coconote[d]	Audio/video recordings or text	Transcripts, podcasts, notes, quizzes	Converts recorded lectures into multimodal study aids
Knowt[e]	Audio recordings or live audio	Transcripts, notes, flashcards	Converts recorded or live lectures into text-based study aids
StudyFetch[f]	PPT, video, PDF	Summaries, study guides	Converts audio or visual lecture content into text-based study aids

[a]https://notebooklm.google
[b]https://wondercraft.ai
[c]https://notegpt.io
[d]https://coconote.app
[e]https://knowt.com
[f]https://studyfetch.com

Clinical Decision Support

Given its ability to rapidly search data and produce succinct responses to user inputs, AI—particularly large language models (LLMs)—have transformative potential in clinical decision-making support (CDS). This is especially the case for trainees, who are still acquiring information necessary to make informed clinical decisions. Broadly, empirical evidence demonstrates considerable promise for AI in this arena, with the strongest evidence for AI in CDS being in image interpretation and diagnostic tasks. For example, the Mammography Screening with AI (MASI) RCT showed that AI-supported mammography resulted in similar cancer detection rates as compared to standard of care (double reading), with lower workload [18]. Text-based reasoning systems similarly show potential. For example, a recent study found that an LLM achieved higher diagnostic accuracy than physicians; however, this study found no differences between physicians using LLM and those using standard resources in terms of both accuracy of diagnosis and time to diagnosis [19]. Accordingly, LLMs require further development and optimization before integration into practice can provide efficient and effective CDS. This need for optimization and validation is embodied by the Epic Sepsis Model (ESM)—an AI-based proprietary model that was integrated into Epic's electronic medical record software. After the ESM showed initial promise, it was implemented at hundreds of hospitals; however, a subsequent validation study found that it had poor discrimination and calibration [20]. Such examples illustrate how, although AI-based CDS tools may seem appealing, they should be met with skepticism and require local validation, bias analysis, and post-development surveillance.

Beyond sepsis prediction, Epic recently integrated a generative AI-based "Summarize" function into its electronic medical record platform. This feature uses large language models to compile concise patient summaries from years of clinical documentation, including progress notes, H&Ps, data entries, and more, so that providers can quickly review a patient's history without manually searching through multiple records. While this represents a significant advancement in streamlining clinical decision-making, it also raises concerns regarding potential mis-summarization, omission of key details, and overreliance on AI-generated text.

Regardless, there are many role-specific opportunities for AI-powered CDS among medical trainees. In the context of UME, LLMs can scaffold clinical reasoning, aid in differential diagnosis, and support knowledge acquisition [21]. Exposure to AI within UME curricula appears to be rapidly expanding, and organizations such as the AAMC have developed helpful resources to aid students, faculty, and administrators [22]. In our experience, ChatGPT seems to be the most heavily used LLM among medical students. Although ChatGPT may, on average, provide accurate information, it remains prone to hallucination (when an AI model generates false information and presents it as fact) and, therefore, may propagate medical misinformation [23]. Accordingly, in our experience, students have begun gravitating toward more evidence-based platforms, such as OpenEvidence. Leveraging content agreements with the American Medical Association (JAMA Network), NEJM Group (The New England Journal of Medicine), and Elsevier Health, OpenEvidence searches reputable journals and society guidelines to provide evidence-based answers to medical questions. As OpenEvidence includes in-text citations, users can readily review relevant sources, ensuring the accuracy of its findings. Also of note, OpenEvidence is HIPAA-compliant [24]. Given the rapidly evolving landscape, it is likely that numerous comparable platforms will emerge in the near future.

AI-powered CDS similarly has relevant applications to GME. Though residents' clinical decision-making skills and medical knowledge are comparatively more advanced than medical students', residents can still leverage AI to improve their clinical performance. As noted previously, LLM assistance can improve diagnostic accuracy, which may be a useful resource for residents to confirm their differentials when working up challenging cases or while on service rotations that may not be in their primary specialty. Further, LLMs may lessen the administrative burden by helping residents draft patient communications (e.g., letters, after-visit summaries, and patient handouts). However, it is important to note that the AMA's 2024 statement on AI use in healthcare recommends disclosing AI use when it directly affects decision-making and advises all AI-generated content to undergo human review and editing prior to implementation [25].

While AI-powered CDS offers clear opportunities in both UME and GME, its use must be approached with both enthusiasm and caution. Such tools may be especially useful for early trainees, who are still honing their clinical skills and knowledge. However, cases such as the ESM underscore the risks of premature deployment of AI-powered CDS tools. As trainees continue to adopt AI-powered CDS tools, it is important to maintain human oversight, local validation, and transparent reporting.

AI in Medical Education Administration

AI is emerging as a tool for medical school administration, with potential applicants spanning from admissions to course organization and workload management. In the context of admissions, AI can help analyze applicant data, streamline the review process, and *potentially* promote consistency. It also can support scheduling and course management by optimizing timetables and avoiding conflicts. Additionally, AI tools can help reduce administrative workload of faculty, allowing them to focus on teaching and patient care. However, these advantages come with challenges, such as concerns regarding data privacy and algorithmic bias, among others. This section will briefly discuss the potential avenues for AI in medical education administration.

Assistance in the Admissions Process

Over the past two decades, the surge in medical school applications has placed an unprecedented strain on admission committees. Allopathic medical school applications have increased by 54% since 2002 [26]; residency programs have concomitantly faced a 71% increase in applications [27]. This has forced institutions to review larger applicant pools while maintaining fairness, consistency, and efficiency. To manage this growing workload, many schools have considered integrating AI tools into their admissions process. For example, some programs have experimented with AI chatbots—autonomous agents designed to mimic human interaction—to transition from static informational websites to interactive platforms that facilitate bidirectional communication with applicants. These chatbots can answer questions, provide candidates with program information, and even streamline processes such as event registration and reminders. One such program implemented at Duke University School of Medicine integrated an AI chatbot into their Pain Fellowship's webpage. Applicants could use this tool to enroll in upcoming events, receive automated reminder emails, and submit inquiries for information. Among those who used the chatbot, 84% reported that they successfully obtained the information they were seeking [28]. These findings suggest that AI chatbots may prove an effective tool to improve applicant engagement while simultaneously reducing the administrative burden placed on program staff.

Some programs have also investigated the possibility of using AI to support decision-making in the screening of medical school applications. For example, the

New York University Grossman School of Medicine employed a virtual algorithm to screen applicants, which demonstrated comparable accuracy to human reviewers. After further testing this algorithm in an RCT, no significant differences were observed between algorithmic and faculty decisions, including among applicants from demographics considered underrepresented in medicine [29]. These findings indicate that AI-assisted screening can replicate faculty decision-making without evidence of additional bias, supporting its potential role in the application screening process. Building on such successes, the American Association of Medical Colleges (AAMC) partnered with Thalamus to provide residency programs with complimentary access to Cortex—an AI-powered platform geared to aid programs with holistic review of residency and fellowship applications. Essentially, Cortex functions to extract key data from applications, helping administrators with the review process. Though no data is peer-reviewed or published, the AAMC asserts this will lead to a 50% reduction in the amount of time program directors must spend screening applicants [30]. At present, the AAMC has exhibited limited transparency about this platform, so it is not currently possible to assess the likelihood of biases or the extent to which programs will become reliant on AI, among other concerns. Though AI may be a viable tool for screening applications, it appears significantly less effective when applied to evaluating applicants' personal statements. For example, a recent study found low agreement between AI-powered and human assessors when tasked to review personal statements, suggesting that human judgment remains critical [31].

It is important to note that, although AI does have some potential benefits for administrators in the admissions process, it also creates some difficult challenges. As an applicant-written personal statement is a critical part of both medical school and residency applications, some have raised concerns about the potential use of generative AI by applicants. Such concerns appear to be well-founded, with survey data reporting that more than 50% of US medical students have used or plan to use generative AI to aid in drafting their personal statements [32]. Such concerns are compounded by the fact that program directors appear unable to accurately distinguish between human- and AI-generated personal statements [33, 34]. This is especially problematic as current plagiarism detection tools cannot accurately identify AI use in personal statements [35, 36].

Assistance in Scheduling and Course Management

AI also shows promise for improving efficiency in scheduling, course management, and faculty evaluation. AI-powered scheduling programs can account for a multitude of variables (e.g., student/faculty availability, and facility use) to produce timetables that minimize conflicts; such programs can further reduce manual administrative burden by dynamically reconciling schedule derangements in response to unanticipated events (e.g., faculty absences). There is some evidence this can effectively be applied to more complex scheduling tasks, such as optimizing student site placement during clinical rotations. For example, an automated scheduling platform was recently shown to effectively integrate student preferences while enhancing fairness and satisfaction within large cohorts [37]. However, it must be noted that no studies have directly compared AI-powered and traditional scheduling in regard to educational outcomes or student satisfaction, so its use should be met with some skepticism until further studies address this gap [38]. AI has also shown promise for faculty assessment in medical education. As AI can efficiently integrate large volumes of data (e.g., resident feedback and faculty productivity), it can rapidly provide faculty with concise, targeted feedback. For example, at the University of Miami Miller School of Medicine, AI has been used to compile common themes in student feedback in concise summaries able to help faculty identify areas for improvement [16].

Workload Reduction

AI-driven training and documentation tools are increasingly being employed to reduce physician and trainee workload while maintaining high standards of clinical care. For example, Cedars Siani employed Virti—an immersive AI-powered learning platform—to balance high staff utilization rates with the need for continued medical education. Virti facilitated virtual simulations for over 800 residents, achieving a massive engagement boost and 50% reduction in in-person training time [39]. Similar programs employing Virti are underway at other major medical centers, including the University of Texas Medical Branch and Weill Cornell Medicine [40, 41].

Beyond training, the growing documentation burden imposed by electronic health records (EHRs) continues to contribute to physician burnout, as both attending physicians and resident physicians spend substantial time entering data. Generative AI tools have emerged as a promising solution, capable of automatically transcribing and summarizing patient interactions into concise SOAP-style notes in real time [42]. At present, numerous institutions have begun piloting AI-powered scribes with varying success [43].

Ethics and Practical Considerations

Bias, Fairness, Equity, and Accuracy

As AI becomes increasingly part of medical education, significant challenges remain pertaining to the issues of bias, fairness, and equity. Importantly, AI systems are only as impartial as the data and programming that shape them—when trained on datasets that reflect incorrect or biased information, AI systems risk perpetuating such biases. In admissions, algorithmic models trained on biased datasets may unintentionally favor applicants from certain demographic or socioeconomic backgrounds. Similarly, AI-based assessment tools can fail to account for cultural or gender differences, leading to inaccurate evaluations. In the clinical context, diagnostic tools trained on data derived from homogenous patient populations may hinder the ability to provide high-quality care to diverse communities.

Moreover, even when scholarly AI models rely on ostensibly reputable data sources, inaccuracies can propagate indirectly if those sources themselves incorporated erroneous or non-scholarly material. Mitigating such risks requires careful design and oversight of AI platforms. Developers should ensure diverse and representative data is used to train AI models, in addition to providing transparent updates about model performance. Most importantly, users must be trained to critically interpret AI-derived information and recognize the limitations of AI platforms.

Data Privacy and Security

At its core, medical education is not only about the transmission of knowledge, but also about cultivating both clinical and non-clinical judgment, professionalism, and trust. Accordingly, though integration of AI into medical education brings immense promise, it also poses several ethical and practical challenges, which must be addressed. Questions pertaining to data privacy, fairness, transparency, and accountability remain central to any discussion of AI in the classroom setting. Likewise, the interplay with practical considerations such as cost, faculty preparedness, and institutional infrastructure will determine whether these tools are sustainable and equitable.

Employing proper data governance—i.e., frameworks, policies, and practices that ensure ethical, secure, and compliant management of data—is foundational to any use of AI in educational or clinical environments. In the United States, existing frameworks such as the Health Insurance Portability and Accountability Act (HIPAA) and Family Educational Rights and Privacy Act (FERPA) establish important safeguards for clinical and educational data. However, HIPAA and FERPA were established long before the advent of AI and have not yet been comprehensively updated to address contemporary challenges. Further, key issues such as algorithmic bias, automated decision-making, and use of data for AI model training fall outside the scope of these acts. As a result, oversight of AI in medical education remains fragmented, relying largely on institutional policies, professional guidelines, and voluntary compliance. In contrast, the European Union (EU) has adopted regulatory frameworks, such as the EU Artificial Intelligence Act, which defines standards for educational institutions and developers, emphasizing the importance of data protection and transparent use [44].

Erosion of Critical Thinking and Judgment

As a key role of medical education is to cultivate critical thinking and sound clinical judgment, some have raised concerns regarding potential impacts AI may have on the development and maintenance of critical thinking skills. Learners may increasingly employ AI to reduce cognitive load (i.e., cognitive off-loading), thereby freeing working memory and cognitive resources for higher order tasks [45]. While beneficial in moderation, delegation of complex functions such as clinical reasoning and decision-making carries inherent risks. These include automation bias (overreliance on AI outputs), de-skilling (erosion of existing competencies), never-skilling (failure to develop essential skills), and mis-skilling (reinforcement of incorrect behaviors through biased or erroneous feedback) [46].

This concern is further compounded by the fact that LLMs behave unpredictably, producing probabilistic outputs without clear insight into their decision-making process. Learners may struggle to distinguish accurate from inaccurate content or fail to critically evaluate algorithmic outputs. Empirical evidence underscores this concern, with a recent study finding that nearly 39% of upper-year medical students failed to recognize erroneous LLM-generated answers to common clinical scenarios, underscoring the real danger of misplaced trust in these systems [47].

To address such issues, several frameworks have been proposed. One such model, DEFT-AI, builds upon the established DEFT framework (Diagnosis, Evidence, Feedback, and Teaching) to promote deliberate appraisal of AI recommendations, structured self-reflection, and the cultivation of adaptive expertise [48,49]. When educators actively supervise learners and require justification of AI-assisted answers, the framework may help preserve or strengthen reasoning skills [48]. Another promising strategy involves integration of AI-specific competencies into medical curricula. For example, consensus-based Delphi studies have been used to emphasize not only technical literacy, but also help learners recognize AI limitations, independently verify AI-obtained information, and evaluate the ethical implications of AI use [50]. Both approaches acknowledge that AI must serve as a scaffold for learning, not a substitute for critical thinking. When supervised and critically evaluated, AI can coexist with the cognitive skills that define the medical profession, lending a new meaning to the adage "trust, but verify."

Accountability

Additionally, the growing use of AI in medical education raises critical questions about accountability and responsibility. When decisions are aided or otherwise influenced by an inanimate AI program, responsibility can begin to blur between developers, institutions, and users. It is important that users remain the final decision-makers and ensure that AI is only used to augment their judgment—not replace it. This requires transparency from both developers and institutions, as regular review and open reporting of AI outcomes will be essential for maintaining trust, integrity, and accountability within medical education.

Conclusion

AI represents a transformative force in medical education and administration, offering unprecedented opportunities to personalize learning, enhance simulation-based training, streamline admissions and scheduling, and reduce administrative workload. By leveraging adaptive algorithms, intelligent tutoring systems, and large language models, AI can tailor instruction to meet learners where they are, supporting diverse educational needs and potentially advancing equity across increasingly diverse trainee populations. Yet, these benefits must be balanced against ethical and practical challenges pertaining to bias, data privacy, and the diminution of critical thinking secondary to overreliance on automation. As medical institutions embrace AI, thoughtful governance, transparency, and faculty oversight will be essential to ensuring that these tools augment rather than replace human judgment. Ultimately, the successful integration of AI will depend not on its capacity to automate, but on its ability to foster a more equitable, efficient, and reflective model of medical education: one that empowers both educators and learners to think critically in an increasingly digital world.

References

1. Zimmerman BJ. Becoming a self-regulated learner: an overview. Theory Pract. 2002;41(2):64–70. Available from: https://www.tandfonline.com/doi/abs/10.1207/s15430421tip4102_2.
2. Azevedo R, Bouchet F, Duffy M, Harley J, Taub M, Trevors G, et al. Lessons learned and future directions of MetaTutor: leveraging multichannel data to scaffold self-regulated learning with an intelligent tutoring system. Front Psychol. 2022;13:813632. Available from: www.frontiersin.org.
3. Krasne S, Stevens CD, Kellman PJ, Niemann JT. Mastering electrocardiogram interpretation skills through a perceptual and adaptive learning module. AEM Educ Train. 2021;5(2):e10454. https://doi.org/10.1002/aet2.10454.
4. Romito BT, Krasne S, Kellman PJ, Dhillon A. The impact of a perceptual and adaptive learning module on transoesophageal echocardiography interpretation by anaesthesiology residents. Br J Anaesth. 2016;117:477–81. Available from: http://vassarstats.net/.
5. Krasne S, Hillman JD, Kellman PJ, Drake TA. Applying perceptual and adaptive learning techniques for teaching introductory histopathology. J Pathol Inf. 2013;4(1):34. Available from: https://www.sciencedirect.com/science/article/pii/S2153353922006551?via%3Dihub.
6. Fazlollahi AM, Bakhaidar M, Alsayegh A, Yilmaz R, Winkler-Schwartz A, Mirchi N, et al. Effect of artificial intelligence tutoring vs expert instruction on learning simulated surgical skills among medical students: a randomized clinical trial. JAMA Netw Open. 2022;5(2):e2149008. Available from: https://jamanetwork.com/journals/jamanetworkopen/fullarticle/2789268.

7. Luo MJ, Bi S, Pang J, Liu L, Tsui CK, Lai Y, et al. A large language model digital patient system enhances ophthalmology history taking skills. npj Digital Med. 2025;8(1):1–12. Available from: https://www.nature.com/articles/s41746-025-01841-6.
8. Brügge E, Ricchizzi S, Arenbeck M, Keller MN, Schur L, Stummer W, et al. Large language models improve clinical decision making of medical students through patient simulation and structured feedback: a randomized controlled trial. BMC Med Educ. 2024;24(1):1–11. Available from: https://bmcmededuc.biomedcentral.com/articles/10.1186/s12909-024-06399-7.
9. Furlan R, Gatti M, Menè R, Shiffer D, Marchiori C, Levra AG, et al. A natural language processing-based virtual patient simulator and intelligent tutoring system for the clinical diagnostic process: simulator development and case study. JMIR Med Inform. 2021;9(4):e24073. Available from: https://pubmed.ncbi.nlm.nih.gov/33720840/.
10. Yilmaz R, Bakhaidar M, Alsayegh A, Abou Hamdan N, Fazlollahi AM, Tee T, et al. Real-time multifaceted artificial intelligence vs in-person instruction in teaching surgical technical skills: a randomized controlled trial. Sci Rep. 2024;14(1):1–11. Available from: https://www.nature.com/articles/s41598-024-65716-8.
11. Giglio B, Albeloushi A, Alhaj AK, Alhantoobi M, Saeedi R, Davidovic V, et al. Artificial Intelligence–augmented human instruction and surgical simulation performance: a randomized clinical trial. JAMA Surg. 2025;160(9):993–1003. Available from: https://jamanetwork.com/journals/jamasurgery/fullarticle/2837234
12. Hicke Y, Geathers J, Rajashekar N, Chan C, Jack AG, Sewell J, et al. MedSimAI: simulation and formative feedback generation to enhance deliberate practice in medical education. 2025 [cited 2025 Oct 10]. Available from: https://arxiv.org/pdf/2503.05793.
13. Augmented Reality Training for Hands-on Learning. VirtaMed [Internet]. [cited 2025 Oct 10]. Available from: https://www.virtamed.com/en/custom-solutions/augmented-reality?utm_source=chatgpt.com.
14. Remember Quick. Remember quick for medical students [Internet]. 2025 [cited 2025 Oct 19]. Available from: https://www.rememberquick.com/medical.
15. Quiz Med AI. How it works [Internet]. 2025 [cited 2025 Oct 19]. Available from: https://www.quizmedai.com/.
16. Boyle P. AI in medical education: 5 ways schools are employing new tools. AAMCNews [Internet]. 2025 [cited 2025 Oct 19]. Available from: https://www.aamc.org/news/ai-medical-education-5-ways-schools-are-employing-new-tools.
17. Wang B. Google Labs. 2024 [cited 2025 Oct 19]. NotebookLM now lets you listen to a conversation about your sources. Available from: https://blog.google/technology/ai/notebooklm-audio-overviews/.
18. Lång K, Josefsson V, Larsson AM, Larsson S, Högberg C, Sartor H, et al. Artificial intelligence-supported screen reading versus standard double reading in the mammography screening with artificial intelligence trial (MASAI): a clinical safety analysis of a randomised, controlled, non-inferiority, single-blinded, screening accuracy study. Lancet Oncol. 2023;24(8):936–44. Available from: https://www.thelancet.com/action/showFullText?pii=S147020452300298X.
19. Goh E, Gallo R, Hom J, Strong E, Weng Y, Kerman H, et al. Large language model influence on diagnostic reasoning: a randomized clinical trial. JAMA Netw Open. 2024;7(10):e2440969. Available from: https://pubmed.ncbi.nlm.nih.gov/39466245/.
20. Wong A, Otles E, Donnelly JP, Krumm A, McCullough J, DeTroyer-Cooley O, et al. External validation of a widely implemented proprietary sepsis prediction model in hospitalized patients. JAMA Intern Med. 2021;181(8):1065–70. Available from: https://pubmed.ncbi.nlm.nih.gov/34152373/.
21. Skryd A, Lawrence K. ChatGPT as a tool for medical education and clinical decision-making on the wards: case study. JMIR Form Res. 2024;8(1):e51346. Available from: http://www.ncbi.nlm.nih.gov/pubmed/38717811.
22. Artificial Intelligence and Academic Medicine|AAMC [Internet]. [cited 2025 Oct 10]. Available from: https://www.aamc.org/about-us/mission-areas/medical-education/artificial-intelligence-and-academic-medicine?utm_source=chatgpt.com.

23. Chelli M, Descamps J, Lavoué V, Trojani C, Azar M, Deckert M, et al. Hallucination rates and reference accuracy of ChatGPT and bard for systematic reviews: comparative analysis. J Med Internet Res. 2024;26:e53164.
24. Wu V, Casauay J. Media review open evidence. Fam Med. 2024;56:1–2. https://doi.org/10.22454/FamMed.2024.587513.
25. American Medical Association. Augmented Intelligence Development, Deployment, and Use in Health Care [Internet]. 2024 [cited 2025 oct 10]. Available from: https://www.ama-assn.org/system/files/ama-ai-principles.pdf.
26. 2024 FACTS: Applicants and Matriculants DatalAAMC [Internet]. [cited 2025 Oct 10]. Available from: https://www.aamc.org/data-reports/students-residents/data/facts-applicants-and-matriculants.
27. Sweet ML, Williams CM, Stewart E, Chudgar SM, Angus SV, Kisielewski M, et al. Internal medicine residency program responses to the increase of residency applications: differences by program type and characteristics. J Grad Med Educ. 2019;11(6):698–703.
28. Yi PK, Ray ND, Segall N. A novel use of an artificially intelligent Chatbot and a live, synchronous virtual question-and answer session for fellowship recruitment. BMC Med Educ. 2023;23(1):152. Available from: https://pmc.ncbi.nlm.nih.gov/articles/PMC10006550/.
29. Triola MM, Reinstein I, Marin M, Gillespie C, Abramson S, Grossman RI, et al. Artificial intelligence screening of medical school applications: development and validation of a machine-learning algorithm. Acad Med. 2023;98(9):1036–43. Available from: https://pubmed.ncbi.nlm.nih.gov/36888969/.
30. AAMC. AAMC-Thalamus Collaboration Information for Programs [Internet]. 2025 [cited 2025 Oct 20]. Available from: https://www.aamc.org/services/eras-institutions/faqs-aamc-thalamus#:~:text=Starting%20July%202025%2C%20all%20ERAS,interface%20and%20experience%20for%20Cortex.
31. Varman PM, Nicholas S, Conner A, Prabhu AS, French JC, Lipman JM. Feasibility of using AI to evaluate general surgery residency application personal statements. J Surg Educ. 2025;82:103655.
32. Smith B, Ramadoss T, D'Amario V, Shoja MM, Rajput V, Cervantes J. Utilization and perception of generative artificial intelligence by medical students in residency applications. J Investig Med. 2025;73(4):338–44.
33. Whitrock JN, Pratt CG, Carter MM, Chae RC, Price AD, Justiniano CF, et al. Does using artificial intelligence take the person out of personal statements? We can't tell. Surgery. 2024;176(6):1610–6.
34. Johnstone RE, Neely G, Sizemore DC. Artificial intelligence software can generate residency application personal statements that program directors find acceptable and difficult to distinguish from applicant compositions. J Clin Anesth. 2023;89:111185.
35. Subillaga O, Coulter AP, Tashjian D, Seymour N, Hubbs D. Artificial intelligence-assisted narratives: analysis of surgical residency personal statements. J Surg Educ. 2025;82:103566.
36. Vaccaro MJ, Sharma I, Espina Rey AP, Lyman N, Palacios C, Zhang Y, et al. Death of the personal statement: a qualitative comparison between human-authored and artificial Intelligence-generated medical school admissions essays. J Am Coll Surg. 2025;242:47–52.
37. Meyer K, Von Jan U, Kitte I, Zuther K, Behrends M. An Automated System to Distribute Students to Clerkships. Stud Health Technol Inform. 2023;305:499–502.
38. Feigerlova E, Hani H, Hothersall-Davies E. A systematic review of the impact of artificial intelligence on educational outcomes in health professions education. BMC Med Educ [Internet]. 2025 Dec 1 [cited 2025 Oct 22];25(1). Available from: https://pubmed.ncbi.nlm.nih.gov/39871336/.
39. Improving medical training with Virti and Cedars Sinai [Internet]. [cited 2025 Oct 10]. Available from: https://www.virti.com/customer-stories/cedars-sinai/.
40. Improving medical training with Virti and Cedars Sinai [Internet]. [cited 2025 Oct 10]. Available from: https://www.virti.com/customer-stories/cedars-sinai/.

41. Transforming Healthcare Training with Virti and uTMB Health [Internet]. [cited 2025 Oct 10]. Available from: https://www.virti.com/customer-stories/utmb-healthcare-training/.
42. Advancing Medical Education at Weill Cornell|Virti [Internet]. [cited 2025 Oct 10]. Available from: https://www.virti.com/customer-stories/weill-cornell/.
43. Janumpally R, Nanua S, Ngo A, Youens K. Generative artificial intelligence in graduate medical education. Front Med. 2024;11:1525604.
44. Leung TI, Coristine AJ, Benis A. AI scribes in health care: balancing transformative potential with responsible integration. JMIR Med Inform. 2025;13:e80898.
45. Risko EF, Gilbert SJ. Cognitive offloading. Trends Cogn Sci. 2016;20(9):676–88. Available from: https://pubmed.ncbi.nlm.nih.gov/27542527/.
46. Schwartzstein RM. Clinical reasoning and artificial intelligence: can AI really think? Trans Am Clin Climatol Assoc. 2024;134:133. Available from: https://pmc.ncbi.nlm.nih.gov/articles/PMC11316886/.
47. Waldock WJ, Lam G, Baptista A, Walls R, Sam AH. Which curriculum components do medical students find most helpful for evaluating AI outputs? BMC Med Educ. 2025;25(1):195. Available from: https://pubmed.ncbi.nlm.nih.gov/39915801/.
48. Abdulnour REE, Gin B, Boscardin CK. Educational strategies for clinical supervision of artificial intelligence use. N Engl J Med. 2025;393(8):786–97. Available from: https://www.nejm.org/doi/full/10.1056/NEJMra2503232.
49. Savaria MC, Min S, Aghagoli G, Tunkel AR, Hirsh DA, Michelow IC. Enhancing the one-minute preceptor method for clinical teaching with a DEFT approach: clinical teaching strategies for infectious diseases. Int J Infect Dis. 2022;115:149–53. Available from: https://pubmed.ncbi.nlm.nih.gov/34883233/.
50. Çalışkan SA, Demir K, Karaca O. Artificial intelligence in medical education curriculum: an e-Delphi study for competencies. PLoS One. 2022;17(7):e0271872. Available from: https://pubmed.ncbi.nlm.nih.gov/35862401/.

Technological Innovations in Medical Education in the Context of COVID-19

Mussa Ibrahim, Piper Cramer, and Melissa Olken

Introduction

The COVID-19 pandemic marked a profound turning point in the history of medical education. Academic institutions across the globe faced the abrupt suspension of in-person instruction, the closure of clinical training sites, and logistical challenges of transitioning thousands of learners and educators to remote formats [1]. These challenges were not merely technical; they were existential. The longstanding pedagogical traditions that had shaped medical training for centuries—face-to-face lectures, bedside rounds, and cadaver-based anatomy—became suddenly unfeasible [2]. In their place emerged a chaotic but ultimately transformative era of technological experimentation, innovation, and adaptation.

The urgency of the crisis exposed systemic limitations in medical education and accelerated long-overdue innovation. While technology had previously been integrated into curricula in limited, supplemental ways, the pandemic made its role central. Institutions were forced to pivot at remarkable speed to adopt online platforms, reconfiguring assessments, incorporating immersive learning tools, and integrating virtual patient-care experiences. For many schools, what might have taken a decade of incremental reform occurred in a matter of weeks.

M. Ibrahim · P. Cramer
Western Michigan University Homer Stryker M.D. School of Medicine, Kalamazoo, MI, USA

M. Olken (✉)
Western Michigan University Homer Stryker M.D. School of Medicine, Kalamazoo, MI, USA

Division of General Medicine, University of Michigan School of Medicine, Ann Arbor, MI, USA
e-mail: Melissa.Olken@wmed.edu

S. S. Chahin et al. (eds.), *Innovation in Medical Education and Clinical Practice*, https://doi.org/10.1007/978-3-032-19116-8_6

This chapter explores how the COVID-19 pandemic catalyzed the integration of diverse technologies across the continuum of medical education not merely as isolated tools, but as interconnected systems of learning. While earlier chapters in this volume explore simulation centers, artificial intelligence, and foundational principles of medical innovation, this chapter builds on those themes by focusing on the real-time application and synthesis of multiple technological approaches during the pandemic.

Specifically, it examines the evolution of hybrid and blended learning models, the deployment of immersive technologies such as virtual and augmented reality in anatomy and procedural training, the rise of telemedicine as both a care modality and a teaching platform, the transformation of assessment and feedback using digital analytics, and the emergence of global and interprofessional collaboration through remote technologies. Case examples illustrate how institutions adapted to shifting demands, and particular attention is given to the ethical, equity, and accessibility challenges that accompanied these changes.

Importantly, this chapter also considers the long-term impact of pandemic-era innovations. While many technologies were adopted reactively, their continued use signals a philosophical shift in medical education. Flexibility, digital literacy, and technological fluency are no longer supplementary skills but essential competencies for modern health care. The boundary between physical and virtual learning spaces has blurred, giving rise to a more fluid, integrated paradigm.

As medical education continues to evolve, the lessons of the COVID-19 pandemic remain critical. The most successful responses were not those that replicated existing practices in virtual format, but those that reimagined how knowledge is delivered, assessed, and applied. In doing so, educators laid the foundation for a more resilient, inclusive, and future-ready system in which technology enhances, rather than replaces, the human elements of teaching and learning. Through this lens, the pandemic stands not only as a disruption but as a critical shift, redefining what it means to educate tomorrow's physicians.

Institutional Agility and the COVID-19 Disruption

The early months of the COVID-19 pandemic tested the structural and philosophical resilience of medical education systems worldwide. Faced with an unpredictable virus, shifting public-health mandates, and an urgent need to maintain educational continuity, medical schools were forced to abandon longstanding norms and innovate rapidly. Institutional agility—the capacity to respond flexibly and effectively to disruption—became not only desirable but essential for survival.

The abrupt cessation of in-person learning in March 2020 presented an immediate challenge: how to deliver core educational content without learner access to classrooms, laboratories, or clinical environments. For many institutions, the first step involved pivoting to video-conferencing platforms such as Zoom, Microsoft Teams, and Webex. Lectures, small-group discussions, and standardized-patient encounters were transitioned online. This transformation occurred globally and within weeks, revealing a capacity for adaptation, at even the most traditional institutions, when driven by necessity.

Agility extended beyond logistics. Curriculum committees and academic leadership reassessed sequencing, graduation requirements, and accreditation standards. Preclinical coursework was restructured to suit virtual delivery, while clinical rotations were paused, shortened, or replaced with simulated or case-based alternatives [3]. Novel electives in pandemic response, telemedicine, and health disparities, which were topics once peripheral, were now deemed indispensable.

Faculty development became critical. Many educators unfamiliar with digital pedagogy required rapid training in online engagement strategies and learning-management systems (LMS). Workshops, peer coaching, and centralized instructional design support enabled faculty to preserve educational quality. Some institutions created "COVID curriculum task forces" comprising faculty, students, and technologists to coordinate responses, monitor outcomes, and iterate rapidly.

The crisis also dismantled institutional silos. Information technology, educational affairs, and clinical leadership teams collaborated more closely than ever, integrating telemedicine into both service and instruction and expanding virtual simulation programs. This fostered a culture of innovation and shared responsibility. Learners themselves drove adaptation. Students designed virtual electives, provided feedback on online formats, and co-taught sessions on digital communication. Their flexibility and creativity sustained institutional momentum.

Despite these successes, challenges persisted: disparities in connectivity, concerns regarding assessment of integrity, and rising faculty burnout. Even so, the overarching themes of the COVID-19 era demonstrated that educational agility, when guided by collaboration and inclusivity, is achievable and essential. The enduring lesson: medical education must be built to withstand disruption, and needs to be learner-centered, flexible, and resilient. Institutional agility is not an emergency reflex but a permanent commitment to innovation.

Blended and Hybrid Learning Models

The pandemic forced a rapid evolution from traditional, classroom-centered instruction to blended and hybrid learning models that merged synchronous, asynchronous, and in-person modalities. This transformation was not simply logistical; it reimagined the roles of both educators and learners.

In the synchronous format, live online sessions on platforms such as Zoom, Microsoft Teams, and Webex replicated the dynamic and interactive nature of in-person lectures. Real-time polling, virtual whiteboards, and breakout discussions were incorporated to sustain learner engagement. Students could ask questions, share screens, and collaborate in small groups, approximating the spontaneity of classroom dialogue.

Meanwhile, asynchronous learning provided flexibility and autonomy. Recorded lectures, curated reading lists, and discussion boards allowed learners to study at their own pace, accommodating different time zones and personal responsibilities. This model proved especially beneficial for international students and those with caregiving obligations, making medical education more accessible than ever before.

The flipped classroom model, in which learners review pre-recorded materials independently and use live sessions for problem-solving, gained significant traction [4]. Rather than passively absorbing information, students attended class prepared to apply knowledge through active discussions, team-based learning, and clinical case analyses. This approach encouraged deeper understanding and critical thinking while keeping learners engaged.

Team-based learning (TBL) and peer collaboration also thrived online. Platforms like Poll Everywhere, Kahoot, and Nearpod enabled interactive quizzes, while digital breakout rooms fostered collaborative problem-solving. Faculty could monitor participation data through LMS analytics, providing targeted feedback to underperforming students and promoting learner accountability.

Learning-management systems such as Canvas, Moodle, and Blackboard became the digital backbone of medical education. These platforms centralized lecture recordings, assignments, announcements, and assessments, offering integrated ecosystems that ensure continuity of instruction. The LMS analytics tools also generated valuable insights: engagement levels, quiz performance, and learning trends became quantifiable in real time.

Nevertheless, the rapid shift in learning models exposed challenges. Students and faculty alike reported Zoom fatigue and decreased interpersonal connection. Variable access to high-speed Internet and suitable devices introduced inequities, particularly among learners from lower socioeconomic backgrounds. Additionally, courses that depend on hands-on skill development, such as anatomic dissection and procedural training, required additional innovative alternatives.

Despite these limitations, hybrid learningyielded enduring benefits. It increased flexibility, scalability, and learner autonomy, aligning education with the digital realities of modern clinical practice. Many institutions, recognizing its success, have since retained hybrid frameworks as a permanent component of their curricula. The pandemic thus accelerated a transformation already underway from passive instruction to dynamic, technology-enhanced learning that meets students where they are.

Immersive Technologies: Practical Integration

Among the most striking developments during the pandemic was the rapid incorporation of immersive technologies such as virtual reality (VR) and augmented reality (AR) into medical education. These tools, once experimental, became essential in replacing suspended clinical and laboratory experiences. Virtual reality provides a fully digital, 3D environment in which learners can interact with anatomical structures or simulate surgical procedures. Augmented reality, by contrast, overlays digital elements onto the physical world, enhancing visualization and interaction. Together, they expanded the boundaries of experiential learning when physical access was restricted [5].

One of the most prominent examples is the HoloAnatomy application developed at Case Western Reserve University, which utilizes Microsoft HoloLens technology to create a lifelike, interactive anatomy experience [6]. Students visualize organs, systems, and spatial relationships in real time, walking around virtual cadavers and manipulating structures through hand gestures. This immersive approach allowed continued anatomy education even when cadaveric dissection labs were inaccessible.

Similarly, the Touch Surgery platform provided procedural simulations for surgical training. Learners could perform VR operations step-by-step with haptic feedback and real-time performance metrics. This tool bridged the gap between theory and practice, enabling safe repetition and skill reinforcement outside the operating room [7].

Emergency medicine programs used VR trauma scenarios to simulate rapid-response decision-making under stress, improving both clinical reasoning and teamwork. In radiology education, AR platforms enabled students to overlay cross-sectional images onto digital patient models, deepening spatial understanding.

Importantly, immersive tools were not meant to replace traditional training but to complement it. Hybrid curricula combined virtual simulations with later in-person reinforcement. This blended approach ensured that learners acquired foundational knowledge before practicing on real patients or specimens.

From an educational theory perspective, VR and AR align with constructivist learning, which emphasizes active, self-directed exploration. Studies have shown that immersive learning may enhance retention, spatial awareness, and confidence, particularly in anatomy and procedural domains [8]. The interactive nature of these tools fosters cognitive engagement and bridges the gap between abstract concepts and tangible experience.

However, implementation posed logistical and ethical challenges. High costs of hardware, limited access in low-resource settings, and motion-sickness concerns restricted universal adoption. Additionally, questions arose about data privacy, as some applications collected performance metrics stored on external servers. Institutions mitigated these risks through centralized purchasing, device sharing, and strict compliance protocols.

Despite these obstacles, the pandemic demonstrated that immersive technologies can democratize experiential learning. Once considered futuristic, they have become integral to modern medical curricula [9]. The ability to practice complex procedures in safe, controlled, and repeatable environments marks a paradigm shift that will continue to expand as technology becomes more accessible.

Clinical Education and Telemedicine

When hospitals restricted student presence in early 2020, clinical education faced an existential crisis. Clerkships, the foundation of experiential learning in undergraduate medical education, were abruptly suspended. The emergence of telemedicine as a mainstream care modality offered an unexpected solution and, for many institutions, a lifeline for continued clinical education.

Telehealth rotations allowed students to engage with patients under faculty supervision [10]. Through HIPAA-compliant platforms such as Zoom for Healthcare, Epic Telehealth, and Doxy.me, learners joined virtual encounters, conducted patient histories, and presented assessments. Supervising physicians observed students in real time and provided direct feedback. This adaptation not only preserved educational continuity for clerkship-level medical students but also reflected the evolving landscape of modern healthcare delivery.

Entire telemedicine curricula were created within weeks. Students completed asynchronous modules on telehealth ethics, patient privacy, and communication strategies. These were followed by teleconsultations where learners practiced establishing rapport, eliciting histories, and managing sensitive conversations virtually. The program also incorporated "shadowing" telehealth sessions across multiple specialties—family medicine, psychiatry, and dermatology, exposing students to a diverse range of virtual care settings. Evaluations showed marked improvements in students' digital professionalism, empathy, and adaptability.

Teaching communication and empathy remotely required rethinking traditional bedside dynamics [11]. Without physical proximity, educators emphasized tone, pacing, and non-verbal awareness; maintaining eye contact through the camera, acknowledging delays, and ensuring patients felt heard. Many programs employed standardized patients trained to simulate virtual interactions, providing a realistic and safe space for learners to practice these skills.

In addition to patient encounters, telemedicine offered new avenues for interdisciplinary collaboration. Students could participate in multi-specialty case discussions or attend virtual tumor boards, often with participants from multiple institutions. These experiences expanded learners' clinical perspectives and professional networks.

Telemedicine's educational value extended beyond the pandemic. Its integration into curricula now prepares students for the future of medicine, where virtual visits and remote monitoring are permanent fixtures [12]. Students graduating post 2020 are expected to demonstrate telehealth competence as part of their core clinical skill set: an educational evolution that aligns with real-world healthcare trends.

Global and Interdisciplinary Collaboration

The pandemic blurred geographic and institutional boundaries, creating unprecedented opportunities for collaboration across nations' healthcare disciplines. Remote technologies transformed local classrooms into global learning communities.

Cross-institutional electives emerged rapidly. Schools partnered to share faculty expertise, offering joint online courses in topics like pandemic preparedness, health equity, and global health systems. This collaborative approach optimized resources and exposed students to diverse perspectives. During the pandemic, many medical schools and global health programs launched virtual international collaborations, enabling students around the world to participate in synchronous seminars, guest lectures, and case-based learning across the globe [13].

International case conferences became a hallmark of this era [14]. Platforms such as Microsoft Teams and Zoom facilitated global grand rounds where clinicians from multiple continents discussed real patient cases. These sessions not only broadened medical understanding but also fostered cultural humility a critical skill for future physicians navigating diverse patient populations.

Interprofessional education (IPE) also expanded in the virtual realm. Nursing, pharmacy, and public health students collaborated with medical trainees on simulated patient scenarios [15]. Using online collaboration tools, teams developed coordinated care plans and reflected on professional roles. Such interactions established mutual respect and interdisciplinary communication skills essential to modern team-based care.

Virtual collaboration also extended into research and innovation. Cloud-based data-sharing tools allowed for multicenter projects and remote mentorship, connecting students with international investigators. The speed and reach of academic networking increased exponentially, accelerating global scholarly exchange.

Although time zones and digital fatigue posed logistical challenges, the benefits of global collaboration outweighed the drawbacks. The shared experience of adapting to crisis forged lasting partnerships. The pandemic revealed that academic medicine thrives when knowledge and mentorship transcend institutional walls, a lesson that continues to shape post-pandemic education.

Digital Assessment and Feedback Tools

Assessment, traditionally anchored in in-person examinations and observed clinical encounters, underwent one of the most dramatic transformations during the pandemic. The need for remote, secure, and equitable evaluation systems prompted a reimagination of how competence is measured [16, 17].

Virtual Objective Structured Clinical Examinations (OSCEs) became a cornerstone of remote assessment during the COVID-19 pandemic [16]. Standardized patients interacted with students via video platforms while faculty observed in real time, using structured rubrics to ensure consistency and fairness. In many programs, sessions were recorded to facilitate feedback and examiner calibration. Studies across multiple institutions demonstrated that virtual OSCEs could effectively evaluate communication, clinical reasoning, and professionalism without compromising rigor [17].

Written examinations transitioned to online proctoring systems. Platforms like ExamSoft and ProctorU used webcam monitoring, browser lockdowns, and artificial intelligence to flag potential irregularities. While these systems safeguarded integrity, they also sparked ethical debates around privacy and surveillance [18]. Many schools implemented reflective professionalism statements and honor codes to foster trust and reduce intrusive monitoring.

Adaptive learning technologies emerged as powerful feedback tools. AI-driven systems such as Firecracker and AMBOSS adjusted content difficulty based on learner performance, providing immediate feedback and analytics on strengths and weaknesses. Faculty leveraged this data to personalize remediation and ensure competency progression.

Real-time analytics transformed assessment from episodic testing to continuous feedback loops. LMS provided dashboards showing attendance, engagement, and assessment trends. Educators could identify struggling students early and intervene with targeted support.

Maintaining equity and fairness remained paramount. As disparities in Internet access and study environments became evident during the pandemic, institutions established accommodations for students with unstable Internet connections or limited access to quiet environments [19, 20]. Flexibility in scheduling, alternative formats for high-stakes exams, and the inclusion of open-book assessments demonstrated that academic integrity and compassion for learners are not mutually exclusive.

Ultimately, digital assessment redefined the purpose of evaluation in medical education. Rather than serving solely as a periodic mechanism to ensure students are prepared to progress to the next phase in learning, assessment became a tool for continuous growth and individualized learning. These shifts align evaluation practices with the broader values of empathy, inclusivity, and lifelong learning.

Accessibility, Ethics, and Equity

The transition to virtual learning during the pandemic exposed longstanding inequities in access to technology, connectivity, and inclusive educational design. The sudden reliance on digital platforms magnified the digital divide, disproportionately affecting students from low-income households, rural regions, and underrepresented backgrounds.

Medical schools responded with targeted mitigation efforts. Many institutions implemented loaner-laptop programs, distributed Wi-Fi hotspots, and extended library hours for socially distanced study. Institutions such as the University of Michigan expanded emergency-aid programs so that students could apply for technology support and high-speed Internet access during the pandemic [21]. These measures supported educational continuity and helped trigger deeper institutional conversations about digital equity as a component of educational justice [19].

Accessibility compliance became a renewed priority. Faculty training sessions focused on creating content compatible with screen readers, providing captions and transcripts for recorded lectures, and using high-contrast visual materials. These efforts aligned with Universal Design for Learning (UDL) principles, which advocate for multiple means of representation and engagement [22]. UDL frameworks benefited all learners, not just those with disabilities, by fostering clarity and inclusivity across learning modalities.

The ethical implications of remote education extended beyond accessibility. Data privacy and surveillance emerged as critical concerns. Proctoring software that tracked gaze movement or recorded rooms raised questions about student dignity and informed consent [18]. Institutions adopted transparent data-use policies and encouraged alternative evaluation methods to reduce reliance on intrusive monitoring.

Additionally, the deployment of artificial intelligence in educational analytics prompted scrutiny of algorithmic bias. Predictive systems used to flag "at-risk" students sometimes reflect systemic inequities. Schools mitigated this risk by pairing AI tools with human oversight, ensuring that decisions about learner performance remained contextual and compassionate.

Finally, the pandemic underscored the importance of ethical scalability, ensuring that innovations benefit all learners rather than amplifying disparities. True progress in educational technology requires not only creativity but conscience: every innovation must be assessed for its inclusivity, privacy, and equity impact.

In the post-pandemic era, digital access, accessibility design, and ethical governance are no longer optional adjuncts. They are foundational responsibilities of academic institutions dedicated to fairness and human-centered progress [22, 23].

Lessons Learned and Future Directions

As in-person instruction resumed, many innovations were maintained. Several technologies and pedagogical strategies adopted during the pandemic have persisted, reshaping the long-term structure of medical education [23].

Hybrid and blended learning models have proven sustainable. Faculty who initially resisted online formats now recognize their value in promoting flexibility and learner autonomy. Institutions continue to use synchronous online lectures, virtual electives, and recorded modules as supplements to in-person education, allowing for more efficient use of faculty time and resources [20, 23].

The pandemic also catalyzed lasting investment in technological infrastructure. Universities built professional studios for recording lectures, expanded high-speed Internet on campuses, and created dedicated departments for digital pedagogy. Simulation centers integrated VR and AR modules, transforming them into multimodal learning hubs that combine virtual and physical experiences [23].

Faculty development remains a cornerstone of this evolution. Educators have shifted from emergency adaptation to intentional innovation. Workshops now focus on advanced online pedagogy, educational data analytics, and accessibility design. The ability to effectively integrate technology is increasingly recognized as an essential competency for modern faculty.

Looking forward, accrediting bodies such as the Liaison Committee on Medical Education (LCME) and the Accreditation Council for Graduate Medical Education (ACGME) are incorporating digital competencies into curricular standards. These include telemedicine skills, data ethics, and virtual collaboration ensuring that graduates are prepared for an increasingly digital healthcare landscape.

Perhaps the most enduring lesson from the pandemic is the recognition that flexibility is strength. Curricula designed with adaptability and inclusivity at their core are better equipped to respond to future crises—whether pandemics, climate events, or technological disruptions [20, 23]. The medical educators of the future must teach not only science and skill but also resilience, equity, and digital fluency.

Conclusion

The COVID-19 pandemic irrevocably transformed medical education, accelerating decades of pedagogical evolution within months. It exposed vulnerabilities while illuminating extraordinary resilience, creativity, and collaboration across the academic community.

Technology, once peripheral, is now foundational to physician training. Yet the true legacy of this transformation lies not in the tools themselves but in the *values* that guided their use: adaptability, inclusion, and humanism. The pandemic reminded educators that innovation is most potent when it enhances empathy, accessibility, and patient-centered care.

The future of medical education will continue to blend the virtual and the physical, the technological and the human. As the world moves forward, the challenge for educators is to sustain the agility born of crisis to ensure that technological progress remains aligned with compassion, ethics, and equity [23]. In this sense, the pandemic was not only a moment of disruption, but a generational turning point, one that redefined what it means to teach, to learn, and, ultimately, to heal.

Glossary

Accessibility Designing learning environments and technologies that accommodate diverse learner needs, including those with disabilities, through universal-design principles and alternative text.

Blended Learning An instructional model combining in-person and online modalities, integrating synchronous and asynchronous formats for flexibility and engagement.

Digital Assessment Use of technology-based platforms for evaluating learner performance, including virtual Objective Structured Clinical Examinations (OSCEs), adaptive testing, and real-time analytics.

Equity in Education Ensuring fair access to educational resources and technologies regardless of socioeconomic or geographic barriers.

Hybrid Curriculum An adaptable educational design that merges traditional classroom instruction with virtual learning experiences.

Immersive Technologies Virtual-reality (VR) and augmented-reality (AR) tools used for simulation, anatomy, and procedural training.

Institutional Agility The ability of academic institutions to respond rapidly and effectively to disruption through flexible policies, innovation, and collaboration.

Learning Management System (LMS) A digital platform (e.g., Canvas, Moodle) that organizes course content, communication, and assessment within programs.

Telemedicine Education Training in virtual patient care and communication using remote technologies to teach clinical reasoning, empathy, and professionalism.

Universal Design for Learning (UDL) A framework that promotes inclusive teaching by providing multiple means of engagement, representation, and expression.

References

1. Rose S. Medical student education in the time of COVID-19. JAMA. 2020;323(21):2131–2. PMID: 32232420.
2. Dost S, Hossain A, Shehab M, Abdelwahed A, Al-Nusair L. Perceptions of medical students towards online teaching during the COVID-19 pandemic: a national cross-sectional survey of 2721 UK medical students. BMJ Open. 2020;10(11):e042378. PMID: 33154063.
3. Sandhu P, de Wolf M. The impact of COVID-19 on the undergraduate medical curriculum. Med Educ Online. 2020;25(1):1764740. PMID: 32400298.
4. Hew KF, Lo CK. Flipped classroom improves student learning in health professions education: a meta-analysis. BMC Med Educ. 2018;18(1):38. PMID: 29544495.
5. Moro C, Štromberga Z, Raikos A, Stirling A. The effectiveness of virtual and augmented reality in health sciences and medical anatomy. Anat Sci Educ. 2017;10(6):549–59. PMID: 28419750.
6. Boillat T, Prithishkumar IJ, Suresh D, Naidoo N. Integrating virtual reality to enhance remote teaching of anatomy during unprecedented times. Anat Cell Biol. 2025;58(1):112–21. PMID: 39623255.
7. Nagendran M, Gurusamy K, Aggarwal R, Loizidou M, Davidson BR. Virtual reality training for surgical trainees in laparoscopic surgery. Cochrane Database Syst Rev. 2013;2013(8):CD006575. PMID: 23980026.
8. Nicholson DT, Chalk C, Funnell WR, Daniel SJ. Can virtual reality improve anatomy education? A randomized controlled study of a computer-generated three-dimensional anatomical ear model. Med Educ. 2006;40(11):1081–7. PMID: 17054617.
9. Sadek O, Baldwin F, Gray R, Khayyat N, Fotis T. Impact of virtual and augmented reality on quality of medical education during the COVID-19 pandemic: a systematic review. J Grad Med Educ. 2023;15(3):328–38. PMID: 37363680.
10. Hilburg R, Patel N, Ambruso S, Biewald MA, Farouk SS. Medical education during the coronavirus disease-2019 pandemic: learning from a distance. Adv Chronic Kidney Dis. 2020;27(5):412–7. PMID: 33308507.
11. Sharma D, Bhaskar S. Addressing the COVID-19 burden on medical education and training: the role of telemedicine and tele-education during and beyond the pandemic. Front Public Health. 2020;8:589669. PMID: 33330333.

12. Kichloo A, Albosta M, Dettloff K, Wani F, El-Amir Z, Singh J, et al. Telemedicine, the current COVID-19 pandemic and the future: a narrative review and perspectives moving forward in the USA. Fam Med Community Health. 2020;8(3):e000530. PMID: 32816942.
13. Moschovis PP, Dinesh A, Boguraev AS, Nelson BD. Remote online global health education among U.S. medical students during COVID-19 and beyond. BMC Med Educ. 2022;22(1):353. PMID: 35538485.
14. Vervoort D, Dearani JA, Starnes VA, Thourani VH, Nguyen TC. Brave new world: virtual conferencing and surgical education in the COVID-19 era. J Thorac Cardiovasc Surg. 2021;161(3):748–52. PMID: 32891447.
15. Khalili H. Online interprofessional education during and post the COVID-19 pandemic: a commentary. J Interprof Care. 2020;34(5):687–90. PMID: 32674721.
16. Chan SCC, Choa G, Kelly J, Maru D, Rashid MA. Implementation of virtual OSCE in health professions education: a systematic review. Med Educ. 2023;57(9):833–43. PMID: 37080907.
17. Cartledge S, Ward D, Stack R, Terry E. Adaptations in clinical examinations of medical students in response to the COVID-19 pandemic: a systematic review. BMC Med Educ. 2022;22(1):607. PMID: 35932046.
18. Coghlan S, Miller T, Paterson J. Good proctor or "big brother"? Ethics of online exam supervision technologies. Philos Technol. 2021;34(4):1581–606. PMID: 34485025.
19. Ramsetty A, Adams C. Impact of the digital divide in the age of COVID-19. J Am Med Inform Assoc. 2020;27(7):1147–8. PMID: 32343813.
20. Rajab MH, Gazal AM, Alkattan K. Challenges to online medical education during the COVID-19 pandemic. Cureus. 2020;12(7):e8966. PMID: 32766008.
21. University of Michigan—Ann Arbor. Emergency financial aid grants to students under the CARES Act. Office of Budget and Planning; 2021. Available from: https://obp.umich.edu/mandatory-reporting/cares-act-reporting/.
22. Burgstahler S. Universal Design in Higher Education: from principles to practice. 2nd ed. Cambridge: Harvard Education Press; 2015.
23. Sandars J, Correia R, Dankbaar M, de Jong P, Goh PS, Hege I, et al. Twelve tips for rapidly migrating to online learning during the COVID-19 pandemic. MedEdPublish. 2020;9(1):82. PMID: 38058947.

Artificial Intelligence Models to Help Process Medical Data

Nikhil Gandikota, Shane Kim, Brady Vibert, Thomas East, and Shamsi Daneshvari Berry

Introduction

Artificial intelligence (AI) is becoming an important part of modern health care, helping doctors process large amounts of medical data, recognize patterns, and make more informed decisions. It is used in many areas such as reading medical images, predicting disease risks, and summarizing patient information. These tools can improve efficiency and accuracy in clinical settings, but they also raise new concerns. Problems like bias in training data, false or misleading outputs known as hallucinations, and a lack of transparency about how results are generated all effect how much AI can be trusted in patient care. When these issues are not addressed, they can lead to unequal treatment, errors, or loss of confidence between patients and providers. Understanding these challenges are important for future healthcare professionals because AI will continue to expand in medicine. Learning how to use it responsibly can help ensure that it supports fairness, accuracy, and trust while improving patient outcomes.

Nikhil Gandikota, Shane Kim, and Brady Vibert are first authors—all individuals equally contributed and were responsible for manuscript production.

N. Gandikota · S. Kim · B. Vibert · T. East · S. D. Berry (✉)
Department of Biomedical Informatics, Western Michigan University Homer Stryker M. D. School of Medicine, Kalamazoo, MI, USA
e-mail: Shamsi.berry@wmed.edu

S. S. Chahin et al. (eds.), *Innovation in Medical Education and Clinical Practice*, https://doi.org/10.1007/978-3-032-19116-8_7

What Is Artificial Intelligence?

Artificial Intelligence (AI) refers to the science and engineering of creating machines capable of performing tasks that typically require human intelligence, such as learning, reasoning, problem-solving, perception, and language understanding. The term was coined in 1956 by John McCarthy, who defined it as "the science and engineering of making intelligent machines" [1].

At its core, AI involves the development of computational models that can represent knowledge, adapt to data, and perform goal-directed actions. Early approaches to AI utilized symbolic reasoning and rule-based systems, where logic-driven "if-then" structures governed decision-making. While these systems laid foundational groundwork, they were limited in scalability and adaptability. Modern AI systems predominantly rely on data-driven methods that enable machines to identify complex patterns and generalize to new scenarios. The most prominent approach is called "deep learning," which uses computational models composed of multiple processing layers to learn hierarchical representations of data. These models capture multiple levels of abstraction, allowing them to excel in tasks such as image classification, natural language understanding, and decision-making in high-dimensional spaces [2].

AI systems using various models, which will be discussed later, extract structured representations from unstructured data by constructing conceptual hierarchies. For instance, given an input such as "generate a question similar to 3+5," an AI model can parse the semantic meaning (addition), assess difficulty (elementary), and synthesize a comparable problem, illustrating the model's ability to abstract and generalize, which represents the hallmark of intelligence that differentiates it from previously built computer-based systems [2].

One of the most well-known examples of a modern-day AI model built with the above algorithm is AlphaGo, a program developed to play the game of Go—a game historically considered one of the most difficult for computers due to its massive search space and the abstract nature of evaluating board positions. Unlike previous rule-based programs, AlphaGo used a combination of deep learning and tree search to master the game in a way that surprised even the AI research community. AlphaGo's architecture relied on two deep neural networks: a policy network, which suggested the most promising next moves, and a value network, which estimated the chance of winning from a given board state. These networks were trained first through supervised learning on thousands of expert human games, then were refined using reinforcement learning by playing millions of games against itself. The system eventually achieved a 99.8% win rate against other Go engines and famously defeated European champion Fan Hui with a score of 5–0 in 2015, as well as international champion Lee Sedol with a score of 4–1 in 2016. This was a major milestone for AI, especially since such a breakthrough was not expected for at least another decade. This accomplishment showed that AI could go beyond rote calculation. It is capable of intuitive, strategic thinking through data-driven training and self-improvement [3].

Most recently, the field of AI has been reshaped by large language models (LLMs), such as OpenAI's GPT models. These models leverage transformer architectures to process and generate human-like language at scale. Trained on vast corpora of text, these models can perform a wide range of tasks, including summarization, question answering, code generation, and reasoning [4]. Their adaptability has made them particularly attractive for medicine, where they can parse unstructured clinical notes, generate patient summaries, support decision-making, and interact conversationally with clinicians and patients [5]. The rapid adoption of such systems in all aspects of human life has highlighted their potential for improving efficiency in addition to their limitations, including hallucination, bias, and interpretability challenges [6].

The field is now advancing toward multimodal and agentic AI systems. Multimodal models integrate diverse forms of input, including text, images, laboratory results, and genomic data, into a single framework, often achieving superior accuracy in clinical prediction and decision support. Agentic AI extends these capabilities further by enabling autonomous action, allowing models to initiate workflows instead of having a human do so, adapt to new tasks with minimal human oversight, and coordinate across interconnected digital health systems [7]. Together, these developments represent a shift away from narrow, task-specific algorithms toward broadly capable, adaptive intelligence with transformative implications for clinical care, public health, and biomedical research [8].

The European Union (EU)'s High-Level Expert Group on AI summed up the benefits of AI very well: "AI is not an end in itself, but rather a promising means to increase human flourishing, thereby enhancing individual and societal well-being and the common good, as well as bringing progress and innovation" [9].

Despite this observation, there is real concern for safety regarding AI implementation, especially within the medical field. As AI advances without sufficient guardrails, developers, deployers, and users can't reliably predict how a system will respond to a given input. Due to the dynamic nature of these systems, the output can change daily. This uncertainty, especially amid unchecked development, raises ethical questions that will be discussed later in the chapter.

In summary, AI represents an interdisciplinary field dedicated to replicating or simulating intelligent behavior in machines. It draws on computer science, mathematics, neuroscience, and cognitive psychology to design systems that adapt, infer, and act autonomously in complex environments. From rule-based expert systems to deep learning, LLMs, and now agentic multimodal platforms, the field has progressed toward increasingly general and versatile forms of intelligence, laying the foundation for its growing role in medicine and beyond.

History of Machine Learning and AI in Medicine

With the rapid advancement of AI since 2020, the integration of AI into medicine has advanced substantially. The first instance of AI use in health care was in the 1970s with the systems called MYCIN and INTERNIST-1, which employed rule-based "if-then" logic to guide antibiotic selection for bacterial infections. Although MYCIN demonstrated strong performance in controlled environments, it failed to achieve clinical adoption due to limited scalability, lack of transparency, and inability to manage the complexity of real-world patient presentations. These shortcomings underscored the need for systems capable of adapting to data rather than relying exclusively on pre-defined rules [10].

The rise of machine learning in the late twentieth century allowed for shift from rule-based systems into probabilistic reasoning systems, like DXplain which incorporated statistical modeling to generate differential diagnoses [11]. As such, Computer-Aided Detection (CAD) tools were introduced in radiology to assist with mammography and chest imaging interpretation [12, 13]. Such models saw wide use in Dermatology, where machine vision tools analyzed skin lesions to distinguish between benign and malignant findings. These early applications demonstrated the feasibility of data-driven modeling, but they remained limited in scope and generalizability.

The development of the deep learning algorithm in the 2000s marked another turning point: convolutional neural networks achieved expert-level performance in image classification, supporting diagnostic advances across radiology, pathology, and dermatology [14]. Recurrent and transformer-based models further extended these capabilities to sequential and textual data, enabling AI to process clinical narratives and patient records with unprecedented accuracy. These innovations led to practical applications such as early detection of sepsis, prediction of hospital readmissions, triage of imaging studies, and stratification of patients by risk for adverse outcomes [15].

With the recent development of large language models such as GPT-3.5, which have demonstrated impressive medical exam performance, AI's role in health care has shifted rapidly [16]. At the same time, GPT has shown a notable capacity to identify and correct its own mistakes, especially when properly guided. With appropriate oversight, clear guardrails, and clinician engagement, the use of AI in medicine looks promising and is likely to continue improving [7].

Current AI Use in Medical Practice

AI is now embedded in clinical practice across a growing number of specialties. In ophthalmology, large language models have reached diagnostic accuracy comparable to established deep learning systems in detecting diabetic retinopathy and macular degeneration, while also lowering the barrier for building decision-support tools

[15]. In mental health, machine learning has been applied to large-scale adolescent health surveys, producing reliable predictions of suicidal ideation and suicide attempts, showing clear potential for earlier detection and intervention. In rehabilitation medicine, AI is being used to monitor movement, customize exercise regimens, and expand telerehabilitation, making physiotherapy more accessible outside the clinic. Likewise, mobile health applications are becoming common in maternal and reproductive care, though inconsistent quality across platforms underscores the need for stronger oversight and regulation [17].

These examples of AI's rapid integration into clinical practice highlight its maturation from proof-of-concept prototypes to tools that can identify problems, interpret patients' conditions, and generate diagnoses based on those findings. Despite its shortcomings, AI continues to be widely used and is now embedded across radiology, pathology, oncology, and population health, supporting early disease detection, imaging triage, and personalized risk assessment [12].

Building on these applications, multimodal and generative AI models have further expanded the field by bringing together diverse data streams into unified frameworks [18]. These systems not only improve diagnostic accuracy but also streamline documentation and enhance clinical decision support. At the same time, the rise of agentic AI marks the next step, with systems capable of initiating clinical tasks, coordinating administrative workflows, and adapting in real time to evolving healthcare environments with minimal human oversight [19].

Concrete examples of this advancement with agentic AI are already visible across care settings. In oncology, "tumor-board co-pilots" synthesize whole-slide pathology, radiology, genomic variants, and Electronic Health Records (EHR) notes to propose staging and evidence-based therapy options with guideline citations, then draft structured notes for clinician review. The increasing amount of molecular data and knowledge about genomic alterations are actively integrated into the current agentic AI models, thereby advancing precision medicine [20, 21]. In pulmonary medicine, an agentic "incidental nodule coordinator" combines CT findings with smoking history and prior reports, retrieves Fleischner guidance, drafts a follow-up plan, places the imaging order, checks prior authorization, books the appointment, and messages the patient, each step requiring clinician approval [21]. In acute care, sepsis early-warning systems stream vitals, labs, and nursing notes to generate an interpretable risk explanation, pre-populate an order set for review, and track time-to-antibiotics as a quality metric [22]. In rehabilitation, smartphone video pose-estimation blended with wearable data personalizes home exercises and auto-summarizes progress for therapists, while patient-friendly instructions are generated in the preferred language [23]. In maternal health, a virtual companion integrates home blood-pressure readings, labs, and symptom logs to flag preeclampsia risk, schedule timely triage, deliver tailored education, and escalate to clinicians when thresholds are crossed [24]. These patterns show how multimodal models raise diagnostic precision while generative and agentic layers reduce documentation burden and reliably move care forward with a human-in-the-loop.

In summary, AI has moved from symbolic systems to machine learning, deep learning, large language models, and now toward multimodal and agentic frameworks. At each stage, its ability to learn, generalize, and adapt has grown more sophisticated. These advances are now converging in health care, where AI is becoming integral for streamlining diagnosis, decision support, patient engagement, and system-level transformation. With clear clinical questions and access to high-quality datasets, clinicians and researchers are increasingly able to design AI tools that address real-world challenges in patient care.

AI Models to Process Medical Data

Patient care requires the management and interpretation of various types of data. This section examines different AI models that can be used to assist physicians in processing these data. General AI principles, including explainability, supervision, and data structure types, are discussed to understand AI in a broad context. Additionally, some general classes of AI models are presented, followed by specific AI models used in the medical field.

General Principles of AI Models

AI models are often described using terms such as explainable or supervised, and their antitheses. Additionally, the data processed by the model may be categorized as structured or unstructured. Understanding these terms is important for understanding the basic descriptions of AI models.

AI models are often deemed explainable or unexplainable based on whether the model's output is accompanied by reasoning. Examples of inherently explainable AI models include regression models and decision trees. The ability to explain a conclusion is beneficial because it increases trust and allows for the refinement of a model [25]. Additionally, many legal and ethical problems arise with the implementation of unexplainable AI models [26]. The predicament of unexplainable AI models is often labeled as the "black-box problem." These models are considered unexplainable due to their nonlinear nature and large number of input parameters. While deep learning models are valuable, their lack of reasoning decreases their utility for making predictions related to very sensitive topics, such as terminal diseases, which are so pervasive in the medical field [27]. However, there have been efforts to increase the explainability of black-box AI models through various methods, such as local interpretations or systematically changing single variables and determining differences in outcomes [28].

When discussing AI models, the terms supervised or unsupervised may be used as descriptor terms for the training process. A supervised model learns from inputs and *known outputs* to determine the relationships between them. Conversely, an unsupervised model learns with inputs and *no outputs*. Unsupervised models are built to identify relationships within the data itself without considering outputs [29].

It is important to understand that supervised models are limited by how a researcher labels the outputs, whereas an unsupervised model is limited by the ability to interpret and verify relationships. To understand these models, an example of colored shapes is shown in Fig. 1. In the colored shapes example, the supervised model neglected colors and only provided outputs based on the categorical labels that the researchers provided to the model. In contrast, the unsupervised model grouped the models based on color and ignored shape. This shows how supervised models can predict outcomes of known interest, and how unsupervised models can categorize based on characteristics that may be overlooked by humans. To shed light on the importance and limitations of the unsupervised model, if a color-blind person were to look at the unsupervised model output, they would see no logic to the model. This displays the ability of the model to look beyond the human scope, while simultaneously revealing the potential for lack of interpretability of the model [29]. Additionally, it is important to note that this example is an oversimplification, and AI models can categorize data based on multiple variables simultaneously [30].

Structured data, often called tabular data, includes information that can be organized in a schema, such as data exchange formats (e.g., XML files), which can be easily interpreted by computers [31, 32]. This contrasts with unstructured data, which lacks a pre-defined format [31]. For example, Hemoglobin A1c (HbA1c) values over the course of many years for a diabetic patient can be structured in a graphical format; therefore, the HbA1c values would be considered structured data. An example of unstructured data is a written summary of an encounter with a patient, such as a History of Present Illness (HPI). Conversely, unstructured data encompasses a significant portion of medical data and includes text, images, and time-series data [33]. However, these data types are often homogenous, and neural

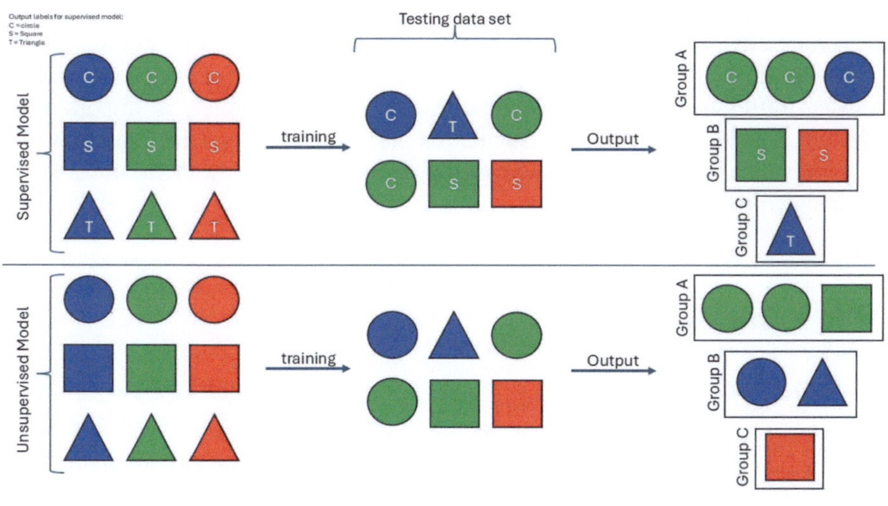

Fig. 1 Supervised Learning versus Unsupervised Learning

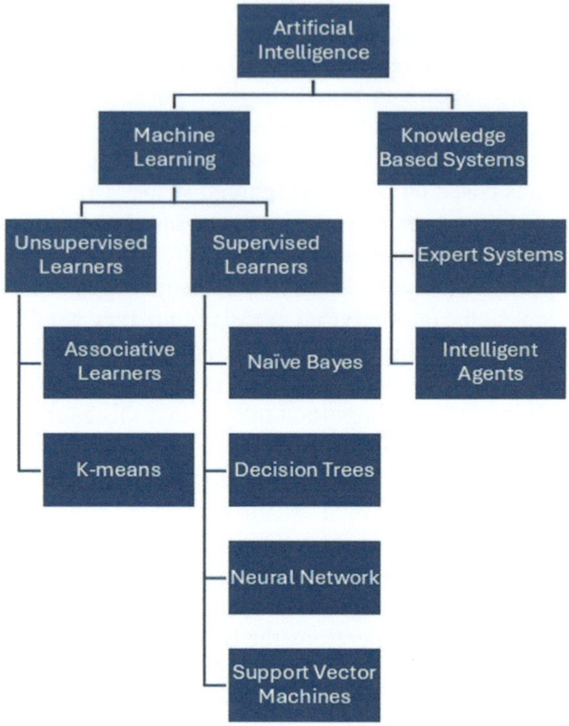

Fig. 2 AI family tree. (Adapted from Kleinstreuer and Hartung [35])

networks are often used to analyze these data because of their ability to make inferences from data with spatial correlations [34].

The family of AI models is vast and diverse, with each model suited for particular functions. Models differ in terms of their efficiency, ease of use, adaptability, interpretability, and other characteristics. A couple of the most popular model groups are included in an AI family tree (Fig. 2) to better understand the relationship between different AI models. Comprehension of these models is important for research, development, and implementation of AI into the physician workflow. The AI family tree is by no means exhaustive but includes many of the most popular models.

AI in Medicine

Medical Images

The medical field utilizes an abundance of visual data to aid in diagnostics. Specifically, the fields of radiology and pathology rely heavily on image processing and analysis. In radiology, some of the most common imaging modalities include ultrasound (US), Computed Tomography (CT), X-Rays, and Magnetic Resonance Imaging (MRI) [36].

As mentioned earlier, images would fall under the categorization of unstructured data and are therefore best processed using Artificial Neural Networks (ANN) [33, 34]. Artificial Neural Networks are composed of layers of artificial neurons and are based on the framework of the human brain. A subtype of ANN, called convolutional neural networks (CNN), is the model of choice for analyzing pixel data [37]. These CNN models have been shown to produce results that are statistically equivalent to those of trained radiologists in specific controlled scenarios. Additionally, radiologists can be more accurate when they use a CNN to assist with diagnosis, compared to radiologists alone [38]. Other potential benefits of integrating AI models into the radiology workflow include increased efficiency and safety [37, 39]. However, there are multiple limitations of AI in radiology, including the necessity of large datasets for training and the potential overfitting of the model [37, 40, 41]. Overall, the data on the efficacy of a CNN compared to radiologists can be variable, but when the technology is used in concert with a trained radiologist, there are substantial benefits [42, 43].

Wearables

With the large-scale use of wearable medical sensors, research is ongoing to optimize the interpretation of time-series data provided by these sensors. Specific types of wearables include smart watches, smart rings, glucose monitors, and smart garments [44, 45].

Time-series data collected from wearable devices are extremely valuable as they allow for the detection of adverse events that could otherwise be missed in short-term studies to monitor pathology (e.g., 24-hour Holter) [44]. These data have historically been processed using statistical models that do not adapt well to complex data. Deep learning models have shown great success in detecting anomalies in time-series data [46]. Additionally, AI models may be used to predict how a lab value will change over time, which could help direct care.

Recurrent Neural Network (RNN) models were shown to be the prevailing AI model for predicting glucose levels 15 and 60 minutes in the future when compared to another neural network model, support vector regression model, and an ensemble model (gradient-boosting system). The RNN model was sufficiently accurate for clinical use for 15-minute predictions, but the 60-minute prediction accuracy did not meet this standard. These models show promise for predicting glucose levels but must be further optimized before clinical implementation [47].

The ability to accurately predict future glucose measurements would increase the precision of closed-loop insulin delivery systems [47]. This increased predictability could potentially allow for more precise intensive diabetes treatment, which has been shown to significantly reduce the risk of cardiovascular disease in patients with diabetes [48].

Ambient AI Scribes

One of the most novel and promising applications of AI in medicine is the use of ambient AI scribes. This process includes the use of a listening device to record patient-provider dialogue. The dialogue is processed using speech recognition, and a Large Language Model then creates a note for the patient. For context, LLMs fall under the neural network family [49]. Initial results show the potential for ambient AI scribes to significantly reduce documentation time for physicians. However, some physicians were considerably less time-efficient with the addition of the AI scribe [50].

Further reductions in documentation time may occur as AI scribe technology improves, and physicians adapt to its integration into clinical practice. Surveys related to physician sentiment about AI scribes show positive views regarding workload reduction and negative views regarding the accuracy and length of the notes [51]. Overall, AI scribes are far from refined, yet the benefits include reducing the workload and, therefore, burnout of physicians.

Summary of AI Models

The medical field is at the precipice of massive reform as AI is integrated into the daily workflow. This technology shows promise for improving accuracy, efficiency, and safety, with applications in various fields of medicine. Understanding the fundamentals of AI will be imperative for future practices to best serve patients. The evolution of AI models will provoke adaptation within the field of medicine, which has the potential to improve patient outcomes and physician quality of work life.

Bias, Hallucinations, and Transparency in Artificial Intelligence Models

In recent years, artificial intelligence (AI) has started playing a more significant role in the medical field, especially when it comes to processing patient data. AI tools are now being used to spot health patterns, help with diagnoses, and even create parts of medical records [52]. These tools are useful because they can go through information quickly and help lighten the workload for healthcare teams. Even though AI has many benefits, it also raises some concerns. The main problems regarding AI include bias, hallucinations, and lack of transparency [53]. These issues affect who receive fair treatment and how much trust people have in AI. That's why it's important for students and future doctors to learn about the risks and use AI carefully in healthcare settings.

Bias in AI occurs when models treat some cases differently because of how they were trained. A good example is an algorithm studied by Obermeyer et al. (2019), which used past healthcare spending to predict future needs. Because Black patients tend to spend less on health care, the model wrongly assumed they were healthier. This led to fewer services being offered to them. Bias like this does not come from bad intentions, but from data that reflects inequality in the real world.

Bias can be hard to see. AI models are often trained on data from one hospital or one population. If most data come from city hospitals, then rural patients might not be represented. Some groups, including older adults, people who speak different languages, or those with disabilities, might also be missing from the data [54]. These gaps affect how well AI performs. The result is that AI might work well for some patients but not others. Bias also shows up when the data does not include confounding variables, like exposure to pollution or poor housing conditions. A model may fail to pick up these risks if it only looks at lab results or past visits (Table 1).

Hallucinations happen when an AI model fabricates information which can result in severe consequences within the healthcare field. A model might write a clinical note with a diagnosis the patient never had or create fake journal citations that sound real. These errors can confuse doctors or students who are still learning. One study showed ChatGPT invented key findings when asked to summarize a medical article. The model sounded confident, but its answer was false [55].

Hallucinations usually happen when AI models are unsure. Instead of saying "I don't know," it fills in the blanks with its best guess. Since it's trained to produce fluent responses, these guesses often sound believable. Even the newer ChatGPT-5 model, which was designed to reduce hallucinations, can still make mistakes [56]. That's why AI should be double-checked by a human. Doctors and students need to review AI-generated information the same way they'd review any other tool which is by using their own judgment.

Table 1 Common types of bias in AI healthcare systems

Bias	Description	Example
Historical bias	Bias is present in the original data	If certain groups historically received less care, AI will learn to continue that pattern
Representation bias	Occurs when the dataset underrepresents certain populations	Common in rural patients or non-English speakers
Measurement bias	When variables are not measured the same way across groups	Example includes pain scores differing by race
Omitted variable bias	Happens when important factors are left out of the model	Environmental risk factors or socioeconomic status
Aggregation bias	When models trained on one group are used for another group without testing how well it works for them	A model trained on younger adult patients is later used to predict disease risk in elderly patients, even though the symptoms and treatment responses are very different

Transparency is another major issue with AI in medicine. As mentioned previously, many AI models are considered black-box models. In medicine, that is a problem. If an AI tool says a patient is at high risk, clinicians need to know why. If there's no explanation, it becomes hard to trust the tool or take an action based on its advice.

Transparency also affects how patients feel. If people find out that an AI tool made a decision about their care, but no one can explain why, it can hurt the doctor-patient relationship [57]. To fix this, developers are working on AI systems that can give reasons for their output. For example, a tool might highlight lab values or symptoms that led to its recommendation. This helps doctors corroborate the AI model's output with reality to confirm accuracy.

Bias, hallucinations, and transparency all tie into the ethics of using AI in health care [58]. Patient privacy is one concern. Even when AI uses deidentified data, there's a risk someone could be identified, especially if they have a rare condition. Many patients do not know if their data is being used at all. Going forward, there should be informed consent when using AI for patient care.

Another ethical issue is accountability. If an AI tool gives bad advice, who is to blame? The doctor who used it? The hospital that bought it? The company that built it? These are hard questions. Right now, most hospitals use AI only to support decisions, not to make the final call. That helps reduce risk, but it doesn't solve the accountability problem entirely.

To use AI safely, education is important [59]. Students and residents should be taught how AI works and how it can fail. They should learn about different types of bias, when hallucinations happen, and why transparency matters. Instead of replacing human decision-making, AI should support it. Doctors still need to think critically and use their own judgment.

In conclusion, AI is a powerful tool in health care, but it comes with real risks. Bias, hallucinations, and lack of transparency can lead to harm if they are ignored. If we want to use AI the right way, we need to build more equitable systems, stay transparent, and always include human oversight. When used responsibly, AI can support better decisions and improve patient care, but it should never take the place of human thinking.

Summary

The implementation of AI within the medical field has created new opportunities for streamlined workflows and improved patient care. The earliest medical AI models followed simple "if-then" structures but have since evolved into agentic models capable of performing tasks without human involvement. However, this rapid advancement raises credible concerns about safety, ethics, and accountability regarding AI in clinical settings. The prevalence of hallucinations, bias, and a lack of model transparency demonstrates the need for rigorous oversight by licensed clinicians. Despite these challenges, AI has shown its capacity for transformative impact by processing medical data in the areas of wearables, imaging, and patient-provider dialogue. With cautious implementation, emphasis on patient safety, and continued physician oversight, AI can serve as a powerful tool to support and enhance physician decision-making while preserving the human judgment essential to patient care.

References

1. McCarthy J. What is artificial intelligence? Stanford University; 2007 (rev.). https://www-formal.stanford.edu/jmc/whatisai.pdf.
2. LeCun Y, Bengio Y, Hinton G. Deep learning. Nature. 2015;521:436–44. Insight Review. https://www.cs.toronto.edu/~hinton/absps/NatureDeepReview.pdf.
3. Silver D, Huang A, Maddison CJ, Guez A, Sifre L, van den Driessche G, Schrittwieser J, Antonoglou I, Panneershelvam V, Lanctot M, Dieleman S, Grewe D, Nham J, Kalchbrenner N, Sutskever I, Lillicrap T, Leach M, Kavukcuoglu K, Graepel T, Hassabis D. Mastering the game of Go with deep neural networks and tree search. Nature. 2016;529(7587):484–9. https://doi.org/10.1038/nature16961. PMID: 26819042.
4. Achiam J, et al. Gpt-4 technical report. arXiv preprint arXiv:2303.08774. 2023.
5. Yu E, Chu X, Zhang W, Meng X, Yang Y, Ji X, Wu C. Large language models in medicine: applications, challenges, and future directions. Int J Med Sci. 2025;22(11):2792–801. https://doi.org/10.7150/ijms.111780.
6. Spotnitz M, Idnay B, Gordon ER, Shyu R, Zhang G, Liu C, Cimino JJ, Weng C. A survey of clinicians' views of the utility of large language models. Appl Clin Inform. 2024;15(2):306–12. https://doi.org/10.1055/a-2281-7092. Epub 2024 Mar 5. PMID: 38442909; PMCID: PMC11023712.
7. Liawrungrueang W. Artificial Intelligence (AI) agents versus agentic AI: what's the effect in spine surgery? Neurospine. 2025;22(2):473–7. https://doi.org/10.14245/ns.2550308.154. Epub 2025 Jun 30. PMID: 40625011; PMCID: PMC12242738.
8. Schouten D, Nicoletti G, Dille B, Chia C, Vendittelli P, Schuurmans M, Litjens G, Khalili N. Navigating the landscape of multimodal AI in medicine: A scoping review on technical challenges and clinical applications. Med Image Anal. 2025;105:103621. ISSN 1361-8415. https://doi.org/10.1016/j.media.2025.103621 (https://www.sciencedirect.com/science/article/pii/S1361841525001689).
9. Stahl BC. Ethical issues of AI. In: Artificial intelligence for a better future; 2021. p. 35–53. https://doi.org/10.1007/978-3-030-69978-9_4. PMCID: PMC7968615.
10. Buchanan BG, Shortliffe EH. Rule-based expert systems: the MYCIN experiments of the Stanford Heuristic Programming Project. Addison-Wesley, Chapter 1; 1984. https://www.shortliffe.net/Buchanan-Shortliffe-1984/Chapter-01.pdf.
11. Barnett GO, Cimino JJ, Hupp JA, Hoffer EP. DXplain. An evolving diagnostic decision-support system. JAMA. 1987;258(1):67–74. https://doi.org/10.1001/jama.258.1.67. PMID: 3295316.
12. Elmore JG, Lee CI. Artificial intelligence in medical imaging-learning from past mistakes in mammography. JAMA Health Forum. 2022;3(2):e215207. https://doi.org/10.1001/jamahealthforum.2021.5207. PMID: 36218833; PMCID: PMC9648493.
13. Chan HP, Samala RK, Hadjiiski LM. CAD and AI for breast cancer-recent development and challenges. Br J Radiol. 2020;93(1108):20190580. https://doi.org/10.1259/bjr.20190580. Epub 2019 Dec 16. PMID: 31742424; PMCID: PMC7362917.
14. Miotto R, Wang F, Wang S, Jiang X, Dudley JT. Deep learning for healthcare: review, opportunities and challenges. Brief Bioinform. 2018;19(6):1236–46. https://doi.org/10.1093/bib/bbx044. PMID: 28481991; PMCID: PMC6455466.

15. Ting DSW, Pasquale LR, Peng L, Campbell JP, Lee AY, Raman R, Tan GSW, Schmetterer L, Keane PA, Wong TY. Artificial intelligence and deep learning in ophthalmology. Br J Ophthalmol. 2019;103(2):167–75. https://doi.org/10.1136/bjophthalmol-2018-313173. Epub 2018 Oct 25. PMID: 30361278; PMCID: PMC6362807.
16. Kung TH, Cheatham M, Medenilla A, Sillos C, De Leon L, Elepaño C, Madriaga M, Aggabao R, Diaz-Candido G, Maningo J, Tseng V. Performance of ChatGPT on USMLE: potential for AI-assisted medical education using large language models. PLoS Digit Health. 2023;2(2):e0000198. https://doi.org/10.1371/journal.pdig.0000198. PMID: 36812645; PMCID: PMC9931230.
17. Kwok WH, Zhang Y, Wang G. Artificial intelligence in perinatal mental health research: a scoping review. Comput Biol Med. 2024;177:108685. ISSN 0010-4825. https://doi.org/10.1016/j.compbiomed.2024.108685.
18. Kaczmarczyk R, Wilhelm TI, Martin R, et al. Evaluating multimodal AI in medical diagnostics. NPJ Digit Med. 2024;7:205. https://doi.org/10.1038/s41746-024-01208-3.
19. Chang LC, Kuo HC, Wang HM, Kuo YC, Wang CT, Chen LC, Hsieh JC. The use of an integrated digital tool to improve the efficiency of multidisciplinary tumor boards-a prospective trial in Taiwan. Cancers (Basel). 2025;17(3):444. https://doi.org/10.3390/cancers17030444. PMID: 39941815; PMCID: PMC11815928.
20. Singh H, Koster M, Jani C, Rupal A, Walker A, Khoory J, Tewari A, Casasola M, Ranker LR, Thomson C. Nodule net: a centralized prospective lung nodule tracking and safety-net program. Respir Med. 2022;192:106737. ISSN 0954-6111. https://doi.org/10.1016/j.rmed.2022.106737 (https://www.sciencedirect.com/science/article/pii/S0954611122000026).
21. Rodríguez Ruiz N, Abd Own S, Ekström Smedby K, Eloranta S, Koch S, Wästerlid T, Krstic A, Boman M. Data-driven support to decision-making in molecular tumour boards for lymphoma: a design science approach. Front Oncol. 2022;12:984021. https://doi.org/10.3389/fonc.2022.984021. PMID: 36457495; PMCID: PMC9705761.
22. Adams R, Henry KE, Sridharan A, et al. Prospective, multi-site study of patient outcomes after implementation of the TREWS machine learning-based early warning system for sepsis. Nat Med. 2022;28:1455–60. https://doi.org/10.1038/s41591-022-01894-0.
23. King SW, Eltayeb M, van Duren BH, Jain S, Kerry J, Pandit HG, Palan J. Wearable sensors to guide remote rehabilitation following knee arthroplasty surgery. Indian J Orthop. 2022;57(5):624–34. https://doi.org/10.1007/s43465-022-00785-3. PMID: 37128555; PMCID: PMC10147850.
24. Chervonski E, Pelegri E, De La Calle F, Mandal S, Graves CA, Colella D, Elmaleh-Sachs A, Nay J, Dapkins I, Schoenthaler A. Cardiovascular health markers with remote team-based hypertension management in a safety-net population. Am J Prev Med. 2025;69(5):108031. https://doi.org/10.1016/j.amepre.2025.108031.
25. Abgrall G, Holder AL, Chelly Dagdia Z, Zeitouni K, Monnet X. Should AI models be explainable to clinicians? Crit Care. 2024;28(1):301. https://doi.org/10.1186/s13054-024-05005-y. PMID: 39267172; PMCID: PMC11391805.
26. Lang M, Bernier A, Knoppers BM. Artificial intelligence in cardiovascular imaging: “unexplainable” legal and ethical challenges? Can J Cardiol. 2022;38(2):225–33. https://doi.org/10.1016/j.cjca.2021.10.009. Epub 2021 Nov 1. PMID: 34737036.
27. Hassija V, Chamola V, Mahapatra A, Singal A, Goel D, Huang K, Scardapane S, Spinelli I, Mahmud M, Hussain A. Interpreting black-box models: a review on explainable artificial intelligence. Cogn Comput. 2024;16(1):45–74.
28. Ali S, Akhlaq F, Imran AS, Kastrati Z, Daudpota SM, Moosa M. The enlightening role of explainable artificial intelligence in medical & healthcare domains: a systematic literature review. Comput Biol Med. 2023;166:107555. https://doi.org/10.1016/j.compbiomed.2023.107555. Epub 2023 Oct 4. PMID: 37806061.
29. Hastie T, Tibshirani R, Friedman J. The elements of statistical learning. 2nd ed. Springer; 2009. p. 1–2, 485–87. https://doi.org/10.1007/978-0-387-84858-7.

30. Jain AK, Murty MN, Flynn PJ. Data clustering: a review. ACM Comput Surv (CSUR). 1999;31(3):264–323.
31. Dekhtiar J, Durupt A, Bricogne M, Eynard B, Rowson H, Kiritsis D. Deep learning for big data applications in CAD and PLM–research review, opportunities and case study. Comput Ind. 2018;100:227–43.
32. Simpson RW, Berman MA, Foulis PR, Divaris DX, Birdsong GG, Mirza J, Moldwin R, Spencer S, Srigley JR, Fitzgibbons PL. Cancer biomarkers: the role of structured data reporting. Arch Pathol Lab Med. 2015;139(5):587–93. https://doi.org/10.5858/arpa.2014-0082-RA. Epub 2014 Oct 2. PMID: 25275812.
33. Kong HJ. Managing unstructured big data in healthcare system. Healthc Inform Res. 2019;25(1):1–2. https://doi.org/10.4258/hir.2019.25.1.1. Epub 2019 Jan 31. PMID: 30788175; PMCID: PMC6372467.
34. Borisov V, Leemann T, Seßler K, Haug J, Pawelczyk M, Kasneci G. Deep neural networks and tabular data: a survey. IEEE Trans Neural Networks Learn Syst. 2022;35(6):7499–519.
35. Kleinstreuer N, Hartung T. Artificial intelligence (AI)-it's the end of the tox as we know it (and I feel fine). Arch Toxicol. 2024;98(3):735–54. https://doi.org/10.1007/s00204-023-03666-2. Epub 2024 Jan 20. PMID: 38244040; PMCID: PMC10861653.
36. Litjens G, Kooi T, Bejnordi BE, Setio AAA, Ciompi F, Ghafoorian M, van der Laak JAWM, van Ginneken B, Sánchez CI. A survey on deep learning in medical image analysis. Med Image Anal. 2017;42:60–88. https://doi.org/10.1016/j.media.2017.07.005. Epub 2017 Jul 26. PMID: 28778026.
37. Najjar R. Redefining radiology: a review of artificial intelligence integration in medical imaging. Diagnostics (Basel). 2023;13(17):2760. https://doi.org/10.3390/diagnostics13172760. PMID: 37685300; PMCID: PMC10487271.
38. Cai JC, Nakai H, Kuanar S, Froemming AT, Bolan CW, Kawashima A, Takahashi H, Mynderse LA, Dora CD, Humphreys MR, Korfiatis P, Rouzrokh P, Bratt AK, Conte GM, Erickson BJ, Takahashi N. Fully automated deep learning model to detect clinically significant prostate cancer at MRI. Radiology. 2024;312(2):e232635. https://doi.org/10.1148/radiol.232635. PMID: 39105640; PMCID: PMC11366675.
39. van Leeuwen KG, de Rooij M, Schalekamp S, van Ginneken B, Rutten MJCM. How does artificial intelligence in radiology improve efficiency and health outcomes? Pediatr Radiol. 2022;52(11):2087–93. https://doi.org/10.1007/s00247-021-05114-8. Epub 2021 Jun 12. PMID: 34117522; PMCID: PMC9537124.
40. Alzubaidi L, Zhang J, Humaidi AJ, Al-Dujaili A, Duan Y, Al-Shamma O, Santamaría J, Fadhel MA, Al-Amidie M, Farhan L. Review of deep learning: concepts, CNN architectures, challenges, applications, future directions. J Big Data. 2021;8(1):53. https://doi.org/10.1186/s40537-021-00444-8. Epub 2021 Mar 31. PMID: 33816053; PMCID: PMC8010506.
41. Katal S, York B, Gholamrezanezhad A. AI in radiology: from promise to practice – a guide to effective integration. Eur J Radiol. 2024;181:111798.
42. Abdullah KA, Marziali S, Nanaa M, Escudero Sánchez L, Payne NR, Gilbert FJ. Deep learning-based breast cancer diagnosis in breast MRI: systematic review and meta-analysis. Eur Radiol. 2025;35(8):4474–89. https://doi.org/10.1007/s00330-025-11406-6. Epub 2025 Feb 5. PMID: 39907762; PMCID: PMC12226709.
43. Kraus M, Anteby R, Konen E, Eshed I, Klang E. Artificial intelligence for X-ray scaphoid fracture detection: a systematic review and diagnostic test accuracy meta-analysis. Eur Radiol. 2024;34(7):4341–51. https://doi.org/10.1007/s00330-023-10473-x. Epub 2023 Dec 15. PMID: 38097728; PMCID: PMC11213739.
44. Dias D, Paulo Silva Cunha J. Wearable health devices-vital sign monitoring, systems and technologies. Sensors (Basel). 2018;18(8):2414. https://doi.org/10.3390/s18082414. PMID: 30044415; PMCID: PMC6111409.
45. Schoenmakers M, Saygin M, Sikora M, Vaessen T, Noordzij M, de Geus E. Stress in action wearables database: a database of noninvasive wearable monitors with systematic technical, reliability, validity, and usability information. Behav Res Methods. 2025;57(6):171. https://doi.org/10.3758/s13428-025-02685-4. PMID: 40360861; PMCID: PMC12075381.

46. Backhus J, Rao AR, Venkatraman C, Gupta C. Time series anomaly detection using signal processing and deep learning. Appl Sci. 2025;15(11):6254.
47. van Doorn WPTM, Foreman YD, Schaper NC, Savelberg HHCM, Koster A, van der Kallen CJH, Wesselius A, Schram MT, Henry RMA, Dagnelie PC, de Galan BE, Bekers O, Stehouwer CDA, Meex SJR, Brouwers MCGJ. Machine learning-based glucose prediction with use of continuous glucose and physical activity monitoring data: the Maastricht Study. PLoS One. 2021;16(6):e0253125. https://doi.org/10.1371/journal.pone.0253125. PMID: 34166426; PMCID: PMC8224858.
48. Diabetes Control and Complications Trial (DCCT)/Epidemiology of Diabetes Interventions and Complications (EDIC) Study Research Group. Intensive diabetes treatment and cardiovascular outcomes in type 1 diabetes: the DCCT/EDIC study 30-year follow-up. Diabetes Care. 2016;39(5):686–93. https://doi.org/10.2337/dc15-1990. Epub 2016 Feb 9. PMID: 26861924; PMCID: PMC4839174.
49. Wiest IC, Ferber D, Zhu J, van Treeck M, Meyer SK, Juglan R, Carrero ZI, Paech D, Kleesiek J, Ebert MP, Truhn D, Kather JN. Privacy-preserving large language models for structured medical information retrieval. NPJ Digit Med. 2024;7(1):257. https://doi.org/10.1038/s41746-024-01233-2. PMID: 39304709; PMCID: PMC11415382.
50. Ma SP, Liang AS, Shah SJ, Smith M, Jeong Y, Devon-Sand A, Crowell T, Delahaie C, Hsia C, Lin S, Shanafelt T, Pfeffer MA, Sharp C, Garcia P. Ambient artificial intelligence scribes: utilization and impact on documentation time. J Am Med Inform Assoc. 2025;32(2):381–5. https://doi.org/10.1093/jamia/ocae304. PMID: 39688515; PMCID: PMC11756633.
51. Shah SJ, Crowell T, Jeong Y, Devon-Sand A, Smith M, Yang B, Ma SP, Liang AS, Delahaie C, Hsia C, Shanafelt T, Pfeffer MA, Sharp C, Lin S, Garcia P. Physician perspectives on ambient AI scribes. JAMA Netw Open. 2025;8(3):e251904. https://doi.org/10.1001/jamanetworkopen.2025.1904. PMID: 40126477; PMCID: PMC11933996.
52. Emsley R. ChatGPT: these are not hallucinations – they're fabrications and falsifications. Schizophrenia (Heidelb). 2023;9(1):52. https://doi.org/10.1038/s41537-023-00379-4. PMID: 37598184; PMCID: PMC10439949.
53. Obermeyer Z, Powers B, Vogeli C, Mullainathan S. Dissecting racial bias in an algorithm used to manage the health of populations. Science. 2019;366(6464):447–53. https://doi.org/10.1126/science.aax2342. PMID: 31649194.
54. Adamson AS, Smith A. Machine learning and health care disparities in dermatology. JAMA Dermatol. 2018;154(11):1247–8. https://doi.org/10.1001/jamadermatol.2018.2348. PMID: 30140971.
55. Wiens J, Saria S, Sendak M, Ghassemi M, Liu VX, Doshi-Velez F, Jung K, Heller K, Kale D, Saeed M, Ossorio PN. Do no harm: a roadmap for responsible machine learning for health care. Nat Med. 2019;25(9):1337–40. https://doi.org/10.1038/s41591-019-0548-6. PMID: 31406307.
56. Goodman B, Flaxman S. European Union regulations on algorithmic decision-making and a right to explanation. AI Mag. 2017;38(3):50–7. https://doi.org/10.1609/aimag.v38i3.2741.
57. Shen Y, Heacock L, Elias J, et al. ChatGPT and other large language models are double-edged swords. Radiology. 2023;307(2):e230604. https://doi.org/10.1148/radiol.230604. PMID: 37705118.
58. Zhang H, Barekati Z, Bozkurt S, et al. Hallucination in generative AI models for health care: a narrative review. J Med Internet Res. 2023;25:e46203. https://doi.org/10.2196/46203. PMID: 37845414; PMCID: PMC10578229.
59. Mehrabi N, Morstatter F, Saxena N, Lerman K, Galstyan A. A survey on bias and fairness in machine learning. ACM Comput Surv. 2021;54(6):1–35. https://doi.org/10.1145/3457607.

Securing Healthcare Data

Alexis Long, Kelly Fan, Max McDonnell, Nishi Patel, Joseph Tomecki, and Ann M. Peiffer

Introduction

As U.S. medical systems began embracing Electronic Health (E-health) and migrated in mass to electronic health records (EHR), the Office of the National Coordinator for Health Information Technology labeled 2014–2023 the "Decade of data" [1]. Medical data is collected within an institution's EHR, an electronic database of patients' personal health records. By transitioning from the need to maintain, store, access, and send physical medical records, this system improves healthcare outcomes, promotes accessibility, and helps to reduce costs [2]. However, privacy and security remain large areas of concern with the amount of health data being generated and stored rising exponentially [2, 3] (see Table 1 for a list of acronym meanings).

E-Health interventions are novel digital technologies developed to meet healthcare demands and can include medical devices, diagnostic algorithms, and other applications [4]. The expansion of data collection and integration through E-Health interventions align closely with the Healthcare 4.0 paradigm, which promotes the digitization of health care to facilitate a more patient-centric approach to medical management [5]. More specifically, Healthcare 4.0 is the application of the current phase of the Industrial Revolution (i.e., Industry 4.0) to the healthcare sector and seeks to utilize advancements in technology to fully automate machines and create virtual environments to deliver enhanced, value-added and cost-effective care [6]. Accompanying the digitization of medical records, a plethora of complex data from

Alexis Long, Kelly Fan, Max McDonnell, and Nishi Patel are first authors—all individuals equally contributed and were responsible for manuscript production.

A. Long · K. Fan · M. McDonnell · N. Patel · J. Tomecki · A. M. Peiffer (✉)
Department of Biomedical Sciences, Western Michigan University Homer Stryker M. D. School of Medicine, Kalamazoo, MI, USA
e-mail: ann.peiffer@wmed.edu

S. S. Chahin et al. (eds.), *Innovation in Medical Education and Clinical Practice*, https://doi.org/10.1007/978-3-032-19116-8_8

Table 1 Acronyms used within this chapter

Acronyms	Full name
AI	Artificial Intelligence
CDSS	Clinical Decision Support Systems
DHL	Digital Health Literacy
DTC	Direct-to-Consumer
E-Health	Electronic Health
EHR	Electronic Health Record
EMS	Emergency Medical Services
ePHRs	Electronic Personal Health Records
FDA	Food & Drug Administration
FTC	Federal Trade Commission
GINA	Genetic Information Nondiscrimination Act
HIPAA	Health Insurance Portability & Accountability Act
HITECH	Health Information Technology for Economic and Clinical Health Act
IoMT	Internet of Medical Things
PGHD	Patient-Generated Health Data
PHI	Protected Health Information
RBAC	Role Based Access Control
SNP	Single Nucleotide Polymorphism
WBAN	Wireless Body Area Network

multiple sources are available as "Big Data" with the technological potential for integrating across multiple devices and systems using analytics and advanced computing [5, 6]. Central to this integration of devices for "Big Data" and Healthcare 4.0 is the concept of the Internet of Medical Things (IoMT), a network of interconnected healthcare devices and systems that gather, analyze, and transmit health data via the Internet without the need for direct human intervention [7]. Through IoMT networks, data from wearable sensors, implantable devices, and remote monitoring applications can be obtained, integrated, and analyzed to inform patient care.

Considerations for the implementation of E-Health interventions within the Healthcare 4.0 framework of "Big Data" include how health-related data are integrated into health management systems in an efficient and secure manner, as well as how patient data can be safely shared with providers and third parties such as researchers, insurance companies, and alternative care providers. Given the sensitivity of patient data, security and privacy safeguards are essential components of the data landscape. IoMT broadly breaks down this landscape into 4 layers: data collection, data transfer, data storage, and data access and use (see Fig. 1). Ensuring trustworthy data flow in each of and among these layers protects patients and allows healthcare organizations to realize the benefits of continuous, data-driven care while being compliant under HIPAA and other federal guidelines regarding the privacy of personal health information. IoMT networks can be developed within a single healthcare organization or extended across multiple organizations and institutional

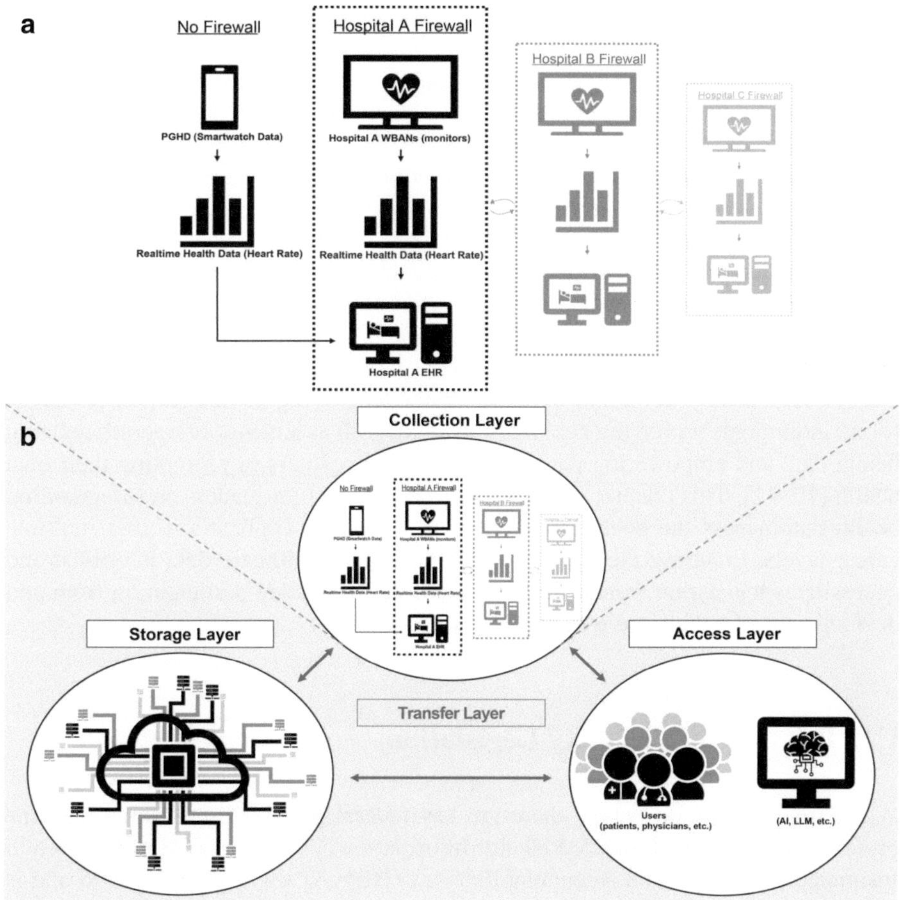

Fig. 1 IoMT Data Landscape. Panel (**a**) WBANS and PGHD can produce real-time health data both within and outside of a hospital's firewall in the data collection layer. Panel (**b**) The data collection layer, storage layer, and access layer all communicate with one another using the data transfer layer of the IoMT framework to implement Healthcare 4.0 E-health interventions

entities. Historically, U.S. health care has been a diverse set of public and private data systems requiring standardization to facilitate the flow of data among various siloed entities [8]. Over the last few decades, the healthcare sector has experienced greater integration of independent physicians into hospital systems [9] indicating a changing landscape in health information technology that supports the potential of Healthcare 4.0 and IoMT opportunities.

A systems-level organization of safeguarding healthcare data is considered for this chapter which takes a wide perspective defining healthcare data within the layers of IoMT. Thus, discussion will extend beyond standard medical record data to include consideration of DNA findings, as well as sensor or wearable device data, which is not currently widespread in institutional EHR systems. Safeguarding "Big

Data" in terms of reliability, security, confidentiality, and patient privacy are major concerns and limitations for expansion into this new age of health care and policies regarding national healthcare practices. Rather than concentrating on the technology used to safeguard data (e.g., encryption, blockchain, and cloud computing), this chapter is centered on answering several questions: where does safeguarding of data happen within the healthcare system; who are the stakeholders and/or responsible parties; how do institutional policies and operations impact the risk to reliability, privacy, confidentiality, and security of the data? A common thread woven throughout is consideration of the patient's perspective, as they are a partner in managing their own health and how they are represented within the healthcare data landscape.

As patients' roles in their own care have increased, greater system-level healthcare education is required to safeguard data as it becomes more patient-centered and accessible. This education falls under the framework of digital health literacy (DHL) for all individuals within the healthcare system, both as a means of operationalizing health data and empowering patients to be active partners in promoting their own health [10, 11]. This chapter seeks to increase the DHL of readers on safeguarding health data across the healthcare system in a manner applicable across multiple career levels. Ensuring the privacy and security of healthcare data is critical and necessitates legislation, hardware advancements, and active participation from and development of healthcare workers and patients.

U.S. Privacy and Security Legislation

While state legislation varies, there are key federal policies establishing baseline protection criteria for Protected Health Information (PHI) in the EHR. The Health Insurance Portability and Accountability Act (HIPAA) was passed in 1996 and is the key piece of legislation that establishes the national standard for PHI protection and confidentiality [12, 13]. HIPAA's Privacy Rule granted patients the right to access, request corrections, and control disclosure of their medical records and PHI. PHI was established as any piece of information that can identify an individual in relation to their medical history. This includes Social Security Numbers, names, birthdays, lab results, and billing information. Only information generated, stored, or transmitted by covered entities—healthcare providers, healthcare plans, healthcare clearinghouses, and their respective business associates—is considered PHI and covered by HIPAA [13].

To bolster confidentiality and the patient's control of PHI disclosure, HIPAA limits who can access, use, and disclose PHI by outlining three key areas for securing PHI: technical, physical, and administrative safeguards [2, 12]. Examples of these safeguards include implementation of a firewall to protect the EHR (technical), limiting access to records by monitoring/restricting computer use (physical), and requiring patient permission to disclose PHI through a signature on a HIPAA authorization form (administrative). Patient consent is mandatory in most situations, but there are exceptions that allow accessing, using, and sharing of PHI for the purposes of treatment, billing, quality improvement assessments and research, hospital accreditation, judicial proceedings, and investigations by law enforcement. However, even in these cases, covered entities must follow the Minimum Necessary Standard and share only the smallest amount of PHI possible for that purpose. To protect patients' privacy in research, HIPAA also created deidentification protocols; these safe harbor protocols require 18 types of identifying information (e.g., names, addresses, contact information, dates, and uniquely identifying characteristics) to be removed from PHI before it can be used [2]. Deidentification and anonymization represent different levels of data security and privacy. Although both are aimed at removing or altering identifiers, the difference is that deidentification reduces the risk for reidentification while anonymization makes it impossible as all identifiers have been removed and the dataset is large enough that the available variables do not single out an individual participant.

The 2009 Health Information Technology for Economic and Clinical Health (HITECH) Act reinforced HIPAA by establishing security breach protocols, including a mandatory reporting requirement for any breaches impacting 500 or more individuals [2, 12]. The HITECH Act incentivized implementation of the EHR across U.S. healthcare providers and required the Centers of Medicaid and Medicare to implement an EHR by 2015 [12]. It also prohibited the sale of identifiable PHI without authorization from the individual and strengthened penalties for violations [13]. While HIPAA and HITECH protect a broad range of identifiable PHI, the protections and regulations only applied to data collected by specified entities [13], meaning there were no protections in place to regulate third party medical devices or health apps.

Due to lack of regulation, numerous medical devices contained glaring vulnerabilities that impacted patients and healthcare delivery. For instance, the Hospira LifeCare Patient Controlled Analgesia and related Hospira infusion systems were able to be remotely accessed through the hospital network, allowing bad actors to disable alarms and change dosages [14]. In response to examples like this, the Food and Drug Administration (FDA) created—and has continually updated—cybersecurity regulations for medical devices in 2014. Under the FDA's "Cybersecurity in Medical Devices: Quality System Considerations and Content of Premarket Submissions" document, medical device manufacturers are required to incorporate built-in protections, identify and fix vulnerabilities before and after their products are released into the markets, list all software components, and demonstrate efforts to address cybersecurity risks during development [15].

Similarly, patients were increasingly using third party health apps and HIPAA's protections are limited, posing major concerns to privacy and security [13]. Third party apps (e.g., menstrual, nutrition, and medication trackers) and many third-party businesses were selling identifiable PHI to other organizations, often without full transparency [13]. To address this gap in regulation, the Federal Trade Commission (FTC) created the Health Breach Notification Rule to further bolster and expand the HITECH breach reporting requirement [15, 16]. As of 2023, this rule outlined reporting requirements for personal health records in health apps, online services, and direct-to-consumer (DTC) services not covered by HIPAA and further expanded the definition of a security breach to include unauthorized sharing and disclosure of information [16]. These FTC reporting guidelines parallel HIPAA breach protocols for covered health entities, who must report to the Department of Health and Human Services. Similar to the HITECH Act, organizations are required to report security breaches impacting 500 or more individuals to the FTC and those impacted within 60 days [16]. All breach notices must be transparent, readily understood, and specify which third parties received the data and what types of health data were compromised [16].

IoMT Layers

Data Collection: EHR data is collected in several different ways that has traditionally started with intake forms and paperwork collected at the beginning of a new patient visit. The provider-patient interaction involving history-taking and physical examination would inform which subsequent EHR data the provider desired to collect such as laboratory or radiological testing. While this data is vital to patient care and positive health outcomes, this form of data collection alone fails to offer a comprehensive and continuous representation of patients and their dynamic health statuses that could be continuously recorded outside of a patient visit. Accomplishing this requires the implementation of IoMT devices into the process of collecting patient health data and offers the capability to collect health data not previously recorded in patients' EHRs. Moreover, much of the data previously collected via intake forms and laboratory testing is now able to be collected through IoMT devices without needing a patient visit. The ability to integrate this new type of health data into patients' charts is established by the data collection layer of the IoMT framework.

Within the data collection layer, wireless body area networks (WBANs) are among the most common technological systems for capturing data. WBANs consist of communicating devices on, in, or around a person that records real-time health data and transmits this information to a central monitoring system. Data collected via WBANs can be integrated into the EHR, enabling providers to remotely monitor patients and track long-term trends of specific physiological parameters. WBANs specifically focus on measuring physiological parameters directly from the human body such as heart rate, heart rhythm, blood pressure, body temperature, and glucose levels by leveraging devices such as smartwatches, pulse oximeters, electrocardiograms, and implanted pacemakers [4]. As such, WBANs are an important mechanism to produce patient-generated health data (PGHD), defined as data that is created, recorded, or gathered by patients outside of clinical encounters to help address a health concern [17]. Ensuring the reliability and validity of incoming PGHD, as well as the secure and private transfer of data into patients' EHRs, is of utmost importance [18]. Moreover, since healthcare professionals often serve as a primary source of information for patients regarding WBANs, they serve an especially important role in safeguarding data within this layer by directing patients to reputable manufacturers meeting FDA and FTC requirements.

Data Transfer: Once raw data is acquired by WBANs or other IoMT devices, it must be securely transferred to a centralized system for storage and access. Data is first accumulated at servers, which can be devices such as mobile phones and laptops [19]. Transmission of information to intermediate servers via gateways and routers often employs networking technologies such as Bluetooth, Bluetooth Low Energy, Near-Field Communication, Radio Frequency IDentification, Zigbee, and Z-Wave [19] and can take place in a variety of environments including the hospital, clinic, or outside of the traditional healthcare setting [20]. Aggregated data at intermediate servers is then transferred to medical servers, often using long-range wireless technologies such as Wi-Fi, Global System for Mobile Communications, and Long Range within an institutional system's firewall [19].

The data transfer layer increases flexibility for patient monitoring from places such as patients' homes, thus enabling early detection of health issues without requiring patients to travel long distances. The use of such technology thus enhances healthcare access in rural or underserved areas [20]. Importantly, however, data transfer that occurs outside of institutional networks also introduces additional security challenges. These environments may rely on unsecured wireless connections or lack standardized security protocols, increasing vulnerability to data interception or unauthorized access [20]. In all steps of data transfer, secure transmission is crucial because unprotected transmission of data is vulnerable to interception and tampering. For example, cyberattackers could alter data in transit or misrepresent patient information, resulting in compromised patient care [21]. End-to-end encryption, secure communication protocols that utilize data encryption and identity verification such as TLS/HTTPS, and cryptographic checks are widely recommended tools used to maintain the integrity and confidentiality of data [22]. Under HIPAA, PHI should be encrypted both when stored and transferred to prevent data breaches [23]. Even without a cyberattack, as institutional systems are linked within U.S. healthcare inconsistently, confusion about patient records can occur such as outdated information being used to populate a patient's record for a new visit. The patient and/or caregiver's ability to verify the medication list and other information is a critical piece to maintaining accurate transmission of data and upholding overall data integrity.

Data Storage: PHI is preserved for later retrieval, analysis, and use within the data storage layer. Storage infrastructures range from hospital servers to distributed cloud platforms, each with unique advantages and disadvantages. Establishing and maintaining an effective security system places a high cost on hospitals and other organizations utilizing an EHR [12]. Cloud computing is an E-Health intervention that offers storage, management, and processing of patient health data, that is unable to be integrated via WBANs alone, through different applications on remote servers accessed via the Internet [4]. This allows different digital databases and approved healthcare applications to be "devices" relaying information into the cloud computing system allowing secure storage and sharing of patient medical information. By uploading and storing data in the cloud, the burden of protecting stored data would be placed on third-party organizations and allows hospitals' security systems to focus primarily on protecting data when it is being uploaded to or accessed from the cloud [12].

Cloud-based systems offer scalability and interoperability, making it a desirable option for integrating PGHD across different platforms. Data tends to be retained within the healthcare system far longer than federal and state policies dictate; however, the U.S. does not have a formalized national strategy for making the decision as to what gets stored and in what manner [24]. Providers often turn to various guidelines on keeping patient records, like the Center for Medicare and Medicaid Services or Bureau of Veterans Affairs; however, regulations also differ based on data modality. Some media such as radiologic images present significant challenges to storage due to their size and the increased cost of storage as file compression is not always a reasonable policy [25]. Regardless, a cloud-based EHR is also vulnerable to data breaches or ransomware that can threaten patient privacy and continuity of care. Health care is one of the most vulnerable industries to data security breaches, which can result in disruption of care and possibly lead to patient deaths [26]. In addition, the risk of security breaches can cause patients to report their health information inaccurately. For example, an estimated 2 million individuals with a mental health disorder do not seek treatment due to privacy concerns in the U.S [2]. A possible solution to these data security concerns is the "cloud bio-security system" [27]. This software acts as a centralized security monitoring and management system that monitors for potential risks, vulnerabilities, and breaches of data during input and output to and from the cloud. Cloud bio-security software records every data input and output from the cloud network allowing for the immediate alerting and response to data breaches according to "playbooks" encoded within the security software [27]. Additional safeguards are also available that can be implemented in conjunction with the central cloud bio-security system to further support the security of stored data and minimize the risk of data breaches from occurring.

Data Access and Use: The sharing and retrieval of stored health data by providers and patients occurs within the final data access and use layer. The security and privacy of stored and shared health data is significantly impacted by the institutional policies and operational procedures that govern how patient health data is stored and shared. Rather than technical failings of security systems, many past security breaches in health information systems have been the result of simple human error or carelessness [28]. Causes of such breaches have been due to things such as provider password sharing, failure to encrypt health data in EHRs, and misplacement of devices that contain identifiable patient health data. Tackling these issues requires the introduction of novel institutional policies and operational procedures to include more rigorous education of providers on how to securely and safely store and share health data as technology continues to evolve, as well as stricter enforcement of penalties for failing to follow stated security precautions. Revisions to the way patients are providing consent to the collection, storage, and sharing of their PHI are also needed to further empower patients to decide how their data is being stored and shared while simultaneously providing the highest standards of data security and protection [28]. Moreover, as technology offering secure storage and sharing of health data continues to evolve, the institutional policies and operational procedures governing how healthcare personnel and patients interact with these technologies and the data they store must evolve alongside.

Patients may access their stored data via electronic personal health records (ePHRs). As a tool to promote patient engagement and empowerment, ePHRs are electronic applications such as patient portals that allow patients to access, manage, and share health information with others [29]. At the same time, ePHRs introduce additional concerns about the privacy and confidentiality of patient information. Patients may worry that sensitive information in their ePHR is easily accessible to researchers, industry members, or insurance companies, preventing them from adopting ePHR use at all [29]. Of those that use ePHR, trust in the privacy and security of the portal is provided by a protected log-in process and is a by-product of the trust in their healthcare provider [30]. While some patients want to share access to ePHRs with a caregiver (e.g., sharing account password and username), some patients desire access limitations requiring a proxy account or access control strategies [29, 31].

The most basic access control strategy is Role Based Access Control (RBAC) where the ePHR system is configured with various roles such as "doctor," "patient," and "administrator," corresponding to a designated set of permissions that dictate what data the role can view or edit [32]. Other forms of access control include Mandatory Access Control and Team-based Access Control, which build on the principles of RBAC. Some hospitals provide proxy accounts for caregivers, which allows them to log in with their own credentials [31] rather than sharing access through the patient's log-in. The design and selection of such access control mechanisms must balance ease of access with strong privacy protections so that patients feel confident in using ePHR tools.

Within the IoMT, Blockchain technology, used in conjunction with cloud computing in the broader setting of institutional firewalls, potentially addresses how data is shared between users in a secure manner, and which users are responsible for sharing such data. Put simply, blockchain securely records data transactions and eliminates the need for a "central authority" to govern these transactions between users [4]. Blockchain achieves this via "smart contracts," self-executing agreements embedded in the blockchain itself which automate consent management and are used to define access rights and data-sharing permissions chosen by the end user (i.e., patient). This design allows a healthcare institution to include the patient's desires in constructing its responsibility of communicating and sharing medical information to approved individuals in a more decentralized, patient-centered manner. Allowing different devices and systems to input and output data into the blockchain enables the patient to decide who the information is shared with, where the data is sent, and what specific data can be shared. The decentralized format allows both patient and provider to share the responsibility of communicating information. Direct patient involvement in the process takes the responsibility of communicating medical data from one person and distributes it among all parties at stake, offering more decision-making power to patients [4].

Blockchain also supports supply chain integrity by improving traceability and transparency of IoMT devices, material supplies, results, and much more. This enables verification of the accuracy, reliability, availability, and trustworthiness of the devices, material, and data being shared, thereby improving patient safety [33].

While promising, blockchain technology does come with certain limitations and concerns in its current capacity. Importantly, scalability is a concern for blockchain use considering the overwhelming amount of health data that is being input and output by this technology [33]. Due to blockchain's decentralized format, ensuring some form of standardized protocols for data exchange between providers, patients, and third party systems must also be addressed. Nevertheless, with improvements and further development, blockchain offers a promising technology to be used to integrate medical information coming from both healthcare providers within a hospital system as well as other entities patients may decide to seek treatment from outside the hospital system such as chiropractors and naturopaths providing a program that both empowers patients, and streamlines many aspects of data-sharing for healthcare professionals.

Healthcare 4.0 Applications Across the Layers

"Smart Health Monitoring" is an E-health intervention synthesizing each of the four layers of data flow and their associated technologies into a practical format to be used in the healthcare setting. This organization of data flow and technologies allows for the immediate integration of medical information into the patient's chart and alerting providers when a critical change in patient condition occurs [34]. In doing so, this takes away the "intermediary" in many situations where physicians rely on lab technicians, nurses, or other members of the care team to continuously monitor vitals or lab results and report critical values to the attending. Other providers may also be added to receive these alerts, allowing for faster response times during medical emergencies and improved patient outcomes.

Practical applications of smart health monitoring include the introduction of emergency medical technicians and paramedics to these technologies, offering an integrated approach of efficient communication and strong data security to confidently take care of patients requiring emergency care in the field. With smart health monitoring, Emergency Medical Services (EMS) can have readily available medical data on their specific patient during transport as the patient's physician, or the patient themselves, may grant access to EMS for pertinent past medical history, drug allergies, diagnoses, and other information that may be critical to know before arriving at the hospital. Additionally, these technologically advanced smart health monitoring systems can be combined to form "smart healthcare systems," utilizing artificial intelligence (AI) and machine learning to track and identify long-term trends in patients' health data to facilitate more accurate diagnoses and personalized treatment plans [34]. While leveraging such technologies can help improve health outcomes, sensitive patient information entered into AI and Large Language Learning Model systems can remain within these systems for long durations and represents a reservoir of data that creates additional challenges regarding consent, ownership, and privacy. One potential programming solution is to use federated learning so that the data never leaves the organization's secured information system yet local data can still be leveraged within these technologies [35].

As more and more of these tools are incorporated into the EHR to utilize digital technology for enhancing patient care, their impact on data security must be considered. Clinical Decision Support Systems (CDSS) analyze patient data within the EHR and produce results that provide clinicians with context relevant to current clinical guidelines, reducing adverse events [36]. The data for such software can be generated from machine learning through training computer models. This makes CDSS a useful tool for making predictions about health outcomes by elucidating patterns in large and complex datasets. Consideration of stakeholders involved with creating these algorithms and the quality of training and testing data is crucial to avoid bias [37]. Integration of these systems within EHRs contributes to data integrity and accuracy challenges that must be addressed when managing the union between AI and health care.

Role of Healthcare Professionals

As E-health interventions take on an increasingly important role in health monitoring and management, developing strategies to protect the privacy and integrity of data collected in these ways has become crucial. Healthcare professionals play an especially important role in safeguarding data within the data collection layer, as they often serve as a primary source of information for patients regarding the collection and handling of PGHD via WBANs. For example, patients may consult their provider to help guide device selection or bring wearable-generated reports with them to the clinic. The clinician's role in providing trustworthy guidance is especially important given that many individuals lack awareness about general privacy and security issues surrounding PGHD. Many wearable device owners usually do not know what types of health data their wearable is transmitting, how the data are encrypted, or who has access to their information [38]. Clinicians should be prepared to educate patients about both the risks and benefits of sharing their health data through WBANs to help them make informed decisions about choosing to use these technologies. Based on how this data is entered into the EHR of the hospital or clinic by the provider (e.g., summary mention in a visit note, report scanned in the system as image versus encoded text) will determine how accessible the PGHD is to automated system queries and/or review by other healthcare providers.

Effective patient education clarifies common misconceptions about the privacy, confidentiality, and security of E-Health interventions. For example, many patients do not know that their data could be sold by wearable device manufacturers to third parties without their knowledge or consent [39]. To address misconceptions about data ownership, clinicians can share that data collected by wearable devices are usually owned by the manufacturer and can potentially be accessed by a cascade of third parties. Patients should also be informed about the risks of data breaches associated with E-Health interventions if applicable. They may not be aware that their personal information can be hacked and that identity theft is possible [40]. Clinicians should help patients understand that although health data collected by sensors or devices may seem benign, data hacks and the theft of medical information can expose them to identity fraud and subsequent financial loss.

In all cases, healthcare providers should approach conversations with patients about PGHD privacy, confidentiality, and security with awareness that their professional authority can shape patients' trust in E-Health interventions. Patients may perceive their provider's recommendation for using a wearable device or monitor as guaranteed assurance of data protection [40, 41]. Clinicians should therefore be well-informed about the privacy and security considerations of E-Health interventions before recommending them to patients. This may necessitate educational programs to improve digital health literacy among healthcare professionals [42]. Such programs can enhance healthcare professionals' ability to recommend E-Health technologies to patients and guide responsible use.

Additionally, healthcare professionals have a crucial role in maintaining the security of PHI and protecting privacy in transfer and storage. The majority of security breaches (73%) compromising health records between 2015 and 2020 were due to unintentional, rather than malicious, insider threats with phishing scams and negligence/carelessness the most common [26]. Phishing is a type of scam that tricks individuals through links or documents sent by a legitimate-looking email into downloading malicious ransomware that compromises security protections, resulting in data breaches [26]. Even just one individual falling victim to this type of attack can compromise the system and result in subsequent attacks. In 2015, Anthem Blue Cross Blue Shield insurance experienced one of the largest cybersecurity breaches in health care, which affected 80 million customers and was caused by phishing attacks [26, 43]. Attending training programs, logging out of computer terminals/applications after use, and updating passwords are some of the fundamental steps required of healthcare workers to protect the privacy of data in the EHR [2, 12, 26]. To help prevent security breaches at these steps, some healthcare security systems have implemented automatic logoff on applications and authentication tokens on log-in [2]. Another critical area is limiting unnecessary access to PHI, which can be achieved through performing audits to periodically check who is accessing charts [26].

Real-Life Applicability: DNA

Genomic information has been integral to the paradigm shift toward delivering precision medicine and advancing scientific discovery within Healthcare 4.0. It equips the healthcare field to tailor treatments for individual variability in disease phenotypes, thus optimizing patient health outcomes. In addition to raw DNA data, genomics offers much to learn about a patient's biology, including RNA and protein data, single nucleotide polymorphisms (SNPs), germline variants, and methylation patterns [44]. Moreover, this abundant information can be systematically leveraged across a group of patients within a research lens to better elucidate disease mechanisms and develop novel therapies. The data represents highly sensitive information unique to a given patient, thereby warranting rigorous oversight over its collection and storage for both clinical and research applications.

In the United States, there exist federal statutes that aim to protect genetic privacy such as the Genetic Information Nondiscrimination Act (GINA) in addition to HIPAA. Despite this, risks remain for unauthorized disclosure of genetic information due to factors such as vulnerabilities in security systems, user error, malicious intent, or blurred boundaries regarding data sharing and ownership. Accordingly, patient anxiety surrounding the security and confidentiality of their personal data is justified [45]. Continuous technological advances and a collective desire to better understand human biology and predict disease mean that genomic information will always remain relevant in health care, highlighting the importance of preserving its security.

The value of genomic data is dependent on the ability to access, share, and interpret it in a manner that is meaningful for patient and population health outcomes. Different types of genomic data carry different risks, but not all genomic data is found within a patient's EHR. DNA, RNA, whole genome sequencing and whole exome sequencing, and germline variants are all considered aspects of genomic data that have high risk for privacy breaches. These modalities have high genome coverage making them more susceptible to privacy breaches and represent frequent ways to collect genetic data in research participants or in third party DNA companies [44]. Research settings often store these larger amounts of participants' genomic data separate from a patient's clinical EHR. Security and privacy are safeguarded primarily at the level of access to the stored data. For genomic data, anonymization is unachievable, as only 30–80 SNPs could be enough to identify an individual [46]. Hence, the possibility for reidentification in the future using genomic data is an unavoidable risk [44]. Consideration of patients involved with research is especially relevant given modern efforts to increase access to large datasets through shared centralized platforms that are linked to clinical EHR systems. As researchers look to collaborate and generate diverse and comprehensive datasets, there is a crucial responsibility to abide by patient expectations regarding how their data can be used as well as maximize patient benefits while minimizing risk.

DNA in the Clinic: DNA data is not typically full genome sequences, as they are too large to be maintained within the EHR, but rather reports summarizing findings of monogenic diseases, risk alleles, carrier status variants, and pharmacogenetic associations. Since these reports present information at the level of specific proteins, PCR-based genotyping, somatic variation, and a low number of SNPs, they pose less privacy risk. However, current protocols greatly differ among U.S. institutions for how genomic information is managed in EHRs. Specifically, the data is often PGHD and presented as a report from a third party with the company's desired format. Hospital systems will scan this information into multiple places across the EHR system and with different modalities, such as PDFs and free text, across institutions [47]. Depending on how these reports are entered, they may or may not be readily searchable or retrievable through digital queries of an institution's medical record such as those used to build CDSS and make population estimates from a clinical dataset. On the other hand, when healthcare providers review these reports, they are provided with access to patient information beyond the scope of their clinical duties that at minimum breach patient confidentiality and could inadvertently influence clinical decisions. Considering that best practice for providers is to access the minimum necessary patient information to carry out their clinical duties, this may conflict with parsing a full genetic report which may be necessary or desired by a patient. Since these genetic reports are often difficult to understand, challenges in meaningfully appreciating the DNA report data could hinder the shared decision-making process and interfere with patient autonomy [48].

Some patients decide to go beyond the traditional healthcare systems in search of services that provide genetic information in a way that is tailored to their specific desires. Patients want more unfiltered access to their genetic information, bypassing the "gatekeeper" clinician, which seems to be a key motivator for patients being drawn to DTC/third party companies [49]. As this patient information is outside of the healthcare system's firewall, it is subject to different data security standards established by the companies themselves. In fact, international transparency guidelines relating to confidentiality and privacy are not routinely met by DTC genetic testing companies [50]. The ultimate consequence of poor regulation of patient data would result in violation of patient privacy with sensitive genetic information about the individual and/or their family members being accessed and misused by unauthorized entities such as insurance companies, mortgage providers, and employers [44]. For example, the DTC genetic testing company 23andMe declared bankruptcy in March 2025 and jeopardized the genetic data of 15 million customers with their plan to sell the company accompanied with their extensive database [51]. Due to the nature of DNA information, risks include the disclosure of sensitive information about family members who did not consent. Accordingly, this raises concerns about data ownership and the extent to which informed consent remains applicable for patients and family members. At the time of writing, U.S. laws do not comprehensively address the privacy and discrimination issues associated with this unique situation. Furthermore, there is great variability in how U.S. states manage privacy regulations, hence many 23andMe consumers are not legally protected at state and federal levels, further exposing their genetic data to risk.

Genomic data will continue to remain an integral part of the healthcare field in our mission to provide patient-centered care. Recognizing the sensitive and unique properties of this type of data helps us understand the need to prioritize its security, privacy, and confidentiality. Additionally, being aware of the different subsets of genomic information and their differing privacy risks enables providers to modify their approach to best fit the needs of their patients. The increasing participation of patients in their own care represents an opportunity to engage in shared clinical decision-making; however, patients must be educated on their shared responsibility in securing their health data. Involvement from other stakeholders, such as third party companies, must be considered with caution as their security regulations may not align with or be as comprehensive as existing federal ones. In conclusion, multiple parties share the obligation to ensure patient genomic data is effectively secured as it is leveraged in medical systems to improve health outcomes and advance scientific discovery.

Summary

- Adoption of E-Health by the healthcare system has prompted the development and use of the Healthcare 4.0 paradigm and IoMT, using "Big Data" to expand and improve the services offered to provide a more patient-centric healthcare model.
- HIPAA and the HITECH act provide foundational regulations and protocols for the U.S. on a broad range of health data and how to respond when data breaches occur.
- Operational procedures and institutional policies greatly impact the security and privacy of health data being stored and shared and therefore must evolve with the changing landscape in health care.
- Flow of health data from the patient to and through the EHR can be understood in four layers: the data collection layer, data transmission layer, data storage layer, and the data access and use layer.
- Supplementing traditional patient health data collected via intake forms and histories, WBANs, PGHD, and genomic information offer new kinds of data being integrated into patient charts that deliver more individualized health care and highlight the need to address privacy and security issues in these evolving systems.
- Smart Health Monitoring integrates the four layers of data flow into a practical format that enables faster updates to patients' charts and communication to their physicians.
- The reliability, security, confidentiality, and privacy of patients and their PHI are main concerns in the new age of health care and in the practices of lawmakers, healthcare entities, and patients. Thus, improving the DHL of healthcare personnel and patients is paramount.

Acknowledgements We would like to thank Dr. Shamsi Berry PhD, Mr. Michael Fusko, and Dr. Alexandra Bayer PhD for comments on earlier drafts of this work.

Competing Interests The authors have no conflicts of interest to declare that are relevant to the content of this chapter.

References

1. Barker W, Gabriel M, Patel V. Health IT buzz. A decade of data: progressing patient-centric care through health IT. 2024 [cited 2025 Oct 2]. Available from: https://www.healthit.gov/buzz-blog/a-decade-of-data-examined/a-decade-of-data-progressing-patient-centric-care-through-health-it.
2. Tertulino R, Antunes N, Morais H. Privacy in electronic health records: a systematic mapping study. J Public Health (Germany). 2024;32(3):435–54.
3. Basil NN, Ambe S, Ekhator C, Fonkem E. Health records database and inherent security concerns: a review of the literature. Cureus [Internet]. 2022 [cited 2025 Aug 13];14(10). Available from: https://pubmed.ncbi.nlm.nih.gov/36397924/.
4. Osama M, Ateya AA, Sayed MS, Hammad M, Pławiak P, Abd El-Latif AA, et al. Internet of medical things and healthcare 4.0: trends, requirements, challenges, and research directions. Sensors. Multidisciplinary Digital Publishing Institute (MDPI). 2023;23:7435.
5. Gupta A, Singh A. Healthcare 4.0: recent advancements and futuristic research directions. Wirel Pers Commun [Internet]. 2022 [cited 2025 Sep 20];129(2):933. Available from: https://pmc.ncbi.nlm.nih.gov/articles/PMC9795952/.
6. Karatas M, Eriskin L, Deveci M, Pamucar D, Garg H. Big data for healthcare industry 4.0: applications, challenges and future perspectives. Expert Syst Appl. Elsevier Ltd. 2022;200:116912.
7. Razdan S, Sharma S. Internet of medical things (IoMT): overview, emerging technologies, and case studies. IETE Tech Rev (Institution of Electronics and Telecommunication Engineers, India). 2022;39(4):775–88.
8. Cheryl U, Bernadette MF, Nerenz DR. Race, ethnicity, and language data: standardization for health care quality improvement. National Academies Press; 2009. 181 p.
9. Luo Q, Black B, Magid DJ, Masoudi FA, Kini V, Moghtaderi A. A more complete measure of vertical integration between physicians and hospitals. Health Serv Res. 2024;59(4):e14314.
10. Boshnjaku A, Krasniqi E, Kamberi F. The emerging need to integrate digital health literacy as a course into health-related and care-related profession curricula. Front Public Health [Internet]. 2025;13. Available from: https://www.frontiersin.org/articles/10.3389/fpubh.2025.1534139/full.
11. Conard S. Best practices in digital health literacy. Int J Cardiol. 2019;292:277–9.
12. Kruse CS, Smith B, Vanderlinden H, Nealand A. Security techniques for the electronic health records. J Med Syst. 2017;41(8):127.
13. McGraw D, Mandl KD. Privacy protections to encourage use of health-relevant digital data in a learning health system. NPJ Digit Med. 2021;4(1):2.
14. CISA. ICS Advisory – Hospira LifeCare PCA Infusion System vulnerabilities (Update A) [Internet]. 2018 [cited 2025 Oct 16]. Available from: https://www.cisa.gov/news-events/ics-advisories/icsa-15-125-01a.
15. Ostermann M, Mathias R, Jahed F, Parker MB, Hudson FD, Harding WC, et al. Cybersecurity requirements for medical devices in the EU and US – a comparison and gap analysis of the MDCG 2019–16 and FDA premarket cybersecurity guidance. Comput Struct Biotechnol J. 2025;28:259–66.
16. Federal Trade Commission. Business Blog. Updated FTC health breach notification rule puts new provisions in place to protect users of health apps. 2024 [cited 2025 Sep 30]. Available from: https://www.ftc.gov/business-guidance/blog/2024/04/updated-ftc-health-breach-notification-rule-puts-new-provisions-place-protect-users-health-apps.
17. Treadwell JR, Reston JT, Rouse B, Fontanarosa J, Patel N, Mull NK. Automated-entry patient-generated health data for chronic conditions: the evidence on health outcomes. Automated-entry patient-generated health data for chronic conditions: the evidence on health outcomes [Internet]. 2021 [cited 2025 Aug 12]. Available from: https://www.ncbi.nlm.nih.gov/books/NBK568443/.

18. Paul PC, Loane J, McCaffery F, Regan G. Towards design and development of a data security and privacy risk management framework for WBAN based healthcare applications. Appl Syst Innov. 2021;4(4):76.
19. Hameed SS, Hassan WH, Latiff LA, Ghabban F. A systematic review of security and privacy issues in the internet of medical things; the role of machine learning approaches. Peer J Comput Sci [Internet]. 2021 [cited 2025 Oct 29];7:e414. Available from: https://pmc.ncbi.nlm.nih.gov/articles/PMC8022640/.
20. Akhtar MN, Haleem A, Javaid M. Scope of health care system in rural areas under medical 4.0 environment. Intell Pharm. 2023;1(4):217–23.
21. Singh N, Buyya R, Kim H. Securing cloud-based internet of things: challenges and mitigations. Sensors (Basel) [Internet]. 2024 [cited 2025 Oct 2];25(1):79. Available from: https://pmc.ncbi.nlm.nih.gov/articles/PMC11723188/.
22. Rasool RU, Ahmad HF, Rafique W, Qayyum A, Qadir J. Security and privacy of internet of medical things: a contemporary review in the age of surveillance, botnets, and adversarial ML. J Netw Comput Appl. 2022;201:103332.
23. Alder S. HIPAA encryption requirements. HIPAA J. 2025 [cited 2025 Sep 30]. Available from: https://www.hipaajournal.com/hipaa-encryption-requirements/.
24. Corn M. Archiving the phenome: clinical records deserve long-term preservation. J Am Med Inform Assoc. 2009;16(1):1–6.
25. Behnam F, Khajouei R, Ahmadian L. The retention duration of digital images in picture archiving and communication systems. Heliyon [Internet]. 2024 [cited 2025 Oct 2];10(6). Available from: https://pubmed.ncbi.nlm.nih.gov/38524536/.
26. Yeo LH, Banfield J. Human factors in electronic health records cybersecurity breach: an exploratory analysis. Perspect Health Inf Manag. 2022;19(Spring):1i.
27. Sachdeva S, Bhatia S, Al Harrasi A, Shah YA, Anwer K, Philip AK, et al. Unraveling the role of cloud computing in health care system and biomedical sciences. Heliyon [Internet]. 2024 [cited 2025 Sep 24];10(7):e29044. Available from: https://www.sciencedirect.com/science/article/pii/S2405844024050758#sec11.
28. Blumenthal D. Implementation of the federal health information technology initiative. N Engl J Med [Internet]. 2011 [cited 2025 Oct 2];365(25):2426–31. Available from: https://www.nejm.org/doi/pdf/10.1056/NEJMsr1112158.
29. Niazkhani Z, Toni E, Cheshmekaboodi M, Georgiou A, Pirnejad H. Barriers to patient, provider, and caregiver adoption and use of electronic personal health records in chronic care: a systematic review. BMC Med Inform Decis Mak [Internet]. 2020 [cited 2025 Oct 2];20(1). Available from: https://pubmed.ncbi.nlm.nih.gov/32641128/.
30. Son EH, Nahm ES. Adult patients' experiences of using a patient portal with a focus on perceived benefits and difficulties, and perceptions on privacy and security: qualitative descriptive study. JMIR Hum Factors. 2023;10:e46044.
31. Latulipe C, Mazumder SF, Wilson RKW, Talton JW, Bertoni AG, Quandt SA, et al. Security and privacy risks associated with adult patient portal accounts in US hospitals. JAMA Intern Med [Internet]. 2020 [cited 2025 Oct 2];180(6):845–9. Available from: https://pubmed.ncbi.nlm.nih.gov/32364562/.
32. Gope P, Amin R. A novel reference security model with the situation based access policy for accessing EPHR data. J Med Syst. 2016;40(11):242.
33. Qahtan S, Yatim K, Zulzalil H, Osman MH, Zaidan AA, Alsattar HA. Review of healthcare industry 4.0 application-based blockchain in terms of security and privacy development attributes: comprehensive taxonomy, open issues and challenges and recommended solution. J Netw Comput Appl. Academic Press. 2023;209:103529.
34. Bhatt V, Chakraborty S. Real-time healthcare monitoring using smart systems: a step towards healthcare service orchestration smart systems for futuristic healthcare. In: Proceedings – international conference on artificial intelligence and smart systems, ICAIS 2021. Institute of Electrical and Electronics Engineers Inc.; 2021. p. 772–7.

35. Wang W, Ferrari D, Haddon-Hill G, Curcin V. Electronic health records as source of research data. In: Neuromethods. Humana Press Inc.; 2023. p. 331–54.
36. Robertson AJ, Mallett AJ, Stark Z, Sullivan C. It is in our DNA: bringing electronic health records and genomic data together for precision medicine. JMIR Bioinform Biotechnol. 2024;5:e55632.
37. Sutton RT, Pincock D, Baumgart DC, Sadowski DC, Fedorak RN, Kroeker KI. An overview of clinical decision support systems: benefits, risks, and strategies for success. NPJ Digit Med [Internet]. 2020 [cited 2025 Aug 21];3(1):1–10. Available from: https://www.nature.com/articles/s41746-020-0221-y.
38. Cilliers L. Wearable devices in healthcare: privacy and information security issues. Health Inf Manag J [Internet]. 2020 [cited 2025 Aug 12];49(2–3):150–6. Available from: https://pubmed.ncbi.nlm.nih.gov/31146589/.
39. Segura Anaya LH, Alsadoon A, Costadopoulos N, Prasad PWC. Ethical implications of user perceptions of wearable devices. Sci Eng Ethics [Internet]. 2018 [cited 2025 Aug 13];24(1):1–28. Available from: https://link.springer.com/article/10.1007/s11948-017-9872-8.
40. Pergolizzi JV, LeQuang JAK, El-Tallawy SN, Varrassi G. What clinicians should tell patients about wearable devices and data privacy: a narrative review. Cureus [Internet]. 2025 [cited 2025 Aug 13];17(3):e81167. Available from: https://pmc.ncbi.nlm.nih.gov/articles/PMC12020962/.
41. Dobson R, Stowell M, Warren J, Tane T, Ni L, Gu Y, et al. Use of consumer wearables in health research: issues and considerations. J Med Internet Res [Internet]. 2023 [cited 2025 Aug 13];25:e52444. Available from: https://pmc.ncbi.nlm.nih.gov/articles/PMC10698659/
42. Brückner S, Sadare O, Fesl S, Scheibe M, Lang C, Gilbert S. Attitudes of healthcare professionals and researchers toward wearable and app derived patient generated health data. NPJ Digit Med [Internet]. 2025 [cited 2025 Aug 13];8(1):1–18. Available from: https://www.nature.com/articles/s41746-025-01568-4.
43. Office of Public Affairs. Member of sophisticated China-based hacking group indicted for series of computer intrusions, including 2015 data breach of health insurer Anthem Inc. affecting over 78 million people. Press Release; 2019.
44. Thomas M, Mackes N, Preuss-Dodhy A, Wieland T, Bundschus M. Assessing privacy vulnerabilities in genetic data sets: scoping review. JMIR Bioinform Biotechnol. 2024;5(1):e54332.
45. Hazin R, Brothers KB, Malin BA, Koenig BA, Sanderson SC, Rothstein MA, et al. Ethical, legal, and social implications of incorporating genomic information into electronic health records. Genet Med. 2013;15(10):810–6.
46. Lin Z, Owen AB, Altman RB. Genomic research and human subject privacy. Science (1979) [Internet]. 2004 [cited 2025 Aug 20];305(5681):183. Available from: https://pubmed.ncbi.nlm.nih.gov/15247459/.
47. Shirts BH, Salama JS, Aronson SJ, Chung WK, Gray SW, Hindorff LA, et al. CSER and eMERGE: current and potential state of the display of genetic information in the electronic health record. JAMIA [Internet]. 2015 [cited 2025 Aug 19];22(6):1231. Available from: https://pmc.ncbi.nlm.nih.gov/articles/PMC5009914/.
48. Carter AB, Abruzzo LV, Hirschhorn JW, Jones D, Jordan DC, Nassiri M, et al. Electronic health records and genomics: perspectives from the Association for Molecular Pathology Electronic Health Record (EHR) Interoperability for Clinical Genomics Data Working Group. J Mol Diagn [Internet]. 2022 [cited 2025 Sep 24];24(1):1–17. Available from: https://www.sciencedirect.com/science/article/pii/S1525157821003275.
49. Hendricks-Sturrup RM, Lu CY. Direct-to-consumer genetic testing data privacy: key concerns and recommendations based on consumer perspectives. J Pers Med. 2019;9(2):25.
50. Laestadius LI, Rich JR, Auer PL. All your data (effectively) belong to us: data practices among direct-to-consumer genetic testing firms. Genet Med. 2017;19(5):513–20.
51. Gerke S, Jacoby MB, Cohen IG. 23andMe's bankruptcy raises concerns about privacy in the era of big data. BMJ [Internet]. 2025 [cited 2025 Aug 21];389. Available from: https://pubmed.ncbi.nlm.nih.gov/40425240/.

Use of Augmented Reality and Virtual Reality for Physician Training and Education Purposes

Chidambaram Nachiappan and Lisa Miller

Introduction to VR and AR in Medical Education

Virtual reality (VR) and augmented reality (AR) represent a shift in medical education by creating an immersive and interactive environment that enhances theoretical knowledge and practical skills. VR provides a fully simulated, computer-generated 3D environment where learners can navigate and work on virtual patients, anatomical structures, or procedural scenarios without causing any physical risk. AR, in contrast, enhances the learner's real-world environment via 3D anatomical models, procedural guides, or diagnostic data, enhancing their perception and enabling real-time integration of information with interactive practice. These technologies complement each other. VR offers a complete immersive experience ideal for repetitive skills practice and procedural rehearsal, while AR supports context-dependent learning and enhances understanding of real-time clinical tasks and bedside procedures [1–4].

The conceptual foundations of VR and AR in medical education date back several decades, with early simulation theories appearing in the 1960s. However, recent technological advancements in graphic processing, sensor accuracy, and display affordability have enabled the widespread adoption in medical education. For example, the miniaturization and cost reduction of head-mounted displays (HMDs), alongside the development of sophisticated tracking systems, have made immersive experiences accessible beyond high-resource centers [1]. Today, nearly all U.S. medical schools have incorporated VR, AR, or both into their curricula, reflecting the technologies' growing importance in standardized medical training and assessment. These advances have allowed institutions around the world to integrate VR and AR

C. Nachiappan · L. Miller (✉)
Western Michigan University Homer Stryker M.D. School of Medicine, Kalamazoo, MI, USA
e-mail: lisa.Miller@wmed.edu

S. S. Chahin et al. (eds.), *Innovation in Medical Education and Clinical Practice*, https://doi.org/10.1007/978-3-032-19116-8_9

into their curriculum, bridging the gap between didactic learning and hands on clinical exposure.

From a pedagogical standpoint, VR and AR align with experiential learning theories. Kolb's experiential learning cycle emphasizes the importance of concrete experience, reflective observation, abstract conceptualization, and active experimentation which VR and AR environments inherently support. Additionally, the teachings through AR and VR are promoted by situated cognition theory, which underscores learning as a function of context. The ability of AR and VR to anchor knowledge within authentic settings can enhance its transfer to clinical practice [5, 6].

VR provides medical educators with a unique opportunity to standardize care and training for rare or complex clinical situations that students and residents may rarely encounter, like managing intraoperative complications or emergency airway management. This controlled repetition of risky procedures helps build muscle memory and procedural fluency while reducing the learners' anxiety. AR can assist with real-time decision-making, such as overlaying vascular anatomy during central line placement or guiding incision lines during surgery, reducing errors, and improving confidence [7]. These applications collectively illustrate the significant learner benefits of integrating VR and AR into medical training.

As the implementation of AR and VR has moved on from early experimentation, the next step is to examine how they can be scaled responsibly, equitably, and effectively in medical education. This chapter will start by analyzing how AR and VR impact cognitive load and learning efficiency. Subsequent sections discuss the specific applications of AR and VR in medical education, before focusing on specialized contexts for AR and VR use, such as in emergency and combat medic training with haptics and multi-user VR. The chapter will then delve into the comparative effectiveness of AR and VR against traditional methods. Finally, the chapter reviews major talking points such as large-scale feasibility and different perspectives, challenges, barriers, and future directions. Together, these sections provide a comprehensive view of the current state and evolving potential of VR and AR in medical education, offering readers both evidence-based insights and a roadmap for practical implementation.

Cognitive Load and Learning Efficiency in VR

Cognitive load is the total amount of mental effort or processing demand placed on a person's working memory at any given moment. It is a central determinant of how effectively trainees acquire skills in medical education when using AR and VR. Cognitive load theory is distinguished by three types of loads. Intrinsic load arises from the inherently difficult nature of the material. Extraneous load is caused by distractions or poor instructional design. Lastly, germane load represents the mental effort needed to build a solid foundation [1]. Efficient instructional design aims to minimize extraneous load, balance intrinsic load, and maximize germane load. This balance is particularly critical in AR- and VR-based training, where the novelty and task complexity can impose significant demands on working memory.

Research has shown that cognitive load is inversely related to learning efficiency in VR. Essentially, when extraneous load is high, learners struggle to process and retain information, leading to impaired performance [8, 9]. This problem is especially pronounced in immersive VR, which can overwhelm novices with sensory input and task complexity. A randomized clinical trial comparing immersive VR to conventional VR using only screen-based simulators in laparoscopic surgery training found that learners had poorer immediate task performance with immersive VR use. These results highlight a paradox. The immersive VR offers realism and engagement at the risk of cognitive overload if not designed with careful attention to learner capacity and extraneous load [9].

However, VR has the potential to reduce intrinsic cognitive overload. The interactive 3D environments can improve spatial visualization and provide intuitive cues that support problem-solving [10]. Such affordances are especially beneficial in anatomy or surgical training, where learners have to develop visuospatial reasoning. Distributed VR practice further diminishes cognitive load by allowing learners to revisit material across multiple sessions, creating a framework to aid memory consolidation [11, 12]. Studies have shown that learners exposed to distributed VR practice performed better and reported lower workload in subsequent dissections or surgical simulations compared to those trained in massed sessions. These findings suggest that structured repetition within VR optimizes the balance between mental effort and retention of skills and concepts.

The degree of immersion should be carefully matched to the learner's experience level and instructional objectives. A systematic review has found that less immersive VR environments were sometimes more effective for knowledge acquisition than fully immersive VR, as mentioned earlier. This is particularly true for beginners [13]. In contrast, advanced learners benefit from higher levels of immersion that reflect the complexity of real-life clinical settings. These findings underscore that the VR instructional design is not universally beneficial, but must be tailored to the learner to minimize extraneous load and maximize germane engagement [14].

Recent innovations have introduced neurophysiological monitoring to address cognitive load challenges directly. Functional near-infrared spectroscopy (fNIRS), a non-invasive brain imaging technique, measures cortical oxygenation changes that correspond to cognitive workload [14]. fNIRS can be integrated with VR, which enables real-time monitoring of trainee brain activity. Aksoy demonstrated that fNIRS could reliably distinguish different workload levels during VR-based training tasks. This suggests the feasibility of adaptive platforms that respond to learner's state [15]. For example, if fNIRS detects signs of overload, the VR system could slow task progression, add instructional cues, or segment the task into simpler components. Conversely, when under-engagement is detected, the platform could escalate complexity to maintain optimal challenge.

The implications of fNIRS integration are profound. Training can become personalized, adapting dynamically to keep learners within their "optimal zone" of cognitive challenge that is neither overwhelmed nor disengaged. This could transform assessment as well. Rather than evaluating performance outcomes alone, educators could assess workload patterns to determine whether trainees are developing efficient problem-solving strategies or relying on inefficient trial-and-error approaches. Over time, such monitoring could yield individualized learning profiles, mapping cognitive progress across different training stages.

Despite its promise, integrating fNIRS with VR faces several limitations. Motion artifacts and noise during active surgical simulations can reduce the accuracy of workload measurements [14]. Additionally, fNIRS equipment adds cost and complexity, which may limit adoption in resource-constrained training programs. Ethical considerations also arise regarding how neurophysiological data are stored, interpreted, and used in evaluating trainees. Transparent guidelines will be needed to ensure that monitoring supports learning rather than penalizing learners for cognitive variability.

Instructional design also remains a key challenge. While VR offers powerful visualization and interactivity, poorly designed modules can impose extraneous load, decreasing its benefits [14]. A learner-centered approach that builds content, uses distributed practice, and aligns immersion levels with training goals is essential for optimizing efficiency [13, 14]. Future research should further investigate how these design principles can be combined with neuroadaptive systems like fNIRS to create scalable, personalized training models.

Both VR and AR have demonstrated strong efficacy in medical education. The effectiveness heavily depends on the instructional designs. VR can impose high cognitive demands, so designing programs that reduce overload and improve retention specific to each learner are of utmost importance. Emerging innovations such as neuropsychological monitoring emphasize the potential for personalized, adaptive training environments. The advances of VR and AR as transformative tools can bridge the gap between theoretical knowledge and clinical proficiency.

Augmented Reality Applications in Medical Training

Augmented reality (AR) has evolved into a versatile tool with applications spanning from foundational anatomy education to complex procedural guidance and simulations of clinical scenarios.

In anatomy education, AR has the ability to transform the traditional 2D textbook into a dynamic 3D exploration of the body. By being able to visualize anatomical structure and allowing interactive manipulation, AR enhances spatial cognition and can deepen understanding of relationships among organs, vessels, and tissues. Studies have shown that learners experience accelerated learning, better retention, and higher satisfaction when using AR supplements or partially replacing cadaveric dissection. It has been found to be especially valuable where specimen access is limited due to cost or ethical considerations [16–19].

Procedural and surgical training benefit immensely from AR's capability to provide layered visual cues and stepwise guidance. For example, AR simulations of laparoscopic surgery can deliver real-time overlays of critical anatomy and instrument paths, which improve precision and reduce cognitive load. Validated metrics such as the Global Operative Assessment of Laparoscopic Skills (GOALS) and Objective Structured Assessment of Technical Skills (OSATS) demonstrate significant skill improvements with AR-based training compared to traditional methods [20–22]. Additionally, AR facilitates autonomous learning by allowing the trainee to practice complex procedures and skills at their own pace while still being able to receive immediate feedback on their performance. In a study by Wolf, complex techniques like extracorporeal membrane oxygenation (ECMO) cannulation were done with learners with the use of AR. The findings showed that the AR instructions significantly improved the accuracy and efficiency of novice learners performing single ECMO cannulation compared to conventional instruction methods, with participants demonstrating fewer errors and higher procedural confidence. These findings support AR as a valuable tool for enhancing the training of complex, high-stakes medical procedures [22, 23].

In radiology education, AR supports immersive visualization of imaging datasets, collaborative interpretation in virtual reading rooms, and procedural planning for interventions. This fosters active learning and helps trainees develop spatial reasoning necessary for complex imaging interpretation and safe image-guided procedures [18].

AR allows for simulations of clinical scenarios that enable realistic, interactive encounters, which can promote clinical reasoning, decision-making, and communication skills. This platform mimics patient variability and unexpected complications, which can prepare learners for the real world. The integration of AR virtual patients into the curriculum is supported by emerging research emphasizing learning design and technical requirements to optimize engagement and knowledge transfer [6, 21].

AR has progressed from an experimental adjunct into a validated education modality and enhances learning across multiple areas of medicine. From improving spatial understanding to clinical reasoning, AR serves to supplement and effectively replace traditional training methods. As the technology continues to mature, AR can become an integral component of medical education and skill development.

Enhancing Procedural and Motor Skills via VR

Virtual reality (VR) has emerged as one of the most useful tools for procedural and motor skills training in medicine and surgery with the capability to provide an immersive, controlled, and repeatable environment to facilitate psychomotor skill acquisition. Unlike traditional training methods, VR allows learners to participate in complex clinical scenarios without putting patients at risk. This safe place allows for deliberate practice and error connection that was otherwise not afforded before.

VR has been used in medicine in many different domains. Clinical and rehabilitation studies consistently demonstrate VR's efficacy in improving fine and gross motor performance across populations. For example, patients with neurological impairments like stroke, cerebral palsy, or traumatic brain injuries have shown gains in upper limb function, hand dexterity, coordination, and range of motion following VR-based therapy [24–26]. In occupation therapy contexts, VR interventions have improved functional outcomes by encouraging repetitive, motivating, and gamified practice that traditional rehabilitation finds difficult to achieve [25]. The benefits extend to healthy learners as they acquire new procedural skills. VR promotes neuroplasticity by combining multisensory integration with active engagement, amplifying recovery and skill acquisition. [26, 27]

At its core, VR training utilizes principles of motor learning like high intensity, task-specific repetition, and multimodal feedback. Manipulating the variables in practice, like difficulty, type of feedback, and practice schedule allows for personalized training. This promotes durable skill retention and transfer to real-world clinical environments [24, 28]. Evidence from behavioral neuroscience suggests that VR enhances learning efficiency by integrating sensory, cognitive, and motor processes in ways that amplify neural adaption [27, 29].

Importantly, the transferability of VR-acquired skills to real-world practice is well-supported. When virtual tasks closely approximate the kinematic and haptic demands of physical procedures, learners demonstrate measurable performance improvements in clinical settings. For instance, surgical residents trained with VR have outperformed conventionally trained peers in cadaveric and operating room environments, displaying greater accuracy, efficiency, and confidence in procedural execution [30–32]. VR modules for procedures like suturing, laparoscopic navigation, and orthopedic fixation can be scheduled for structured repetition, which fosters procedural fluency while minimizing the variability in the quality of training [32, 33].

Another advantage of VR lies in its ability to enhance learner engagement and motivation, both critical to mastering procedural skills that often require repetitive practice. Learners have found immersive simulations to be more stimulating and enjoyable, while reducing fatigue and sustaining practice intensity [8]. Furthermore, VR systems capture rich, quantitative performance data such as movement trajectories, kinematics, error rates, and completion times. This data can be used to provide objective, individualized feedback to improve the learner's skills [30, 34, 35]. These metrics not only enhance formative assessment but also help standardize evaluation across learners, improving fairness and transparency in competency-based training.

Social and collaborative VR adds an additional dimension to skill development. Techniques such as virtual co-embodiment and multi-user environments enable synchronous interaction among learners. VR allows for simulation of interprofessional collaboration through team-based procedural training and peer-assisted learning [31, 35]. This is particularly relevant in surgical teams and emergency medicine, where teamwork and communication are as essential as individual technical proficiency.

Concrete examples of VR applications illustrate its expanding scope. Suturing simulators replicating needle tissue interaction dynamics have been shown to enhance haptic sensitivity and fine motor coordination, providing beginner surgeons with an opportunity to rehearse fundamental skills before patient contact [33]. VR modules also allow learners to practice stepwise sequences for full procedure rehearsal. The modules provide integrated feedback, reinforcing procedural fluency and confidence. In orthopedics, VR applications for arthroscopy and pedicle screw placement have demonstrated improved technical performance and patient outcomes in controlled studies, highlighting VR's value as an adjunct to operative training [31, 32].

Overall, VR represents a paradigm shift in medical training, combining motor learning science with immersive technology to accelerate skill acquisition, improve patient safety, and standardize procedural education. As evidence accumulates and hardware continues to advance, VR's role in procedural and motor skills training is set to expand from supplemental tool to essential component of clinical education.

Emergency and Combat Medic Training with Haptics and Multi-user VR

AR and VR have proven to be valuable in enhancing anatomical learning, surgical training, and motor skill development. The qualities that make them so useful can be applied in high-pressure environments as well, where precision and rapid decision-making are paramount. In this section, the use of AR and VR will be analyzed when used in emergency and combat situations. It will explore the emerging tool, as haptic feedback and multi-user VR platforms are being adapted to better prepare clinicians for providing care in extreme conditions.

Preparing emergency responders and combat medics requires a balance of technical skill mastery, resilience under stress, and the ability to function within a highly coordinated team. Traditional methods utilize mannequins, standardized patients, and sometimes live tissue exercises, but they usually fall short of replicating the sensory inputs, immediacy, and distributed teamwork that are key to real-world emergencies. Recent innovations in VR, haptic technologies, and multi-user platforms transform how medics can acquire and retain lifesaving skills. These approaches emphasize tactile realism, collaborative problem-solving, and adaptive learning.

The most critical gap in traditional VR training is lack of tactile sensation. That is where the introduction of haptic feedback comes into play. Casualty care involves performing interventions for hemorrhage control, airway management, and needle decompression, which heavily rely on cues from touch. Haptic simulators bridge this gap by providing force feedback, resistance, and texture simulation, allowing learners to practice psychomotor skills in environments similar to reality. Studies have found that the inclusion of haptics improves performance outcomes, reduces error rates, and accelerates learning curves, making skills more transferable to real combat situations [36, 37].

Evidence from combat medicine emphasizes the value of tactile realism in training. Senior special operations medics, for example, consistently rate tactile fidelity as one of the most important features of live tissue training, underscoring its role in confidence-building and procedural competence [38]. Similarly, recent research has shown that combat medics perceive a high-fidelity haptic simulator as superior to a mannequin only or VR only training for complex procedures [39].

This evidence indicates that haptics is a necessary component of combat medic training. By integrating immersive VR with tactile realism, training programs can improve procedural competence, reduce errors, and enhance the learner's experience and confidence.

Haptics improves an individual's skill acquisition, but medical emergencies also depend on team performance. Resuscitation protocols such as Advanced Cardiovascular Life Support (ACLS) require real-time collaboration, leadership, and role clarity. Traditionally, such training demands trainees to be in the same area, limiting accessibility for geographically dispersed teams. Multi-user VR platforms enable ACLS training where participants can join simulated scenarios from remote locations. The platforms support voice communication, avatar-based patient and teammate interaction, role assignments, and shared decision-making. The tool effectively recreates the dynamics of an actual resuscitation team.

A prospective study by Katz et al. demonstrated that voice-based VR ACLS modules achieved comparable learner satisfaction and non-technical skill acquisition to high-fidelity, in-person simulations, while reducing training costs, instructor workload, and time requirements [40]. These findings highlight the practical benefits of VR, particularly for systems that must train a large number of providers across distributed settings.

Multi-user VR also facilitates standardization and scalability. Unlike traditional simulations, where variability in instructor style or resource availability may influence outcomes, VR scenarios are highly reproducible. This is particularly advantageous for military and disaster medicine contexts, where consistent training across dispersed units ensures continuity during deployment. Systematic reviews further support VR's role in mass casualty training, suggesting that extended reality tools can prepare first responders for complex, large-scale emergencies [41]. Longitudinal studies confirm that immersive multi-user VR can effectively train large student groups in emergency protocols, sustaining engagement and performance over time [42].

These findings highlight the potential for multi-user VR to improve ACLS and emergency training. The reproducibility and consistency in teaching, regardless of location or logistical barriers, ensure that civilian and military teams are prepared to respond cohesively.

With the haptic and multi-user innovations, the outcomes of responders trained by VR need to be examined more closely. Randomized controlled trials and systematic reviews have consistently demonstrated that VR is at least as effective as or sometimes superior to traditional methods for teaching resuscitation protocols.

A recent randomized controlled trial found that fully immersive VR training with automated feedback improved immediate knowledge acquisition and supported higher retention under stress compared to traditional methods [41]. Similarly, VR training has been shown to enhance long-term skill retention, with one study reporting improved cardiopulmonary resuscitation (CPR) acquisition and maintenance at 12 months compared to mannequin-based training [43]. These findings are both supported more broadly as the American Heart Association explicitly acknowledges the role of VR and gamified learning to improve knowledge acquisition, CPR skills, and learner engagement [44]. A systematic review further highlights that VR consistently enhances learner engagement and perceived training effectiveness across healthcare professionals [45].

Together, this evidence suggests that VR is not merely a supplement but a viable alternative to traditional resuscitation training, capable of supporting knowledge retention, psychomotor skill performance, and learner motivation.

By integrating these technologies into medical education, training programs can produce medics who are better prepared, more confident, and more adaptable in the face of emergencies on the battlefield or in the hospital.

Comparative Effectiveness and Systematic Reviews

Building on individual study findings, it is essential to considering evidence at a broader scale. Systematic reviews and meta-analyses provide this perspective, clarifying the overall effectiveness and limitations of AR and VR in medical education.

Meta-analyses and systematic reviews have consistently shown that VR and AR are at least as effective as traditional methods for knowledge acquisition in medical education. There is growing evidence that immersive approaches can outperform conventional instruction in certain skill-based and engagement domains. While short-term knowledge improvements and learner satisfaction are well-documented in the literature, the evidence remains heterogeneous, and gaps persist in understanding long-term outcomes and application of knowledge in the real world.

Across different domains, VR training has shown small to moderate improvements in knowledge and skill outcomes compared with traditional instruction. A systematic review and meta-analysis by the Digital Health Education Collaboration reported that VR modestly improves post-intervention knowledge and cognitive skills compared to both conventional and other digital education methods. However, the certainty of evidence was rated as moderate, and findings for learner attitudes and satisfaction were mixed [46].

Other more targeted reviews stipulate particular strengths in areas that require procedures like surgery. A recent meta-analysis in orthopedic education found that VR significantly improved knowledge, surgical design ability, and clinical operation score. It also enhanced engagement and satisfaction when compared to traditional teaching [47]. Similarly, reviews of surgical education have illustrated that VR-based training generally outperforms didactic instruction and is comparable to supervised operative experiences. However, there are instances where VR may be less effective, like in laparoscopic dry lab practice. One reason for this may be because learners still need to physically manipulate laparoscopic instruments without the VR overlay to develop tactile familiarity and fine motor control. This suggests that VR should be used in tandem with traditional teaching methods [48].

Some large-scale systematic reviews also reinforce these findings. Recent large-scale reviews consistently conclude that VR-based education improves knowledge and psychomotor outcomes across medical and nursing student populations, particularly in procedural skill training [13]. These reviews also report that immersive approaches enhance learner motivation and engagement while improving overall learning outcomes [49, 50].

Evidence with AR is more mixed, particularly in anatomy education. A systematic review reported no significant difference in knowledge outcomes when comparing AR to traditional methods. However, AR was perceived as more engaging and motivating [51]. More recent syntheses highlight the unique strengths of AR in its ability to support 3D visualization and spatial understanding. For instance, it has been demonstrated across multiple reviews that AR consistently increases learner motivation and satisfaction, especially when used as a supplement to conventional anatomy didactics [52]. Similar findings are seen in other reviews, which emphasize AR's decision-support role in higher education when integrated alongside established teaching modalities [53].

Meta-analyses of immersive technologies also note synergistic effects when VR and AR are used together. Immersive technologies have been shown to improve performance in physiology and anatomy assessments when compared to traditional resources, particularly when both modalities are used complementarily [54]. These results align with broader reviews concluding that the greatest benefits of immersive technologies are realized when they are used as supplements and not substitutes for the established curriculum [49, 52].

Overall, systematic reviews indicate that VR and AR are viable adjuncts and possible alternatives to conventional teaching. The strongest evidence supports VR for procedural skills and engagement, while AR has shown promise in anatomy and spatial learning contexts. Across both modalities, learners report higher satisfaction and motivation compared to traditional methods [52].

Large-Scale Feasibility and Gender Perspectives

While earlier sections outlined the benefits of AR and VR in medical education, their true value depends on how these tools can be implemented equitably and sustainably. This section turns to issues of feasibility and access, considering the challenges that shape their broader adoption.

Transitioning VR and AR from pilot projects to large-scale immersive curricular tools requires evaluation of feasibility, usability, and learner acceptance across diverse populations. Recent studies highlight that immersive technologies have been well-received by medical students, particularly with increased motivation, improved understanding, and increased confidence. A large-scale feasibility study examined the application of screen-based 3D visualization and AR mirror tools in anatomy education. Students were divided into groups using traditional textbooks, tablet-based 3D visualizations, and screen-based AR interfaces. The exercise involved muscle identification and painting directly on a partner's skin based on the learning tool used. The study revealed that digital platforms outperformed traditional textbooks in learner engagement and perceived intuitiveness [55, 56].

However, technical hurdles such as alignment inaccuracies in AR overlays and hardware calibration difficulties can impede seamless learning experiences, especially with complex interactive interfaces like AR mirrors. These issues highlight the importance of user-centered design and iterative refinement based on learner feedback [55].

Interestingly, several studies have reported variations in how learners experience and benefit from VR-based education. Factors such as prior exposure to digital tools, comfort with immersive environments, and even gender have been shown to influence outcomes. The review noted gender differences in VR learning outcomes, though the underlying causes remain unclear. The authors did not identify a definitive explanation, suggesting that factors such as prior gaming experience, spatial ability, and technology familiarity might play a role. More studies are needed to explore these differences further. This variability underscores the importance of designing inclusive VR training environments that accommodate diverse learner needs [55, 57].

From an institutional perspective, the scalability of immersive technologies depends on overcoming financial constraints, technical infrastructure challenges, and faculty development needs. Training educators to integrate VR/AR meaningfully into teaching and assessment workflows is critical. Interdisciplinary collaboration among educators, technologists, and cognitive scientists can help create pedagogically sound and technically robust immersive modules. Additionally, establishing standardized frameworks to evaluate long-term educational and clinical impacts will support evidence-based expansion of these tools [55, 57].

Challenges, Barriers, and Future Directions

Despite substantial evidence supporting the educational benefits of VR and AR in medical education, their widespread adoption faces multiple challenges, from equity to financial, technical, and logistical barriers, highlighting the complex factors that influence the adoption of immersive technologies in medical education. Understanding these barriers is crucial for creating effective implementation strategies and guiding future innovations.

Technical limitations remain among the most significant obstacles to integration of VR and AR. Hardware constraints like limited processing power, display resolution, and battery life can reduce usability and learner comfort [55, 58]. Software challenges like compatibility, interoperability, and stable Internet can disrupt immersive experiences, especially in multi-user or cloud-based setting [18, 58].

Users may encounter cybersickness, like nausea or eye strain, which undermines engagement and learning [18, 59]. Beyond the user issues, integrating VR and AR with existing educational systems and clinical platforms is complex, adding to institutional demands.

The financial costs of implementing VR and AR are substantial even though their prices have been trending downward. There is a high initial investment required for the advanced hardware, haptic devices, and software on top of the ongoing expenses for updates, maintenance, and technical support [18, 52, 54, 60]. Many institutions lack the resources to deploy immersive technology at scale, limiting its accessibility. Cost-effectiveness data is limited, making it difficult for administrators to justify spending compared to conventional teaching methods.

Pedagogical barriers include lack of standardization, validated guidelines to assess AR- and VR-based learning [55, 60]. Many studies demonstrate different methodologies, small sample size, and risk bias which complicates interpreting results for long-term education outcomes [46, 55]. Additionally, content often lacks localization for different cultural or education contexts [6, 61]. Faculty must also design VR and AR experiences that align with their course objectives, requiring time and sometimes specialized training.

Human factors influence adoption and sustained engagement with immersive technologies. Educators as well as students may exhibit hesitancy due to the unfamiliarity regarding educational value of AR and VR [18, 59]. Beyond cost and infrastructure, ergonomic issues such as discomfort with head-mounted devices and concerns about distracting from patient-centered care can further complicate implementation. These practical barriers, though often overlooked, can affect user acceptance and long-term integration in both educational and clinical settings [57].

Disparities in access to VR and AR technology raise concerns of equity, especially in areas with limited resources [1, 61]. Without targeted strategies, the digital divide may exacerbate the inequalities in medical education already present, privileging learners in well-funded institutions. Addressing access requires low-cost hardware solutions, open-source content, and scalable training platforms to ensure inclusivity.

Future innovations aim to address these multifactorial challenges. Artificial intelligence (AI) can enable personalized adaptive learning, which can optimize cognitive load in individual learners. Multi-user cloud-based platforms expand collaborative training opportunities. Enhanced haptics promise more accurate tactile feedback, improving skill transfer to real-world clinical scenarios [55, 59]. Efforts toward global collaboration, content localization, and open-source development can mitigate equity and access issues. Continuous research is essential to establishing evidence-based best practices, optimize structural design, and evaluate long-term outcomes in medical education contexts.

Conclusion

The integration of VR and AR into medical education represents more than just a technological advancement. It reflects a shift toward learning environments that are immersive, adaptive, and learner-centered. VR and AR have demonstrated the ability to bridge the gap between theoretical knowledge and clinical proficiency, offering controlled opportunities to practice rare or high-stakes procedures, refine spatial reasoning, and develop psychomotor skills. These technologies are not inherently superior, but their strength lies in how they can complement traditional methods and be tailored to the learner's needs. The balance among immersion, cognitive load, and instructional design is imperative if this type of teaching is to be effective. Additionally, immersive training environments support teamwork and collaboration, allowing learners to work together on complex scenarios and practice coordinated decision-making skills, which is especially relevant in contexts like combat medic training.

Equally important is the recognition that technology alone does not guarantee educational impact. Large-scale feasibility studies and gender analyses highlight that adoption of AR and VR is shaped by usability, learner perception, and equitable access. Technical challenges intersect with human factors and institutional readiness reinforces the idea that successful implementation requires thoughtful planning and iterative design. When thought out, this technology can transform learning from anatomy to complex clinical scenarios like combat medic training.

Systematic reviews underscore that VR excels in procedural skill acquisition, while AR excels in spatial learning and decision support. The broader lesson is that these technologies work at their best as part of a cohesive curriculum rather than in isolation. As medical education evolves, there is an opportunity and responsibility to harness these tools in a way that is effective, accessible, and adaptive for all learners.

VR and AR are not merely alternatives to traditional training. They open new spaces where learners can test ideas, make mistakes without harm, and refine their craft in ways that once seemed out of reach. Immersion on its own is not enough. It must be coupled with thoughtful pedagogy and equitable access. If these elements come together, medical education can move toward a model of training that feels more authentic, more inclusive, and more closely attuned to the realities of patient care.

References

1. Arjomandi Rad A, Subbiah Ponniah H, Shah V, et al. Leading transformation in medical education through extended reality. Adv Exp Med Biol. 2023;1421:161–73. https://doi.org/10.1007/978-3-031-30379-1_7.

2. Taghian A, Abo-Zahhad M, Sayed MS, Abd El-Malek AH. Virtual and augmented reality in biomedical engineering. Biomed Eng Online. 2023;22:76. https://doi.org/10.1186/s12938-023-01138-3.
3. Petrakis A, Koumakis L, Kazantzaki E, Kondylakis H. Transforming healthcare: a comprehensive review of augmented and virtual reality interventions. Sensors (Basel). 2025;25(12):3748. https://doi.org/10.3390/s25123748.
4. Uruthiralingam U, Rea PM. Augmented and virtual reality in anatomy education. Adv Exp Med Biol. 2020;1235:89–101. https://doi.org/10.1007/978-3-030-37639-0_5.
5. Tene T, et al. Virtual reality and augmented reality in medical education: an umbrella review. Front Digit Health. 2024;6:1365345. https://doi.org/10.3389/fdgth.2024.1365345.
6. Chahartangi F, Zarifsanaiey N, Mehrabi M, Ghoochani BZ. Integrating augmented reality virtual patients into healthcare training: a scoping review of learning design and technical requirements. PLoS One. 2025;20(7):e0324740. https://doi.org/10.1371/journal.pone.0324740.
7. Iqbal AI, Aamir A, Hammad A, Hafsa H, Basit A, Oduoye MOO, Anis MW, Ahmed S, Younus MI, Jabeen S. Immersive technologies in healthcare: an in-depth exploration of virtual reality and augmented reality in enhancing patient care, medical education, and training paradigms. J Prim Care Community Health. 2024;15:21501319241293311. https://doi.org/10.1177/21501319241293311.
8. Young JQ, Van Merrienboer J, Durning S, Ten Cate O. Cognitive load theory: implications for medical education: AMEE Guide No. 86. Med Teach. 2014;36(5):371–84. https://doi.org/10.3109/0142159X.2014.889290.
9. Frederiksen JG, Sørensen SM, Konge L, Svendsen MB, Nobel-Jørgensen M, Bjerrum F, et al. Cognitive load and performance in immersive virtual reality versus conventional virtual reality simulation training of laparoscopic surgery: a randomized trial. Surg Endosc. 2020;34(3):1244–52. https://doi.org/10.1007/s00464-019-06887-8.
10. da Silva Soares R, Ramirez-Chavez KL, Tufanoglu A, et al. Cognitive effort during visuospatial problem solving in physical real world, on computer screen, and in virtual reality. Sensors (Basel). 2024;24(3):977. https://doi.org/10.3390/s24030977.
11. Andersen SAW, Konge L, Sørensen MS. The effect of distributed virtual reality simulation training on cognitive load during subsequent dissection training. Med Teach. 2018;40(7):684–9. https://doi.org/10.1080/0142159X.2018.1465182.
12. Andersen SA, Mikkelsen PT, Konge L, Cayé-Thomasen P, Sørensen MS. Cognitive load in distributed and massed practice in virtual reality mastoidectomy simulation. Laryngoscope. 2016;126(2):E74–9. https://doi.org/10.1002/lary.25449.
13. Kim HY, Kim EY. Effects of medical education program using virtual reality: a systematic review and meta-analysis. Int J Environ Res Public Health. 2023;20(5):3895. https://doi.org/10.3390/ijerph20053895.
14. Birbara NS, Pather N. Instructional design of virtual learning resources for anatomy education. Adv Exp Med Biol. 2021;1317:75–110. https://doi.org/10.1007/978-3-030-61125-5_5.
15. Aksoy M, Izzetoglu M, Baysoy E, Agrali A, Kitapcioglu D, Onaral B. Performance monitoring via functional near infrared spectroscopy for virtual reality based basic life support training. Front Neurosci. 2019;13:1336. https://doi.org/10.3389/fnins.2019.01336.
16. Zammit C, Calleja-Agius J, Azzopardi E. Augmented reality in anatomy education. Clin Anat. 2022;35(6):824–7. https://doi.org/10.1002/ca.23920.
17. Romand M, Dugas D, Gaudet-Blavignac C, Rochat J, Lovis C. Mixed and augmented reality tools in the medical anatomy curriculum. Stud Health Technol Inform. 2020;270:322–6. https://doi.org/10.3233/SHTI200175.
18. Lang M, Ghandour S, Rikard B, et al. Medical extended reality for radiology education and training. J Am Coll Radiol. 2024;21(10):1583–94. https://doi.org/10.1016/j.jacr.2024.05.006.
19. Olexa J, Cohen J, Alexander T, Brown C, Schwartzbauer G, Woodworth GF. Expanding educational frontiers in neurosurgery: current and future uses of augmented reality. Neurosurgery. 2023;92(2):241–50. https://doi.org/10.1227/neu.0000000000002199.

20. Barsom EZ, Graafland M, Schijven MP. Systematic review on the effectiveness of augmented reality applications in medical training. Surg Endosc. 2016;30(10):4174–83. https://doi.org/10.1007/s00464-016-4800-6.
21. Xiong J, Dai X, Zhang Y, Liu X, Zhou X. Augmented reality for basic skills training in laparoscopic surgery: a systematic review and meta-analysis. Surg Endosc. 2025;39(1):307–18. https://doi.org/10.1007/s00464-024-11387-5.
22. Celdrán FJ, Jiménez-Ruescas J, Lobato C, Salazar L, Sánchez-Margallo JA, Sánchez-Margallo FM, González P. Use of augmented reality for training assistance in laparoscopic surgery: scoping literature review. J Med Internet Res. 2025;27:e58108. https://doi.org/10.2196/58108.
23. Wolf J, Wolfer V, Halbe M, Maisano F, Lohmeyer Q, Meboldt M. Comparing the effectiveness of augmented reality–based and conventional instructions during single ECMO cannulation training. Int J Comput Assist Radiol Surg. 2021;16(7):1171–80. https://doi.org/10.1007/s11548-021-02408-y.
24. Levin MF, Weiss PL, Keshner EA. Emergence of VR in physical therapy. Phys Ther. 2015;95(3):415–25. https://doi.org/10.2522/ptj.20130579.
25. Bell J, Decker B, Eichmann A, Palkovich C, Reji C. Effectiveness of virtual reality for upper extremity function and motor performance of children with cerebral palsy: a systematic review. Am J Occup Ther. 2024;78(2):7802180180. https://doi.org/10.5014/ajot.2024.050374.
26. Levac DE, Huber ME, Sternad D. Learning and transfer of complex motor skills in virtual reality: a perspective review. J Neuroeng Rehabil. 2019;16(1):121. https://doi.org/10.1186/s12984-019-0587-8.
27. Wankhede NL, Koppula S, Ballal S, Doshi H, Kumawat R, Raju SS, et al. Virtual reality modulating dynamics of neuroplasticity: innovations in neuro-motor rehabilitation. Neuroscience. 2025;566:97–111. https://doi.org/10.1016/j.neuroscience.2024.12.040.
28. Capriotti A, Moret S, Del Bello E, Federici A, Lucertini F. Virtual reality: a new frontier of physical rehabilitation. Sensors (Basel). 2025;25(10):3080. https://doi.org/10.3390/s25103080.
29. Darekar A. Virtual reality for motor and cognitive rehabilitation. Curr Top Behav Neurosci. 2023;65:337–69. https://doi.org/10.1007/7854_2023_418.
30. Markwell LT, Cochran K, Porter JM. Off the shelf: investigating transfer of learning using commercially available virtual reality equipment. PLoS One. 2023;18(10):e0279856. https://doi.org/10.1371/journal.pone.0279856.
31. Clarke E. Virtual reality simulation—the future of orthopaedic training? A systematic review and narrative analysis. Adv Simul (Lond). 2021;6:2. https://doi.org/10.1186/s41077-020-00153-x.
32. Lohre R, Bois AJ, Pollock JW, Lapner P, McIlquham K, Athwal GS, Goel DP. Effectiveness of immersive virtual reality on orthopedic surgical skills and knowledge acquisition among senior surgical residents: a randomized clinical trial. JAMA Netw Open. 2020;3(12):e2031217. https://doi.org/10.1001/jamanetworkopen.2020.31217.
33. Choi KS, Chan SH, Pang WM. Virtual suturing simulation based on commodity physics engine for medical learning. J Med Syst. 2012;36(3):1781–93. https://doi.org/10.1007/s10916-010-9638-1.
34. Haar S, Sundar G, Faisal AA. Embodied virtual reality for the study of real-world motor learning. PLoS One. 2021;16(1):e0245717. https://doi.org/10.1371/journal.pone.0245717. PMID: 33503022; PMCID: PMC7840008.
35. Chang Y-H, Chang H-S, Li H-P, Chen H-C. Effects of collaborative training using virtual co-embodiment on motor skill learning. IEEE Trans Vis Comput Graph. 2023;29(5):2345–56. https://doi.org/10.1109/TVCG.2023.3238924.
36. Gao K, Wiederhold BK, Kong L, Wiederhold MD. Methodology case study of haptics in combat medic training. Stud Health Technol Inform. 2013;191:53–7.
37. Kumar A, Saudagar AKJ, Kumar A, Alkhrijah YM, Raja L. Innovating medical education using scalable VR with AI-driven haptics. Sci Rep. 2025;15(1):26360. https://doi.org/10.1038/s41598-025-10543-8.

38. Bukoski A, Uhlich R, Bowling F, Shapiro M, Kerby JD, Llerena L, Armstrong JH, Strayhorn C, Barnes SL. Perceptions of simulator- and live tissue-based combat casualty care training of senior special operations medics. Mil Med. 2018;183(suppl_1):78–85. https://doi.org/10.1093/milmed/usx136.
39. Bailey SKT, Brannick MT, Bowling F, et al. Comparing simulation modalities for combat casualty care training. Mil Med. 2024;189(7–8):e1738–44. https://doi.org/10.1093/milmed/usad460.
40. Katz D, Shah R, Kim E, Park C, Shah A, Levine A, Burnett G. Utilization of a voice-based virtual reality advanced cardiac life support team leader refresher: prospective observational study. J Med Internet Res. 2020;22(3):e17425. https://doi.org/10.2196/17425.
41. Otero-Varela L, Cintora-Sanz AM, Espinosa S, Redondo M, Uzuriaga M, González M, García M, Naldrett J, Alonso J, Vazquez T, Blanco A, Cardós-Alonso MDC. Extended reality as a training method for medical first responders in mass casualty incidents: a protocol for a systematic review. PLoS One. 2023;18(3):e0282698. https://doi.org/10.1371/journal.pone.0282698.
42. Einloft J, Meyer HL, Bedenbender S, Morgenschweis ML, Ganser A, Russ PG, Hirsch MC, Grgic I. Immersive medical training: a comprehensive longitudinal study of extended reality in emergency scenarios for large student groups. BMC Med Educ. 2024;24(1):978. https://doi.org/10.1186/s12909-024-05957-3.
43. Zhang N, Ye G, Yang C, Zeng P, Gong T, Tao L, Zheng Y, Liu Y. Benefits of virtual reality training for cardiopulmonary resuscitation skill acquisition and maintenance. Prehosp Emerg Care. 2024:1–7. https://doi.org/10.1080/10903127.2024.2416971.
44. Cheng A, Magid DJ, Auerbach M, Bhanji F, Bigham BL, Blewer AL, Dainty KN, Diederich E, Lin Y, Leary M, Mahgoub M, Mancini ME, Navarro K, Donoghue A. Part 6: resuscitation education science: 2020 American Heart Association guidelines for cardiopulmonary resuscitation and emergency cardiovascular care. Circulation. 2020;142(16_suppl_2):S551–79. https://doi.org/10.1161/CIR.0000000000000903.
45. Trevi R, Chiappinotto S, Palese A, Galazzi A. Virtual reality for cardiopulmonary resuscitation healthcare professionals training: a systematic review. J Med Syst. 2024;48(1):50. https://doi.org/10.1007/s10916-024-02063-1.
46. Kyaw BM, Saxena N, Posadzki P, et al. Virtual reality for health professions education: systematic review and meta-analysis by the Digital Health Education Collaboration. J Med Internet Res. 2019;21(1):e12959. https://doi.org/10.2196/12959.
47. Li T, Yan J, Gao X, et al. Using virtual reality to enhance surgical skills and engagement in orthopedic education: systematic review and meta-analysis. J Med Internet Res. 2025;27:e70266. https://doi.org/10.2196/70266.
48. Co M, Chiu S, Cheung H. Extended reality in surgical education: a systematic review. Surgery. 2023;174(5):1175–83. https://doi.org/10.1016/j.surg.2023.07.015.
49. Ryan GV, Callaghan S, Rafferty A, Higgins MF, Mangina E, McAuliffe F. Learning outcomes of immersive technologies in health care student education: systematic review of the literature. J Med Internet Res. 2022;24(2):e30082. https://doi.org/10.2196/30082.
50. Liu JYW, Yin YH, Kor PPK, Cheung DSK, Zhao IY, Wang S, Su JJ, Christensen M, Tyrovolas S, Leung AYM. The effects of immersive virtual reality applications on enhancing the learning outcomes of undergraduate health care students: systematic review with meta-synthesis. J Med Internet Res. 2023;25:e39989. https://doi.org/10.2196/39989.
51. Bölek KA, De Jong G, Henssen D. The effectiveness of the use of augmented reality in anatomy education: a systematic review and meta-analysis. Sci Rep. 2021;11(1):15292. https://doi.org/10.1038/s41598-021-94721-4.
52. García-Robles P, Cortés-Pérez I, Nieto-Escámez FA, García-López H, Obrero-Gaitán E, Osuna-Pérez MC. Immersive virtual reality and augmented reality in anatomy education: a systematic review and meta-analysis. Anat Sci Educ. 2024;17(3):514–28. https://doi.org/10.1002/ase.2397.
53. Rodríguez-Abad C, Fernández-de-la-Iglesia JD, Martínez-Santos AE, Rodríguez-González R. A systematic review of augmented reality in health sciences: a guide to decision-making in

higher education. Int J Environ Res Public Health. 2021;18(8):4262. https://doi.org/10.3390/ijerph18084262.

54. Moro C, Birt J, Stromberga Z, Phelps C, Clark J, Glasziou P, Scott AM. Virtual and augmented reality enhancements to medical and science student physiology and anatomy test performance: a systematic review and meta-analysis. Anat Sci Educ. 2021;14(3):368–76. https://doi.org/10.1002/ase.2049.
55. Mergen M, Meyerheim M, Graf N. Reviewing the current state of virtual reality integration in medical education – a scoping review. BMC Med Educ. 2024;24(1):788. https://doi.org/10.1186/s12909-024-05777-5.
56. Einloft J, Bedenbender S, Michelsen M, Meyer HL, Russ PG, Heidtmann A, Hirsch MC, Grgic I. Structured exposure achieves high acceptance of immersive technology among medical students and educators. Cyberpsychol Behav Soc Netw. 2024;27(6):363–71. https://doi.org/10.1089/cyber.2023.0297.
57. Mahling M, Wunderlich R, Steiner D, Gorgati E, Festl-Wietek T, Herrmann-Werner A. Virtual reality for emergency medicine training in medical school: prospective, large-cohort implementation study. J Med Internet Res. 2023;25:e43649. https://doi.org/10.2196/43649.
58. Jung C, Wolff G, Wernly B, Bruno RR, Franz M, Schulze PC, et al. Virtual and augmented reality in cardiovascular care: state-of-the-art and future perspectives. JACC Cardiovasc Imaging. 2022;15(3):519–32. https://doi.org/10.1016/j.jcmg.2021.08.017.
59. Bruno RR, Wolff G, Wernly B, Masyuk M, Piayda K, Leaver S, et al. Virtual and augmented reality in critical care medicine: the patient's, clinician's, and researcher's perspective. Crit Care. 2022;26(1):326. https://doi.org/10.1186/s13054-022-04202-x.
60. Williams A, Sun Z, Vaccarezza M. Comparison of augmented reality with other teaching methods in learning anatomy: a systematic review. Clin Anat. 2025;38(2):168–85. https://doi.org/10.1002/ca.24234.
61. Mondal H, Mondal S. Adopting augmented reality and virtual reality in medical education in resource-limited settings: constraints and the way forward. Adv Physiol Educ. 2025;49(2):503–7. https://doi.org/10.1152/advan.00027.2025.

Education-Centered Medical Home

Kayla Johnson and Roger W. Apple

Medical Home

Although the concept of the medical home has evolved over the course of several decades, the goal to improve patient care remains unchanged. The medical home was introduced by the American Academy of Pediatrics (AAP) to address a barrier to effective health supervision for children with chronic disease or serious illness [1]. A centralized source of pediatric records, a medical home, was proposed to decrease record duplication and gaps in services due to a lack of communication and care coordination among various medical providers. In the late 1970s, the AAP policy statement referred to the medical home as a method to ensure continuity of care in which medical data for a child was stored together and accessible to physicians [1].

Subsequently, the medical home in primary care began to focus on the needs of the child and family in relation to their familial and environmental context. The medical home was conceptualized as a family-centered, community-based, comprehensive model that coordinated care and utilized community resources [1]. A training manual that included interdisciplinary collaboration and collaboration between pediatricians and families was created to address barriers to implementation of the medical home. In 1992, the AAP defined the medical home as "accessible, continuous, comprehensive, family-centered, coordinated, and compassionate" care directed by a physician familiar to the patient and the family [1 , p. 1475]. Medical schools with pediatric residency programs began to use the medical home as the foundation for training in community pediatrics. The medical home concept developed from a centralized source of medical records to a method of interdisciplinary

K. Johnson · R. W. Apple (✉)
Western Michigan University Homer Stryker M.D School of Medicine, Kalamazoo, MI, USA
e-mail: Kayla.Johnson@wmed.edu; Roger.Apple@wmed.edu

S. S. Chahin et al. (eds.), *Innovation in Medical Education and Clinical Practice*, https://doi.org/10.1007/978-3-032-19116-8_10

care that focuses on the patient, utilizes the community, and enhances the quality of patient care.

Research evidence demonstrates the effectiveness of a medical home on patient care. Primary care orientation is associated with lower costs for health services and better health outcomes [2]. Research also suggests that better primary care reduces racial disparities and improves health care for other disadvantaged populations. Improvements in health care as a result of the medical home in primary care are as follows [2]:

- Better recognition of problems/needs
- More accurate and timely diagnosis
- More consistent appointment keeping and treatment advice
- Fewer emergency department visits
- Fewer hospitalizations
- Lower health care costs
- Better prevention
- Better monitoring
- Fewer drug prescriptions
- Fewer unmet needs
- Increased satisfaction

The advanced medical home model was proposed by the American College of Physicians [3] in the year 2006 to address the issues in the health care system in the United States. Developed from the original model, the advanced medical home aimed to provide patient-centered, economical, longitudinal care guided by a primary care physician on a team of health care professionals [3]. Components of the advanced model include (1) individualized care with the use of evidence-based medicine and clinical decision support tools at the point of care, (2) implementation of the Chronic Care Model for patients with and without chronic health problems (the Care Model), (3) a plan for medical care developed by the patient and their families, (4) health care provided in person and out of the office with various methods of communication, (5) quality indicators to monitor health status improvements, (6) the implementation of confidential health information technology, (7) and programs that offer feedback and guidance on the practice and physician. The ACP recommended that the advanced medical home be implemented into medical education and training to better prepare primary care physicians for practice. Medical school training in ambulatory settings for fourth year medical students would be designed with a patient-centered and service-oriented approach that informs patient care [3]. Inpatient and outpatient care is often provided from a multidisciplinary team of nurses, social workers, care managers, dietitians, physical and occupational therapists, speech pathologists, psychologists, and other health care professionals. The advanced medical home teaches the importance of cohesive collaboration on a health care team and led to the development of the patient-centered medical home.

Patient-Centered Medical Home

The patient-centered medical home (PCMH) was developed in the year 2007 as a model of primary care across all age groups. The PCMH is defined as a team that is meaningfully involved with the local community to improve the health of community members [4]. Access to primary care, continuity or comprehensive patient care over time, reimbursement reform, and practice innovations are components of the PCMH [5]. The reimbursement system is the way in which the medical home is incentivized to physicians and patients [3, 4]. Physicians receive reimbursement from system-based care while patients receive the benefits of patient-centered care. Practice innovations such as enhanced access, team-based care, population management, care coordination, care management, systems-based approach to quality, and health information are the tools utilized to help reach the goals of the model [5]. Enhanced access in primary care involves open scheduling, expanded office hours in addition to the ability to reach an on-call provider 24/7, and communication with the patient through patient portals. Team-based care consists of multi-disciplinary teams in which medical assistants, social workers, and other health care related professionals have a prominent role in patient care and quality improvement. Population management is the identification of patients that have care gaps with electronic patient registries. Care coordination involves referral management, transition care, and relationships between different care providers. Care management includes assessment, care planning, support of patient self-management, evidence-based practice protocols, and medication management. A system-based approach to quality and safety is one in which a leadership team facilitates quality improvement with performance measurements and patient feedback. Finally, health information technology consists of electronic medical records, provider order entry on the computer, and quality measurement and reporting tools. To guide desired outcomes such as practice innovations, the seven joint principles of the PCMH were developed by a group of national medical associations (Table 1). Both PCMH and inspired models such as The Family Health Team in Ontario follow the principles closely [6] The PCMH is defined by the joint principals and practice innovations that contribute to effective patient-centeredness in primary care.

Outcomes from several programs that implemented the PCMH provide support for the positive impact of the various components such as enhanced access, continuity of care, chronic disease management, other quality outcomes, and patient satisfaction [5, 7]. One randomized control study investigated the quality and efficiency of small medical practices that transitioned to the PCMH [8]. Over the course of 2 years, physicians in the intervention condition, a new PCMH, achieved a larger increase in hypertension blood pressure control and breast cancer screenings compared to the control. Additionally, each physician in the intervention condition reduced the amount of patient visits to the emergency department in comparison to an increase of visits for physicians in the control. A reduction in emergency department visits and hospital admissions is characteristic of many PCMH models [7]. Systematic reviews suggest moderately strong evidence for improved patient

Table 1 Joint principles of the patient-centered medical home

Personal physician	A physician who provides first contact, continuous, and comprehensive care during an ongoing relationship for each patient
Physician-directed medical practice	The personal physician leads a team of health care and health-care-related professionals who take responsibility for the ongoing care of patients.
Whole person orientation	The personal physician provides care for the health-care needs of the patients and with other professionals arranges acute care, chronic care, end-of-life care, and preventative services.
Care is coordinated and/or integrated	Across all elements of the complex health care system of community of the patient, registries, information technology, health information exchange, and other modalities assure that patients receive the indicated care when, where, and how they would like in a culturally and linguistically appropriate manner.
Quality and safety	Continuous quality improvement is managed with performance measurement and improvement, client feedback, patient and family participation in quality improvement activities, information technology, and the use of evidence-based medicine and clinical decision support tools to enhance patient-centered outcomes demonstrated by a voluntary recognition process.
Enhanced access	More availability to care through open scheduling, expanded hours, and new options communication options for patients, their personal physical, and practice staff.
Payment	A framework in which the payment structure adds value to patients within a patient-centered medical home and to the work of the physician.

Adapted from the American College of Physicians [6]

experiences, preventative care, health care outcomes and patient satisfaction for low-income patients, and reduction in health care disparities across process and outcome measures [9–11]. The successful integration of the PCMH into medical practice is not the only way in which the model has been incorporated.

Medical schools integrate the PCMH into their curriculum to provide education that informs clinical skills and practice. A system named Care by Design (CBD) at the University of Utah Community Clinics implemented components of the PCMH such as advanced access, care teams with a physician and medical assistants (MAs), and planned care [12]. During the first year of medical school, students worked as MAs in the clinics in preparation for clinical clerkships in the M-3 year and a primary care track in the M-4 year. Within CBD, primary care residents participated in continuity clinics in outpatient practices. Residents and faculty also worked on quality improvement (QI) projects. The Family Medicine Center (FMC) at the University of Southern California provided clinical services in the context of a PCMH [12]. Resident training included activities to improve client care, quality metrics, and QI projects. Similarly, third year medical students at the Eastern Virgina Medical School participated in a simulated PCMH [13]. Students felt more prepared to collaborate with the patient, effectively address the emotional concerns of a patient, implement feedback from the doctor and behavior faculty, and desired to improve communication with the patient. The PCMH design demonstrates the benefit of a patient-centered approach for medical school students in preparation for clinical practice. Despite implementation of the PCMH in medical school curriculum, a new curricular medical home model was developed to enhance student exposure and experience with a longitudinal integrated clerkship.

Longitudinal Clerkship

A longitudinal integrated clerkship (LIC) is an approach in medical education to improve learning and patient experiences over a period of time much longer than traditional block rotations. LICs are characterized by longitudinal relationships with patients, preceptors, the clinical setting, and integrated multidisciplinary opportunities over the course of 6–12 months [14]. There are several advantages to a LIC in primary care. Students are able to further understand the patient experience, provide patient care, and care coordination. Continual exposure to core content across multiple disciplines enhances learning because students encounter the same clinical problems repeatedly. As a result, LIC students meet most core clinical competencies for their year and reach peak knowledge across multiple disciplines by the end of the year [15]. Longitudinal placement allows students to acclimate to the clinical setting and focus on content and clinical skills rather than adapt to new settings and disciplines [14]. Students also have more time to understand health issues in the social context of the patients and provide follow up with the patient and their families. Follow ups are a component of continuity of care in which medical students have a continuous relationship with the patient and manages care for the duration of the health problem [16]. Other aspects of continuity in LICs are of supervision, curriculum, idealism, peers, and systems. Continuity also includes the relationship between the preceptor and student. In fact, another aspect of LICs that contribute to learning is how students interact with faculty. Students can observe the professional behavior and values modeled by faculty mentors throughout the clerkship and receive feedback that promotes personal and professional development [14, 15]. Evidence from measures on patient-centeredness and traditional assessments suggest that students in LICs are more patient-centered and perform equally to their non-LIC peers [14]. To foster continuity and patient-centered care, a blended model of the LIC structure and PCMH developed into the Education-Centered Medical Home in 2011.

Education-Centered Medical Home

The education-centered medical home (ECMH) is a LIC based on the PCMH for medical students of all years. The curriculum consists of five PCMH principles that correspond to PCMH and ECMH learning and continuity objectives (Table 2) [17]. A LIC design allows for continuity among patients, peers, and preceptors which can positively influence development of core competencies, relationships between

Table 2 PCMH principles that correspond to PCMH/ECMH learning and continuity objectives [17]

Integrated PCMH principles	PCMH/ECMH learning objectives	PCMH/ECMH continuity objective
Continuity with a personal physician	Achieve continuity of care	I look forward to going to my ECMH clinic
Team-based care	Manage a patient panel	I feel ownership for my ECMH patients
Care coordination and integration	Provide care for "high-risk" patients	I am achieving continuity with my ECMH patients
Quality and safety	Educate patients on self-care	I am enjoying having continuity with my ECMH patients
Enhanced access	Track and coordinate care	Continuity has affected my perspective on patient care
	Measure health outcomes; improve performances	I am able to balance my classwork with my ECMH responsibilities

students and patients, professional development, understanding of the relationship between the social context and health, care fragmentation, and chronic disease management [17]. The PCMH is not longitudinal and can contribute to gaps in continuity. Discontinuity in medical education is attributed to alternating training blocks in ambulatory structures, misaligned schedules between students and preceptors, and short-term relationships between students, preceptors, and patients [18]. A lack of continuity can negatively affect multiple areas of medical practice such as clinical skills, patient-centeredness, quality improvement, adequate feedback for learners, and teamwork. To achieve continuity in medical education, Henschen and colleagues created the ECMH, a longitudinal model, to increase student awareness and knowledge of the PCMH curricular model [17].

At the Northwestern University Feinberg School of Medicine, ECMH clinics with a faculty preceptor and the curriculum were developed with three educational objectives [17]. One, increase continuity experiences with patients, preceptors, and peers within a LIC. Two, exemplify patient-centered care principles with effective coordinated care for complex clients, education for self-care, and overall improved quality of clinical care. Three, position students to approach care as health coaches and coordinators. Students also attended ECMH Grand Rounds to discuss topics related to PCMH principles [17]. The longitudinal ECMH curriculum consists of various roles and responsibilities for preceptors and students alike.

Educational Design

The ECMH is designed to span the course of all 4 years of medical school curriculum. During the 4 years, students develop clinical skills, provide preventative care, active management of acute and chronic disease management, and implement health systems science [19–21]. Students experience interprofessional collaboration facilitated by the ECMH as a member of a team of professionals from multiple different disciplines that coordinate care [22, 23]. ECMH curriculum consists of a team of 16 students with an equal number of students from each year [20]. M1/M2 students are paired with M3/M4 students and jointly see patients under the supervision of a preceptor who approves management and clinical decisions [17]. The students are assigned to one preceptor in the EMCH clinic with whom they foster a longitudinal relationship. On the contrary, an individual preceptorship (IP) from the traditional medical education curriculum spans 2 years. IP M2 students individually meet with an attending biweekly while M3 students participate in a primary care outpatient clerkship for 4 weeks with a different attending [20]. In the ECMH, students and faculty jointly develop a continuity panel with patients considered medically or socially complex, high-risk, or patients without a primary care provider [17]. These patients may require three or more office visits per year, hospitalization, have one or multiple chronic conditions, or are at risk of deterioration [20]. In fact, some preceptors may specifically assign students to challenging patients, individuals whose physical concerns are accompanied with mental health or emotional problems [24]. Students indicate that working with challenging clients helps them grow as physicians. IP students see the panel of patients assigned to the preceptor [25]. Clinic expectations for both clerkships are different as ECMH students are encouraged to discuss health maintenance topics with patients and implement motivational interviewing in office and over the phone. IP students are only encouraged to discuss health maintenance topics during clinic. Over the course of ECMH curriculum, students interact closely with the preceptor, patients, and other students.

Students work together and provide feedback to one another and receive informal and formal feedback from the preceptor. Informal reflection with their preceptor about challenging patients or situations also commonly occurs [24]. Students take the time to make meaning of reactions to certain experiences in the clinic and discuss actions to take in the future if something similar arises. The ability to reflect is an important trait for professional competence and indicative of transformative learning. Comfortability with sharing thoughts and feelings with a preceptor and receiving feedback from peers may be the result of longitudinal relationships.

In the ECMH, 6–8 students attend clinic per week and work in pairs under the supervision of a preceptor, whereas one student attends clinic in the IP and only receives clinical feedback from the preceptor. Both ECMH preceptors and M3/M4 students teach and provide feedback [25]. During clinic, preceptors provide feedback on clinical skills and medical decision making [25]. Preceptors also complete yearly evaluations twice per year for ECMH students over the course of the 4 years of medical school. Similarly, IP or additional preceptors complete twice yearly evaluations. The more experienced students serve as peer and team educators and in the moment provide evidence-based answers to clinical questions posed by their junior partner [17, 26]. ECMH students believe that the expectation of the model is to teach other students at every patient encounter [27]. M3 and M4 level students often provide advice and feedback about medical knowledge, clinical skills, and how to achieve success in medical school. Students that transition from M2 to M3 also feel a responsibility to act as a clinical role model and provide positive peer learning experiences for less experienced students. The more senior students also receive education, feedback, and recommendations from one another [26]. ECMH students are provided stable mentorship from peers on the basis of clinic work. Mentors in medical education teach students how to provide care for patients with complex psychosocial needs and prepare them for life as a physician [22]. Due to the nature of the EMCH clerkship, students have multi-year engagement with consistent faculty and peers and a longitudinal relationship with a panel of patients.

Continuity is a component of the patient–physician relationship. Beyond peer education duties, ECMH M3 and M4 students assume the role of outreach manager and contact patients to discuss laboratory or radiology studies, consultations, and clinical status [17, 26]. Clients that establish care within the EMCH are called to gauge clinical progress, follow-up on any issues and receive help with appointments, scheduling overdue appointments or tests, and meeting with specialists [15, 25]. All telephone calls are documented in the medical record and new medical content is discussed with the preceptor. As the outreach manager within an ECMH, students monitor quality metrics. Students use the QI curriculum within the ECMH to monitor clinic performance and improve quality of care when necessary [22]. Students in an ECMH are able to track core quality of care metrics and manage QI projects for the continuity panel [25]. IP students are not able to track QI metrics because of an inconsistent patient panel. Steps taken toward continuity such as follow-up and QI are unique to the ECMH compared to the IP. There are, however, similarities between both clerkship models.

Similarities of the models are evident for the characteristics of the curriculum. M1/M2 curriculum for both models consists of 30 biweekly site visits that alternate with standardized clinical skills workshops [25]. Attendance at the ECMH clinic biweekly is expected and each ECMH session starts with a team huddle focused on patient care issues and educational goals. Additionally, students in both clerkships in the M3/M4 attend 26 site visits and complete didactics, OSCE, and the NBME primary care shelf exam. ECMH students schedule the site visits during other clerkships whereas the IP site visits occur during a 1-month PCC rotation with multiple different preceptors.

Integration of the ECMH with core features of the PCMH not only contribute to continuity but values-based care. The features include access, care coordination, QI, and population health. Patients in the ECMH clerkship had more phone contact, exchanges through the patient portal, and clinic visits with students [20]. Students also indicated that they connected patients with services and coordinated care for concerns beyond the purpose of the visit [26]. O'Neil and colleagues measured quality improvement with an ECMH "Quality Scorecard" with measures related to chronic disease management and adult and pediatric preventive care measures [28]. Prior to implementation, students also received didactic and training modules for QI skills. ECMH clinics used the scorecards to review performance and strategize how to immediately implement clinical improvement. Performance on quality measures that compared to pre-ECMH baselines were improved according to the increased number of exams, screening rates, medical attention to diabetic nephropathy, and use of steroids for asthma [28]. Population health is evident with consideration of social and financial factors in patient care and patient information continuity in which students attempted to understand the patient from the context of the community [24, 29]. Patient-centeredness in the ECMH model allows for values-based care as students recognize the values of the patient, considers patient preferences in medical decisions, and prioritizes how the patient perceives an illness [29]. The purpose of the ECMH is to prepare students for real-world clinical practice in which the PCMH principles and value-based care will be demonstrated.

Outcomes and Evidence for Success of the ECMH

The ECMH has an impact on learning competence and satisfaction with knowledge, skills, identity formation, and professionalism. Students who participate in an ECMH feel more confident in regard to learning and continuity objectives [17]. Patient-centered communication skills, diagnostic assessment, and treatment management planning among other skills grow with experiences of continuity with patients [20, 24, 26]. ECMH students demonstrate increased professional and primary care self-efficacy as a result of active clinical roles and training experiences [20, 25]. Students feel like a member of the clinical team rather than an observer and engage more with the learning environment [26]. This contributes to high satisfaction with primary care experiences and the ECMH learning environment [20, 25]. For this reason, a very high percentage of ECMH students recommend the curriculum to incoming medical students [20, 25]. ECMH students are also more likely to show interest in a primary care career [25]. Satisfaction with the outcomes of the ECMH model are related to efficacy of the model itself.

Patient-centered and team-based care contributes to the efficacy of ECMH objectives. Students have high patient-centered attitudes, establish more patient relationships, and active involvement in patient care compared to IP students [20, 25]. Because of the longitudinal nature of the ECMH, more meaningful relationships are developed among students and primary care patients [20]. Students appear to have a sense of responsibility for patients and take on the role of a care manager to provide counseling and coordinate follow-up [26]. Care is approached from the biopsychosocial perspective in which primary care is oriented around the patient and their lives, rather than the presenting concern [21]. Therefore, the ECMH primary care clinic is perceived as more patient-centered and effective compared to the traditional curriculum in primary care [20]. Not only do students report that they achieve continuity of care with patients, but preceptors also agree that students achieve continuity and enjoy the curriculum [17, 20]. Team-centered approaches to care consist of peer and preceptor interactions. ECMH students report greater peer and preceptor support on patient-centered tasks [25]. Students also feel better prepared for team-based, collaborative, and patient-centered settings. A benefit of patient-centered and team-based care in the ECMH are improved patient-level outcomes.

Patient-level outcomes include quality of care and continuity of care metrics. ECMH clinics provide students the opportunity to have their own experiences with providing care to patients over time. Longitudinal relationships with continuity patients develop and allow students to get to know the patient better and advocate for patient care [21, 26]. To improve the quality of care, ECMH students use clinical quality metrics and implementation of quality improvement principles [20, 21]. An effect of quality of care on patient level outcomes is an increase of patient engagement in the clinic and the ability to see patients for follow-up visits more frequently [20]. Other examples of patient outcomes that increase with the ECMH are cancer screenings and administration of the influenza vaccine. Continuity of care metrics indicate that the role of health coach taken on by students can increase chronic disease management [20]. Rewarding relationships with patients and satisfactory patient level outcomes can lead students to career in primary care and implement QI in the ECMH.

The ECMH consists of workforce pipeline development and QI engagement. Longitudinal experiences within the ECMH may encourage students to pursue a career in primary care and primary care specialties [21]. Because of costs associated with student education in ambulatory settings, some medical programs do not provide students the opportunity for LICs. However, medical students could perform the roles of community health care workers and other clinic employees that are solicited for hire if the students themselves follow up with clients and perform care management services [30]. The ECMH can prepare students for continuity management roles in primary care and decrease costs for clinical practices or ambulatory settings. Other strategies that contribute to cost effectiveness of the ECMH in medical schools, clinics, and practices, is management and assessment of quality metrics, community engagement, and ECMH learning objectives for quality improvement [30]. Indeed, almost 70% of students agree or strongly agree that reviewal of quality of care for patients is valuable [28]. Almost 80% agree that future implementation of ECMH quality metrics will be valuable. Medical students in one ECMH reviewed quality metrics which led to a QI project for improvement of type 2 diabetes mellitus (T2DM) [31]. Students were educated on the quality metrics through a project summary then conducted audits on patients with T2DM. Based on the information from the audit, continuity personalized care plans were created to schedule patients, plan tests at upcoming visits, and follow up on medication adherence and care plans. The results of the QI project indicate that adherence to the annual diabetic eye exam increased and patients had a clinically significant decrease among several clinical indicators [31]. Inclusion of medical students in ECMH clinics to practice continuity and quality engagement may lead to a career in primary care and even reduce the workload of preceptors.

Preceptors in ECMH clinics have the ability to manage the workload alongside other professional responsibilities. Traditionally, medical programs have difficulty with the recruitment and retention of clinical faculty and training them in competency-based assessment [23]. Some clinics do not have the number of faculty preceptors necessary to manage ambulatory learning. Available ambulatory faculty are often preoccupied with other interests and the addition of a care home such as the ECMH may contribute to an additional workload and stress. A solution to this dilemma is LICs such as the ECMH, in which students are integrated into residency clinics [23]. Not only is one preceptor assigned to a team of students, but the students also provide teaching and mentoring to each other. The preceptors and students also share the same panel of patients which can help offset the additional amount of time preceptors need to supervise ECMH students. In fact, three of four preceptors in an ECMH program agreed that they could balance the ECMH alongside other professional responsibilities and indicated desire to continue with the ECMH clinics [19, 20].

Challenges and Lessons Learned

Location is one barrier to implementation of a LIC or the ECMH. LICs that are established in rural areas may require placement in remote locations that may negatively impact the mental health of the students [32]. However, students may have the opportunity to make more connections within a tight knight community. Rural communities appear to adapt well to LICs because local leaders and officials understand the value of health-related outcomes for the community and the benefit of LICS for the local economy and community members [33].

Additionally, LIC family medicine preceptors in rural areas report the development of trusting relations with students, person-centered teaching opportunities, and learning goals related to student career goals [19]. LICs are historically implemented in rural, underserved areas but should not be restricted to rural regions [33]. LICs are adaptable in urban areas and have been implemented in larger, urban locations, and teaching hospitals. A downside is that urban areas are more at risk of higher turnover of health care staff which can disrupt continuity among students and preceptors [32]. While this may be true, preceptors in an urban LIC feel responsible for student learning and appreciate student growth. Despite the history of LICs in rural areas, much of the current research on the ECMH takes place at larger more urban institutions. This research demonstrates community engagement and continuity between students and preceptors [20, 24, 26]. The ECMH can be adaptable across urban and rural locations as well as large and small institutions.

Other barriers include institutional buy-in, faculty bandwidth, and scheduling constraints. The traditional curriculum of block training is familiar to physicians and perhaps considered the best approach to clinical training by some [33]. Therefore, buy-in from faculty, academics, health services and regulators, patients, and students may be difficult when a change is proposed in a medical program. Associated costs and funding of a LIC compared to block rotations are often a concern of stakeholders. Programs may fear that removal of blocks may result in knowledge gaps and may be more difficult to administer [18, 19]. Plus, some organizations may not understand the purpose of a LIC or lack experience training students with continuity or other aspects of a longitudinal care [32]. The barrier is that faculty will also need to undergo training and new faculty at some locations may be necessary. Preceptors and administration must also dedicate more time to implement, organize, and manage a LIC. Clinic related barriers such as preceptors not being readily available in the clinic or too busy while in the clinic interferes with the ability to see the patients of students [34]. Scheduling is another clinic barrier in which residents and attendings cannot coordinate schedules and schedulers may be unaware of coverage arrangements. Guidelines on how to establish and maintain a sustainable LIC such as focus on building relationships, clearly articulate and manage learning outcomes and expectations promote communities of practice, and ensure good initial and ongoing faculty development, minimization of preceptor workload, and strong institutional leadership among others can help address barriers to implementation of LICs like the ECMH [32, 33]. Barriers to LICs disrupt implementation into medical education and clinics but equity considerations should not be abandoned.

LICs should ensure access for underserved populations and promote learning diversity. Underserved populations could include patients that are uninsured and do not qualify for federal or statement programs but demonstrate financial need [35]. CommunityHealth Chicago is a free volunteer-based ECMH clinic that serves an uninsured population. The patients at the clinic are also low-income and predominately ethnic and racial minorities [36]. Distributed education materials are multilingual to provide effective patient care for non-English speakers. ECMH students often have a panel of patients in diverse health care settings and integrate learning objectives from multiple specialties which promotes learning diversity [18, 20]. The ECMH feature of continuity is considered most beneficial for vulnerable health populations [36]. ECMH clinics provides the opportunity to work with a variety of populations and gain hands-on experience with community health and continuity.

Innovation and Future Directions

Digital Health and Telemedicine Integration

Digital health during the ECMH clerkship can increase patient-centered care and digital competency. Medical schools do not incorporate digital health training into the curriculum although the health care system is digitized [37]. The point of digital health in health care is to advance universal health coverage with quality, accessible, and affordable services [38]. Digital health encompasses electronic health records, telehealth, wearable devices, mobile apps, and artificial intelligence (AI) in clinical practice [39]. Chandrashekar suggests that digital health be a preclinical course requirement that includes types of digital health technologies, theoretical frameworks for evaluation of the technologies, and an introduction to how technologists communicate [37]. The context of the course would be clinical scenarios. Other topics may include health data infrastructure, basics of AI, clinical decision support systems, basics of electric health records, digital ethics, impact of digital health on patient-provider relationships, and telemedicine [39]. Digital health plays a prominent role in medicine but could be introduced earlier in medical school curriculum along with telemedicine.

Telemedicine integration should also occur pre-clerkship and during the ECMH. Training of telemedicine during pre-clerkship should inform students on how to use relationship-centered language as an effort toward patient-centered care [40]. Digital health literacy is imperative in the current age of technology in medicine and should be a learning and professional competency [37]. Not only should telemedicine with hands on experience be taught prior to the clerkship, telemedicine can be integrated longitudinally [40]. An example of telemedicine in the ECMH would be the incorporation of telemedicine visit training in the first year of the clerkship. Continual use of telemedicine during the 4 years of curriculum provides students the opportunity to further develop telemedicine skills.

Expansion to Other Disciplines and Learner Types

Core components of the ECMH could be applied to other disciplines to enhance student learning. Within medical education, the ECMH model of peer teaching and other curricular components can be applied to inpatient settings. Peer mentoring and supervision has been successfully applied to nursing education in clinical settings [28]. A version of ECMH for nurses can contribute to professionalism, leadership and teaching skills, and the effective preparation for the workforce. The PCMH has been implemented with physician assistant (PA) students 45). PA students at urban clerkship sites with more components of the PCMH expressed more interest in perusal of a primary care career due to their experience. Students reported positive experiences with team-based learning and interprofessional collaboration. The ECMH could be expanded to PA programs and other disciplines that require experiential learning with patients. Interestingly, a community-based education model was implemented in medical sciences education for students in pathobiology [41]. Students in the community-oriented group were taught a pathobiology course that focused on prevalent and important infectious diseases in the local area. Students in the control group were taught pathobiology according to the original curriculum. The group with community orientated medical education received an overall total grade better than the control group. Components of the ECMH may also benefit the education of other disciplines in the classroom in addition to clinical skills acquired at clerkships.

Community Engagement and Population Health

Community describes the geographical area within which people reside and can also refer to culture or ethnicity in more urban areas [42]. Medical education in the community occurs in remote, rural, suburban, and urban academic medical centers. Community oriented medical education (COME) is characterized as students learning about the community as part of clinical learning environments and the impacts of community on patient care for those from different cultural and social backgrounds [42]. Similar to patient-centered care in the ECMH, COME transitioned into community engaged medical education in which medical schools have a reciprocal relationship with the community. To promote community engagement, representatives from the ECMH must have a conversation with members and leaders from the community to understand one another. The community would also be involved in the activities, missions, priorities, and outcomes of the medical school. From there, individual sites can align ECMH learning objectives with the specific health care needs of the surrounding community. This will provide students the ability to learn skills that help guide practice in specific community settings. Community engagement can have an effect on the practice the student pursues as a career.

Community engagement within ECMH also affords students the opportunity to learn more about social determinants of health. A strategy for medical schools to integrate community engagement is to identify local public health data and identify health concerns [43]. Community mentors can also provide students with information about the community, provide insight into local health concerns, and oversight of the program [42]. Within the ECMH, the health needs of the community would then be described and measured. Students and preceptors can identify the causes and develop effective measures to address the needs. Measures may include community projects that focus on finding solutions for community health issues. Chandratre et al. also describe 12 tips for medical schools to utilize for community engagement [43]. Notable tips are to make connections with individuals in the community, develop community engaged projects that relate to student goals, identify evidence-based practices that address community concerns, and discuss metrics that are currently used by community partners to determine if more quality metrics should be implemented [43].

Research and Evaluation Opportunities

There are multiple research and evaluation opportunities for the ECMH. The impact of authentic LICs and curriculum structure on career choice is an area that can be furthered studied [21]. In relationship to careers, future research can expand a longitudinal clerkship model like the ECMH to various health related professions to determine the efficacy of the curriculum in other educational programs and clinical experiences. Just as each profession is different, each ECMH is different due to location, available resources, the practice, patient populations and challenges faced [28]. QI research across multiple institutions can better determine the treatment effect of the ECMH model on patient care. In the same way, the structure of the ECMH is not uniform across different clerkships which could account for differences in student perceptions of the ECMH. Research can explore the generalizability of the clerkship structure, student roles in primary care clinics, and further investigate student perceptions [26]. Research at different ECMH sites from different institutions and regions may result in more representative attitudes and perceptions of students across various measures such as patient-centered care [29]. The ECMH model is often compared to the traditional curriculum or individual preceptorship. Despite differences amongst the models in regard to continuity and patient-centeredness, the actual structure of what contributes to the differences is unclear. Future research is needed to better understand the differences between continuity in both models and how clerkships can be better structured for student learning [26]. Both ECMH and IP models positively impact professional efficacy, a component of burnout, although ECMH students experience greater gains [21]. However, more research can help investigate factors that reduce other aspects of burnout such as high levels of exhaustion and cynicism as a result of medical school curriculum [25]. Research on burnout in medical school can contribute to an alternate curriculum within the ECMH model to address those factors once identified. With the advancement of digital technology, research opportunities for the ECMH include the evaluation of student competency outcomes following digital health and telemedicine curriculum pre-clerkship. Research should also investigate the impact of longitudinal implementation of digital health on patient outcomes and the physician-patient relationship. Finally, much of the research on the ECMH looks at the result of the model on patient care outcomes. Future research could investigate patient satisfaction by way of patient perception of care from an ECMH compared to a traditional clerkship and the impact that patients notice on their health and wellbeing.

Conclusion

The Education-Centered Medical Home (ECMH) is a longitudinal integrated clerkship (LIC) that developed from the concepts of the medical home and Primary Care Medical Home (PCMH). With a focus on patient-centered care and PCMH principles and learning objectives, the model achieves continuity in primary care practices. Continuity is achieved through longitudinal relationships among peers, preceptors, and patients. Over the course of 4 years, students work closely on a team with peers, a preceptor, and interdisciplinary health care professionals. Feedback from the preceptor and peers help build clinical skills and improve practice and experience with team-based care. Commitment to continuity, quality metrics, and quality improvement projects help improve patient outcomes. Indeed, patient outcomes across multiple ECMH clinics have improved and demonstrate the benefit of continuity and student dedication to patient-centered care. Despite the benefit of the ECMH on medical education and the patient experience, there are barriers to implement a LIC but suggestions are offered to counter any concerns. As ECMH clerkships continue to grow, consideration of future directions for research can contribute to the effectiveness and efficiency of the education-centered medical home.

References

1. Sia C, Tonniges TF, Osterhus E, Taba S. History of the medical home concept. Pediatrics. 2004;113(Supplement_4):1473–8.
2. Starfield B, Shi L. The medical home, access to care, and insurance: a review of evidence. Pediatrics. 2004;113(Supplement_4):1493–8.
3. American College of Physicians. The advanced medical home: a patient-centered, physician guided model of healthcare. American College of Physicians; 2006.
4. Stange KC, Nutting PA, Miller WL, Jaén CR, Crabtree BF, Flocke SA, et al. Defining and measuring the patient-centered medical home. J Gen Intern Med. 2010;25(6):601–12.
5. Arend J, Tsang-Quinn J, Levine C, Thomas D. The patient-centered medical home: history, components, and review of the evidence. Mt Sinai J Med J Transl Pers Med. 2012;79(4):433–50.
6. Rosser WW, Colwill JM, Kasperski J, Wilson L. Progress of Ontario's family health team model: a patient-centered medical home. Ann Fam Med. 2011;9(2):165–71.
7. Grumbach K, Grundy P. A review of the evidence from prospective evaluation studies in the United States. Patient-Centered Primary Care Collaborative; 2010.
8. Fifield J, Forrest DD, Burleson JA, Martin-Peele M, Gillespie W. Quality and efficiency in small practices transitioning to patient centered medical homes: a randomized trial. J Gen Intern Med. 2013;28(6):778–86.
9. Jackson GL, Powers BJ, Chatterjee R, Prvu Bettger J, Kemper AR, Hasselblad V, et al. The patient-centered medical home. Ann Intern Med. 2013;158(3):169–78.
10. Van den Berk-Clark C, Doucette E, Rottnek F, Manard W, Prada MA, Hughes R, et al. Do patient-centered medical homes improve health behaviors, outcomes, and experiences of low-income patients? A systematic review and meta-analysis. Health Serv Res. 2018;53(3):1777–98.
11. Anderson DR, Olayiwola JN. Community health centers and the patient-centered medical home: challenges and opportunities to reduce health care disparities in America. J Health Care Poor Underserved. 2012;23(3):949–57.
12. Magill MK, Baxley E. Patient care, education, and scholarship in the patient-centered medical home. Fam Med. 2013;45(4):235–9.
13. Margolies SO, Cowan R, Rehfuss MC, Britton B. The patient centered medical home and medical school education: an innovative interprofessional education model. J Interprofessional Educ Pract. 2018;10:41–3.
14. Hauer KE, O'Brien B, Poncelet AN. Longitudinal, integrated clerkship education: better for learners and patients. Acad Med. 2009;84(7):821.
15. Greenhill J, Poncelet AN. Transformative learning through longitudinal integrated clerkships. Med Educ. 2013;47(4):336.
16. Hudson JN, Poncelet AN, Weston KM, Bushnell JA, Farmer EA. Longitudinal integrated clerkships. Med Teach. 2017;39(1):7–13.
17. Henschen BL, Garcia P, Jacobson B, Ryan ER, Woods DM, Wayne DB, et al. The patient centered medical home as curricular model: perceived impact of the "education-centered medical home". J Gen Intern Med. 2013;28(8):1105–9.
18. Warm EJ, Desai SS, Bowen JL. Navigating the discontinuity crisis in medical education. N Engl J Med. 2025;392(24):2447–57.
19. Evans DB, Henschen BL, Poncelet AN, Wilkerson L, Ogur B. Continuity in undergraduate medical education: mission not accomplished. J Gen Intern Med. 2019;34(10):2254–9.
20. Henschen BL, Bierman JA, Wayne DB, Ryan ER, Thomas JX, Curry RH, et al. Four-year educational and patient care outcomes of a team-based primary care longitudinal clerkship. Acad Med. 2015;90(11):S43.
21. Henschen BL, Shaunfield S, Golden BP, Gard LA, Bierman J, Evans DB, et al. From passive gatekeeper to quarterback: evolving perceptions of primary care among medical students in longitudinal outpatient clerkships. J Gen Intern Med. 2022;37(3):608–14.

22. Han ER, Yeo S, Kim MJ, Lee YH, Park KH, Roh H. Medical education trends for future physicians in the era of advanced technology and artificial intelligence: an integrative review. BMC Med Educ. 2019;19(1):460.
23. Fazio SB, Chheda S, Hingle S, Lo MC, Meade L, Blanchard M, et al. The challenges of teaching ambulatory internal medicine: faculty recruitment, retention, and development: an AAIM/SGIM position paper. Am J Med. 2017;130(1):105–10.
24. Asgarova S, MacKenzie M, Bates J. Learning from patients: why continuity matters. Acad Med. 2017;92(11S):S55.
25. Henschen BL, Liss DT, Golden BP, Cameron KA, Bierman JA, Ryan ER, et al. Continuity with patients, preceptors, and peers improves primary care training: a randomized medical education trial. Acad Med. 2020;95(3):425.
26. Golden BP, Henschen BL, Gard LA, Ryan ER, Evans DB, Bierman J, et al. Learning to be a doctor: medical students' perception of their roles in longitudinal outpatient clerkships. Patient Educ Couns. 2018;101(11):2018–24.
27. Yang MM, Golden BP, Cameron KA, Gard L, Bierman JA, Evans DB, et al. Learning through teaching: peer teaching and mentoring experiences among third-year medical students. Teach Learn Med. 2022;34(4):360–7.
28. O'Neill SM, Henschen BL, Unger ED, Jansson PS, Unti K, Bortoletto P, et al. Educating future physicians to track health care quality: feasibility and perceived impact of a health care quality report card for medical students. Acad Med. 2013;88(10):1564–9.
29. Henschen BL, Ryan ER, Evans DB, Truong A, Wayne DB, Bierman JA, et al. Perceptions of patient-centered care among first-year medical students. Teach Learn Med. 2019;31(1):26–33.
30. Curry RH. Meaningful roles for medical students in the provision of longitudinal patient care. JAMA. 2014;312(22):2335.
31. Aristova M, Shaw M, Hendel E, Tschoe M. Longitudinal medical student collaborative care in primary care patients with type 2 diabetes. PRiMER. 2024;8:16.
32. Brown ME, Anderson K, Finn GM. A narrative literature review considering the development and implementation of longitudinal integrated clerkships, including a practical guide for application. J Med Educ Curric Dev. 2019;6:2382120519849409.
33. Bartlett M, Couper I, Poncelet A, Worley P. The do's, don'ts and don't knows of establishing a sustainable longitudinal integrated clerkship. Perspect Med Educ. 2020;9(1):5–19.
34. Forman JH, Robinson CH, Krein SL. Striving toward team-based continuity: provision of same-day access and continuity in academic primary care clinics. BMC Health Serv Res. 2019;19(1):145.
35. Russi AE, Bhaumik S, Herzog JJ, Tschoe M, Baumgartner AC. Impact of an education-centered medical home on quality at a student-volunteer free clinic. Med Educ Online. 2018;23(1):1505401.
36. Mesa AS, Tschoe M. Comparison of quality metrics in an education-centered medical home with local and national benchmarks. Med Educ Online. 2022;27(1):2073806.
37. Chandrashekar P. A digital health preclinical requirement for medical students. Acad Med. 2019;94(6):749.
38. World Health Organization. WHO guideline. Recommendations on digital interventions for health system strengthening. Geneva: World Health Organization; 2019.
39. Khurana MP, Raaschou-Pedersen DE, Kurtzhals J, Bardram JE, Ostrowski SR, Bundgaard JS. Digital health competencies in medical school education: a scoping review and Delphi method study. BMC Med Educ. 2022;22(1):129.
40. Hassan S, Cheng BT, Zhao J, Mohammed TO, Mahmoud A, Uchida TL. Comment on: twelve tips for the integration of medical students into telemedicine visitsMed Teach. 2022;44(3):337.
41. Assadi SN. Community oriented medical education for learning of pathobiology. Health Scope [Internet]. 2016;5(3). Available from: https://brieflands.com/journals/healthscope/articles/20151.

42. Strasser R, Worley P, Cristobal F, Marsh DC, Berry S, Strasser S, et al. Putting communities in the driver's seat: the realities of community-engaged medical education. Acad Med. 2015;90(11):1466.
43. Chandratre S, Norrbom C, Zeman C, Prunuske A. Strategies to integrate community engagement in medical student education. J Reg Med Campuses [Internet]. 2021;4(2). Available from: https://pubs.lib.umn.edu/index.php/jrmc/article/view/3600.

New and Innovative Ideas in Health Equity/ Cultural Humility

Technology as a Tool for Improving Patient Safety

Allen Terteryan, Ali Baidoun, and Mahesh Shrestha

Introduction

Patient safety is a central element of quality healthcare delivery. Technological advancements now play a critical role in preventing medical errors and improving outcomes throughout the care continuum. The adoption of advanced technological solutions has changed how healthcare providers address safety challenges. These solutions offer significant opportunities to reduce adverse events, support clinical decision-making, and strengthen patient monitoring. In recent years, healthcare systems globally have increasingly recognized the value of digital health technologies in addressing persistent safety issues and improving both efficiency and patient satisfaction.

A lot of preventable harm can be blocked by the right product, used at the right moment. In practice, these "physical" tools work in a few predictable ways: they reduce pathogen exposure (antiseptics and cleansing systems), mechanically interrupt pathophysiology before it starts (compression devices for VTE), or improve the interface between long-term hardware and the body (dressing kits and materials that

A. Terteryan
Western Michigan University Homer Stryker M.D. School of Medicine, Kalamazoo, MI, USA
e-mail: allen.terteryan@wmed.edu

A. Baidoun
Department of Pediatrics and Adolescent Medicine, Western Michigan University Homer Stryker M.D. School of Medicine, Kalamazoo, MI, USA
e-mail: ali.baidoun@wmed.edu

M. Shrestha (✉)
Department of Pediatrics and Adolescent Medicine, Western Michigan University Homer Stryker M.D. School of Medicine, Kalamazoo, MI, USA
e-mail: Mahesh.shrestha@wmed.edu

S. S. Chahin et al. (eds.), *Innovation in Medical Education and Clinical Practice*, https://doi.org/10.1007/978-3-032-19116-8_11

lower driveline infections). The literature points to a simple pattern: When a product removes friction for the team and fits naturally into the workflow, safety improves.

Over the last decade, a lot of progress on prevention has come not just from fancy gadgets but also from simple, repeatable techniques built into everyday care. Things like structured rounds, postoperative checklists, aseptic "bundles," and risk-based prescribing rules all aim to make the safest action the default one. The literature shows that when teams standardize these steps and place them at the right moment in the workflow, routine care gets safer.

Tools have also started playing a bigger role in preventing medical errors before they happen. Technologies like clinical decision support systems (CDSS), real-time dashboards, electronic quality measures, and patient-facing apps are being used more often to catch things early and help care teams stick to evidence-based practices. These tools are also helping uncover weak spots in clinical workflows that might not have been obvious otherwise.

Healthcare technology has advanced significantly, now including smart infusion devices, electronic health records (EHRs), AI-based clinical decision support systems, and remote patient monitoring platforms. These technologies serve as essential safeguards against medical errors and patient harm. Contemporary literature provides substantial evidence for their safety benefits when implemented appropriately. For example, smart infusion pumps and EHR-integrated computerized physician order entry (CPOE) systems reduce medication errors [1–3]. Minimally invasive approaches and closed-loop systems decrease procedural risks and physiological instability [4–6]. Continuous monitoring technologies facilitate earlier detection of clinical deterioration [7]. Telehealth and remote monitoring platforms lower hospital readmissions by supporting proactive management of post-discharge complications [8–10].

Technology enables patients and their families to access educational resources and self-management tools, which support safer engagement in care processes [11, 12]. Despite these benefits, technology is not a universal solution and may introduce new safety challenges. Usability problems, inadequate integration with clinical workflows, and alert fatigue can compromise safety by encouraging workarounds or leading to the omission of critical information [13, 14]. For instance, in a bustling emergency room, a nurse fatigued by constant alerts on patient monitoring systems might miss a critical warning that a patient is developing sepsis, leading to delayed intervention and potentially serious outcomes. Additionally, emerging technologies such as AI present risks related to bias, transparency, and validation that require thorough evaluation and mitigation, particularly when used with vulnerable populations such as children [15, 16].

To truly make healthcare technology as safe as possible, we need to consider it from multiple vantage points. This includes regularly evaluating system performance, designing tools that are intuitive for both healthcare providers and patients (and their families), offering comprehensive training, and ensuring equitable access while maintaining a focus on ethical standards [2, 15]. While the research is clear on finding equilibrium between pioneering technological advances and maintaining vigilance, it is paramount to recognize the challenges at the frontline, such as workflow disruptions or cultural resistance, which can impact adoption and execution. Bridging the gap between innovation and bedside application requires using advanced systems alongside human oversight and solid contingency plans, expanding telehealth in a way that continues to offer coordinated care with accessible escalation support when necessary, and employing AI in clinical settings without overshadowing the essential judgment of human clinicians and ensuring algorithms are equitable for all [8, 13, 15].

When it comes to children, it's especially important to adjust and think carefully about how we use technology, so it fits their stage of development and meets their unique health and safety needs [3, 10, 12, 16]. Overall, bringing technology into healthcare has clearly made patient care safer. It's helped care become more reliable, proactive, and centered around what patients need. Tools and devices help prevent injuries, tech-driven approaches reduce mistakes and make procedures less unpredictable, and digital systems enable care and monitoring to reach far beyond the hospital or clinic. Looking ahead, there's even more promise with things like AI, better connectivity, and digital tools tailored to each person. For all these changes to really help everyone, it's vital that doctors, nurses, tech experts, and leaders work together, making sure new tech is rolled out fairly and thoughtfully, with a constant focus on keeping every patient, especially kids, as safe and healthy as possible.

We have divided this book chapters into 3 distinct sub-headings (a) Use of technology in prevention or prophylaxis, (b) Use of technology during treatment phase of patient, and (c) Use of technology after treatment.

Use of Technology in Prevention or Prophylaxis

Physical Product Prophylaxis

Mechanical prevention of venous thromboembolism (VTE) is a good example. Sequential compression devices (SCDs) are standard when chemoprophylaxis is delayed or contraindicated, but they only work if they're actually on—and stay on. A surgeon-led initiative in neurosurgery used small, practical levers (visual cues, order-set tweaks, accountability) and drove real bedside uptake of SCDs, showing that product effectiveness is inseparable from ease of use and team habits [17]. These projects are reminders that VTE prevention is less about which sleeve your hospital buys, and more about how reliably that sleeve is on the patient.

That said, design still matters. Earlier comparison work clarified how different compression platforms generate and transmit pressure; choosing a device that delivers the intended hemodynamic effect for your population isn't trivial [18]. And comfort/portability aren't cosmetic—patients and clinicians keep low-profile devices on longer. A miniaturized compression unit used in trauma achieved better adherence simply because it was less obtrusive in day-to-day care [19]. Put together, the message is straightforward: Pick compression that people will use, build it into daily checks, and measure device-on time—not just orders.

Device–tissue interfaces are another place where physical products quietly change outcomes. For Left Ventricular Assist Device (LVAD) patients, driveline exit-site infections remain stubbornly common. A scoping review points to several product-level choices that appear to lower risk: silicone–skin interfaces outperform velour at the exit site; octenidine outperforms merbromin as a cleanser; and standardized, pre-packed dressing kits improve consistency and staff satisfaction [20]. Equally useful are the "doesn't help" findings: chronic suppressive antibiotics didn't reduce infection and were associated with more hospitalizations/exchanges, and swapping to smaller needles or add-on anchors didn't clearly move the needle [20]. Frequency of dressing change showed mixed results; in practice, the kit components and the aseptic steps likely matter more than the calendar. The overall lesson is practical: standardize the kit and the surface chemistry, and the day-to-day burden on staff goes down while safety goes up.

Technique Prophylaxis

One of the clearest examples is the daily ward-round prompt card. Johnston et al. built a short, "every patient, every day" tool that nudges teams to confirm basics—treatment plans, antibiotic review, venous thromboembolism (VTE) assessment, and direct communication with patients. After rollout, hospitals saw substantial, measurable gains across those exact items [21]. The lesson is straightforward: When the checklist sits at the bedside, the right actions happen more reliably, with minimal friction.

Some risks are highly procedure-specific and need codified "safe technique." In laparoscopic cholecystectomy, three decades of data synthesized by the SAGES Safe Cholecystectomy Task Force show that consistent use of defined safety steps has coincided with a meaningful drop in major bile duct injury rates over time [22]. The message isn't that one maneuver fixes everything; it's that disciplined identification of anatomy, timely escalation when conditions are unsafe, and adherence to standardized steps together prevent rare but devastating harm.

Simple technique also matters in infection prevention. The Anaesthetists Be Cleaner (ABC) trial protocol targets a handful of high-yield behaviors—context-appropriate hand hygiene, filtered IV drug preparation, and cleaner work surfaces during anesthesia—to curb postoperative infections [23]. It's intentionally practical: Pick the few actions with the biggest impact and implement them with a stepped-wedge design so sites can adopt in sequence without disrupting care.

Risk stratification is a core preventative technique too. A study of elderly inpatients in a Saudi tertiary center found that while most high-risk patients received VTE prophylaxis, a sizable share of low-risk patients were exposed to unnecessary anticoagulation, highlighting the need to anchor prescribing to validated scores like Padua and to build hard stops against overuse [24]. Complementing that, a review by Chindamo and Marques argues for pairing thrombosis risk with bleeding risk up front and choosing pharmacologic vs mechanical prophylaxis accordingly [25]. In short: Don't just ask "who needs chemoprophylaxis?"—also ask "who might it harm?" and act on both answers.

Software/Digital Technology Prophylaxis

CDSS (clinical decision support systems) platforms, in particular, show a lot of promise. In one randomized trial, Huang et al. found that an AI-powered CDSS cut hospital-acquired VTE nearly in half by helping providers stick to thromboprophylaxis guidelines [26]. Another study by George et al. showed that integrating CDSS into the VA's EHR helped improve appropriate prescribing while cutting back on unnecessary meds in high-risk patients [27]. These results point toward CDSS being more than just a convenience; they're changing how clinicians make decisions.

Electronic clinical quality measures (eCQMs) are also being used to drive safer care without overwhelming providers. In a rapid-cycle improvement project, Mohsen et al. used eCQMs to improve VTE prophylaxis rates and saw meaningful gains [28]. Taha et al. paired similar tools with a structured approach to clinical reasoning and ended up boosting prophylaxis rates from 87% to over 98% in a single year [29]. These kinds of gains show that with the right setup, digital systems can really scale up safety efforts without adding more burden.

Dashboards are another strong area. In one study, Shaw et al. looked at a pediatric ICU dashboard that tracked consent status, med reconciliation, and catheter use. Just having those metrics visible helped reduce unnecessary catheter days and speed up the consent process [30]. Another dashboard project, CERTAINp, raised prophylaxis-related discussions and helped ICU teams go from 57% to full adherence with safety protocols [30]. This kind of visibility seems to really help teams stay on track.

Of course, not every tool delivers. Klemann et al. studied a perioperative support tool meant to help with Postoperative Nausea and Vomiting (PONV) prevention, but even with it in place, only about half of patients got the right prophylaxis [31]. This shows that it's not just about having technology; it has to be used the right way, and it must match how real clinical teams actually work.

Use of Technology During Treatment of a Patient

When patients are being treated, there's a lot going on, and decisions have to be made quickly, treatments can be urgent, and many different health professionals need to work together. With all this happening, the risk of mistakes can go up. That's where technology really steps in as a safety net. It adds extra layers of protection to help prevent things from going wrong and to make treatments more accurate and effective. Advanced technology has changed the way healthcare teams keep patients safe, with tools like real-time monitors, decision-support systems, and automated systems working together to reduce risks and improve outcomes.

Smart Infusion Systems and Medication Safety

Smart infusion pumps with dose-error reduction software (DERS) have really changed the game in keeping patients safe during treatment. These advanced devices use detailed drug lists with set limits and safety checks to help stop medication mistakes, a problem that's been all too common (and dangerous) in healthcare. There's a lot of solid research backing up just how much safer these smart pumps can make things: Studies and reviews have shown that, when used correctly and integrated into healthcare teams' daily routines, they can lead to dramatic reductions in medication errors [1–3].

But smart infusion systems aren't just about reducing mistakes; they also make the whole process of administering medicine smoother and more reliable. For example, these devices warn you right away if a dose exceeds the safe limit, keep detailed records that help teams spot trends and make improvements, and help ensure medication is administered consistently across different parts of a hospital. Still, making the most of this technology isn't always easy. There can be issues, such as staff growing tired of too many alerts, disruptions to how things usually work, and the need to train everyone thoroughly so the tech is used correctly [1, 13].

The integration of smart infusion systems with electronic health records and computerized provider order entry systems marks the next step in medication safety technology. By automatically populating pump settings from digital prescriptions, these systems help reduce transcription errors and streamline documentation of medication administration. Studies demonstrate that integrated systems can not only further decrease medication errors compared to standalone smart pumps but also boost workflow efficiency and lessen the administrative strain on nursing staff [3, 14]. This advancement in interoperability simplifies the medication process, leading to a more cohesive healthcare environment.

Minimally Invasive Surgical Technologies

Recent developments in minimally invasive surgical techniques, facilitated by advanced technological platforms, have significantly improved surgical safety by lowering procedural risks, decreasing tissue trauma, and enhancing patient outcomes. The integration of robotic-assisted surgical systems, advanced imaging modalities, and precision instruments allows surgeons to conduct complex procedures with superior visualization, greater dexterity, and less invasiveness than conventional open surgery [4, 5].

Minimally invasive technologies provide safety benefits across various surgical specialties, as evidenced by reduced complication rates, shorter recovery periods, and improved long-term patient outcomes. Robotic surgical systems specifically enhance procedural precision by eliminating tremors, enabling scaled motion control, and providing three-dimensional visualization that exceeds manual capabilities in specific scenarios. These features result in measurable safety improvements, such as decreased blood loss, lower infection rates, and reduced incidence of surgical site complications [4, 5].

The adoption of minimally invasive surgical technologies necessitates thorough evaluation of surgeon training requirements, procedural learning curves, and risks of technology-related complications. Research highlights the necessity of comprehensive training programs, standardized procedural protocols, and continuous quality monitoring to maximize safety benefits and reduce associated risks [4, 5].

Closed-Loop Control Systems

Closed-loop control systems are changing how we monitor patients and manage treatments. They automatically adjust care based on real-time feedback from the body. This approach is especially helpful in critical care and for people with chronic conditions like diabetes or heart disease, where precise management is important. By combining continuous monitoring with automated delivery, these systems respond quickly to a patient's needs and reduce the need for constant manual adjustments [6].

The artificial pancreas system for diabetes management is the most established example of closed-loop technology in healthcare. This system integrates continuous glucose monitoring with automated insulin delivery to achieve optimal glycemic control. Clinical trials indicate that artificial pancreas systems significantly improve glucose management and reduce the risk of hypoglycemic events, marking a substantial advancement in diabetes care safety [6]. The demonstrated success of closed-loop systems in diabetes has led to the investigation of similar technologies for other conditions, such as blood pressure management, sedation control, and fluid balance optimization.

To implement closed-loop systems safely, it is important to focus on system reliability, fail-safe features, and human oversight. These systems can improve treatment precision and responsiveness, but they also bring new risks, such as sensor errors, algorithm issues, and connectivity problems. Managing these risks requires thorough validation and ongoing monitoring [6]. Clinicians must be prepared with contingency plans for instances when sensor data are missing or conflicting, ensuring that human judgment remains a crucial part of the decision-making process.

Electronic Health Records and Clinical Decision Support

Electronic health record systems that incorporate clinical decision support functions have become essential for improving patient safety. They offer real-time access to comprehensive patient data, automated safety verifications, and evidence-based treatment guidance. By serving as centralized repositories for patient information, these systems enable healthcare providers to make informed decisions and reduce the likelihood of errors caused by incomplete or inaccurate data [2].

EHR systems offer several safety benefits, including improved medication reconciliation, allergy checks, drug interaction screening, and adherence to clinical guidelines. Clinical decision support tools can provide real-time alerts on safety concerns, recommend evidence-based treatments, and help coordinate care across providers. Studies show that well-designed EHRs with strong decision support can lower medical errors and help providers follow safety protocols [2].

Implementing EHR systems introduces challenges with usability, workflow integration, and technology-related errors. Common issues include alert fatigue, documentation burden, and over-reliance on automation, all of which may compromise patient safety if left unaddressed. Successful EHR adoption requires thoughtful system design, thorough user training, and continuous improvement informed by user feedback and safety outcomes [2].

Pediatric Applications of Safety Technology

Using safety technologies in pediatric healthcare brings both challenges and opportunities. Children have different developmental stages, unique physiological needs, and often rely on their families for care. Because they may not be able to describe their symptoms clearly and may depend on adults for decision-making, safety solutions must be tailored and tested specifically for children, taking into account their age, development, and the care they receive.

Pediatric-Specific Smart Infusion Technology

Safe implementation of smart infusion technology in pediatric care requires drug libraries, dosing algorithms, and safety settings specifically designed for the unique needs of children at various developmental stages. Pediatric patients are at increased risk of medication errors due to weight-based dosing, frequent dilution of medications, and narrow therapeutic ranges for many drugs [3, 14].

Smart infusion systems for pediatric patients include age-specific and weight-based dosing limits, specialized drug concentrations, and safety alerts tailored to the risks of pediatric medication administration. Research indicates that pediatric-specific smart pump implementations significantly reduce medication errors in children and improve nursing staff workflow efficiency [3, 14]. The complexity of pediatric dosing calculations and the frequent dose adjustments required by patient growth and development necessitate continuous system maintenance and updates.

Integrating pediatric smart infusion systems with electronic health records and computerized provider order entry systems enhances safety by automating weight-based dose calculations, verifying dosing parameters in real time, and thoroughly documenting medication administration. These systems also reduce cognitive workload for healthcare providers and ensure consistent application of pediatric safety checks [3, 14].

Remote Monitoring and Telehealth for Pediatric Patients

Remote monitoring and telehealth technologies have the potential to enhance pediatric patient safety by enabling continuous observation of children with chronic illnesses, supporting timely intervention for acute health issues, and assisting families in managing complex medical care at home. These technologies are especially beneficial for pediatric populations as they reduce the frequency of hospital visits, lower the risk of healthcare-associated infections, and facilitate care within the home environment [10, 12].

Implementing pediatric remote monitoring systems requires attention to age-appropriate interfaces, effective family engagement, and the specific communication needs of children and caregivers. Successful telehealth programs use child-friendly technologies, offer thorough family education and support, and ensure strong communication between families and healthcare providers [10, 12].

Studies show that well-designed pediatric telehealth programs can lead to better health outcomes, lower healthcare use, and greater family satisfaction. Still, these programs work best when technology is accessible, families are comfortable with digital tools, and telehealth is integrated with traditional care [10, 12].

Artificial Intelligence and Predictive Analytics in Pediatric Care

The integration of AI and predictive analytics in pediatric healthcare presents significant opportunities for early detection of clinical deterioration, prediction of adverse events, and optimization of treatment protocols. Pediatric-specific AI systems must account for distinct physiological patterns and developmental variations across age groups, which require specialized algorithms and rigorous validation methods [16].

Predictive analytics systems designed for pediatric sepsis detection constitute a leading application of AI in pediatric safety. Research indicates that these systems can facilitate early sepsis identification in children by analyzing vital signs, laboratory results, and clinical indicators. Early warning alerts generated by these systems support timely intervention and may reduce the risk of progression to severe sepsis or septic shock [16].

The implementation of AI systems in pediatric care necessitates rigorous algorithm validation, effective bias mitigation, and integration with clinical expertise. The rapid physiological changes and developmental variations characteristic of pediatric patients pose challenges for AI development, requiring comprehensive testing and validation protocols [16]. To ensure these AI systems account for developmental variability, several validation checkpoints can be incorporated. First, developmental benchmarking should be used to align the algorithms with key growth milestones. Second, diverse data sets reflecting the spectrum of pediatric development must be employed to train and test the AI systems, reducing the risk of bias. Lastly, iterative peer reviews with pediatric specialists should be conducted to continually assess and refine the AI's accuracy and reliability in real-world scenarios.

The advancement of pediatric safety technology is expected to focus on increasingly personalized approaches that account for developmental stage, individual risk factors, and family context. As these technologies advance, it is essential to balance technological innovation with the core human elements of pediatric care, such as the therapeutic relationship among providers, children, and families, to effectively enhance pediatric patient safety [10, 12].

Ongoing evaluation should incorporate pediatric outcome measures that assess both clinical safety endpoints and patient and family experiences. The participation of multidisciplinary teams, including child life specialists, developmental experts, and family advisors, is critical to ensure that technologies address the specific needs of children and their families [10, 12].

Technology After Treatment/During Recovery

The post-acute treatment period, whether at home, in rehabilitation facilities, or during outpatient follow-up, is a critical phase for patient safety. Adverse events such as infections, medication errors, and preventable hospital readmissions often occur during this transition as patients assume greater responsibility for self-management. Technology increasingly bridges care gaps and supports safety throughout recovery. This section reviews (a) physical devices that support recovery, primarily home monitoring tools, (b) technology-enabled approaches such as telerehabilitation and virtual follow-ups, and (c) digital health tools, including comprehensive recovery platforms and mobile health applications.

Much like the technologies applied during a patient's hospital stay, a range of new tools has emerged to support safer recovery after discharge. For instance, remote monitoring devices can alert care teams to concerning changes in vital signs at home, allowing for early intervention if problems arise [7]. Mobile apps that remind patients to take their medications help improve adherence to treatment plans, while secure messaging platforms and telehealth systems make it easier for patients and healthcare providers to stay connected and address issues quickly [8, 9, 11, 32]. Research has shown that these innovations can significantly reduce the risk of hospital readmissions and support better recovery outcomes. When evaluating these technologies, it is important to consider how well they engage patients, whether they are accessible and usable across different populations, and how they protect health information outside of traditional clinical settings [7, 9, 11].

Physical Devices for Post-treatment Care

Home monitoring devices: Remote patient monitoring (RPM) has become an important part of keeping patients safe after they leave the hospital. With RPM, people use devices at home, such as wireless blood pressure cuffs, digital scales, pulse oximeters, or glucose monitors, to track their health and send that information directly to their healthcare team. This setup makes it possible for doctors and nurses to catch early signs of trouble, such as high blood pressure, sudden weight gain in patients with heart failure, or unstable blood sugar levels, and step in before things get worse [7]. Studies have shown that RPM can help patients stick to their care plans, lower the chances of having to go back to the hospital, and reduce emergency room visits, especially for those with chronic illnesses or recovering from surgery [7, 9]. Many patients also say they feel more at ease knowing that their health is being watched, even when they are at home [7].

The success of remote patient monitoring (RPM) depends on several practical considerations. First, the devices must be accurate and dependable, since unreliable data can lead to either unnecessary alarms or missed health concerns. Patients also need to use these devices correctly and regularly, but if the equipment is difficult to use or inconvenient, they may not follow through as needed. Problems with internet or Bluetooth connections can also prevent information from reaching healthcare providers, possibly giving a misleading sense of security. In addition, healthcare teams must have strong systems for handling and reviewing the large amounts of data generated, and they need to be ready to respond quickly if something unusual appears. Protecting patient privacy is also essential when personal health data are sent from home. Even with these challenges, RPM programs that combine dependable devices and responsive support from clinical staff have shown that they can offer valuable extra protection for patients after they leave the hospital [7, 9].

Techniques for Recovery and Follow-Up

Telerehabilitation

For many patients, rehabilitation continues well after they leave the hospital. Telerehabilitation uses technology such as video calls, virtual reality, and other telehealth tools to deliver physical, occupational, or speech therapy at a distance. This method has made it much easier for people to access therapy, especially those who live far from clinics, have difficulty getting around, or lack reliable transportation [33]. Multiple systematic reviews and meta-analyses have shown that telerehabilitation can be just as effective as in-person therapy for improving movement, reducing pain, and enhancing quality of life. This holds true for a variety of situations, including recovery after a stroke or orthopedic injuries [33, 34]. Many patients also report that they appreciate the added convenience that telerehabilitation brings [33].

From a safety standpoint, telerehabilitation allows therapists to monitor and guide patients as they perform exercises in their own homes. This can reduce the risk of injury that might occur if patients exercise on their own without supervision. It also helps patients avoid the risks that come with traveling to a clinic, such as accidents or exposure to illness [34]. Of course, telerehabilitation does have its limits. Some treatments that require hands-on techniques cannot be done remotely, and it can sometimes be tough to ensure a patient is performing an exercise perfectly just by watching via a video connection. Patients also need to have access to the right technology and be comfortable using it. Even with these challenges, research shows that telerehabilitation is a safe and effective way to maintain rehabilitation, help patients stay on track, and support better recovery for many people [33, 34].

Virtual Follow-Up Visits

The replacement of traditional in-person clinic visits with virtual follow-ups via video or telephone has become increasingly prevalent for post-treatment monitoring. Virtual follow-ups provide greater convenience for patients by reducing travel requirements during recovery and decreasing the risk of exposure to infections in clinical environments [8, 35]. Evidence from randomized controlled trials and systematic reviews demonstrates that, for many procedures and conditions, virtual follow-ups yield clinical outcomes, complication detection rates, and patient satisfaction comparable to those of in-person visits [8, 9]. In the postoperative period, telehealth interventions have been linked to significant reductions in hospital readmission rates and emergency department visits, likely due to earlier identification and management of complications [9].

Virtual follow-ups do not work for every situation. If a patient needs a physical exam or a procedure like suture removal, they should come in for an in-person visit. Clinicians need to know when virtual care is not enough and when to recommend an in-person appointment [8]. For patients who are a good fit, though, virtual visits offer a safe and effective way to stay connected, track recovery, and quickly address any concerns after treatment [8, 9, 35].

Remote Patient Education

Clear patient education is vital for safe recovery and helps people manage their health at home. Technology now allows educational materials to be delivered remotely, going beyond what can be taught in a single discharge session. This includes scheduled video or phone check-ins with healthcare providers, patient portals with custom resources and videos, interactive apps, and automated text reminders [9]. Learning at home helps patients better understand their medications, recognize warning signs, care for wounds, and follow activity guidelines. Studies show that structured remote education can boost adherence to care plans and may lower the risk of complications or readmission [9]. Ongoing access to digital resources and repeated reminders support safer self-care after leaving the hospital.

Digital Health Tools for Post-treatment Care

Digital Recovery Platforms

Usually delivered through apps or web portals, they are now widely used to support patients after hospital care. These tools offer personalized care plans, symptom tracking, educational materials, and direct messaging with providers [9, 36]. Features like checklists and reminders help patients stay on track, and symptom monitoring can alert clinicians to problems early [9]. Studies show these platforms reduce hospital readmissions and emergency visits [9]. Their success depends on user-friendly design, good integration with health records, and strong patient engagement [36]. When thoughtfully implemented, digital platforms help keep recovery safer and more organized [9, 36].

Mobile Health Apps

In addition to institution-specific platforms, a diverse range of mobile health (mHealth) applications is available for independent patient use or upon clinical recommendation to support post-treatment health management. These applications include medication reminder tools, symptom tracking diaries, physical therapy and fitness monitors, mental health support apps, and chronic disease management solutions [11, 32]. Evidence-based mHealth applications improve patient safety by increasing medication adherence, which is essential for preventing complications [11, 32]. Meta-analyses demonstrate that app-based interventions produce statistically significant improvements in adherence rates across multiple chronic conditions [11]. Symptom tracking applications enable patients to identify and report health changes promptly. Furthermore, research documents additional benefits, including improved disease control and increased patient engagement [32].

Clinicians are essential in directing patients to validated, reliable apps. The unregulated app market leads to inconsistent quality and evidence, potentially compromising safety. Data privacy and security remain significant concerns, and maintaining long-term user engagement with mHealth apps is challenging [11, 32]. However, when carefully selected and integrated into a comprehensive care plan with provider oversight, mHealth apps can effectively support self-management, improve adherence, and enhance communication throughout recovery and ongoing health maintenance [11, 32]

Telehealth for Post-treatment Monitoring

Telehealth serves as the enabling infrastructure for many post-treatment safety initiatives, including virtual visits, remote monitoring, and telerehabilitation. Its impact comes from providing timely access to clinical advice and support during recovery [8, 35]. Patients can quickly connect with providers about symptoms or concerns, which can prevent minor issues from escalating into serious complications that require acute care. This accessibility is especially valuable for patients with mobility limitations or those in remote areas. As previously noted, systematic reviews consistently link telehealth interventions in the post-discharge period with reduced readmissions and emergency care utilization [9]. Integrating with the patient's primary care team and maintaining strong data privacy protocols are essential for safe and effective implementation [8, 35]. Telehealth extends the reach of the healthcare system into patients' homes, providing a continuous safety net during recovery.

Conclusion

Technology plays a vital role in improving patient safety throughout the care continuum and across all age groups. Smart devices, connected clinical techniques, and advanced digital health systems help prevent medical errors and patient harm. Recent high-quality studies highlight the safety benefits of these technologies when used effectively. Smart infusion pumps and EHR-integrated CPOE systems reduce medication errors [1–3]. Minimally invasive procedures and closed-loop systems lower procedural risks and physiological instability [4–6]. Continuous monitoring enables earlier detection of clinical deterioration, while telehealth and remote monitoring reduce hospital readmissions by supporting proactive post-discharge care [7–10]. Technology also empowers patients and families with accessible education and self-management tools, encouraging safer involvement in care [11, 12].

However, this review makes it clear that technology is not a catch-all solution and can pose its own safety concerns. Problems such as complicated interfaces, poor fit within clinical routines, and alert fatigue may unintentionally compromise safety by causing staff to miss important details or develop workarounds [13, 14]. Newer tools, including artificial intelligence, pose additional challenges such as bias, lack of transparency, and the need for thorough validation. These issues become even more important when caring for vulnerable groups such as children [15, 16]. As a result, truly maximizing the safety benefits of healthcare technology requires ongoing outcome assessment, thoughtful design centered on users, strong training for both healthcare professionals and patients or families, and a commitment to ethical practices and fair access for all [2, 15].

The evidence shows that it is important to balance new technology with careful oversight. Success comes from using smart systems alongside strong human supervision and backup plans, expanding telehealth while ensuring care is well coordinated and escalated when needed, and using AI tools while still relying on clinicians' judgment and ensuring algorithms are fair [8, 13, 15]. For pediatric patients, it is especially important to adapt these technologies to their developmental stage and to meet their specific health and safety needs [3, 10, 12, 16].

Across product categories, a few patterns keep showing up. Prevention works best when the product is the easiest path (pre-packed kits, portable compression, etc.). Measurement needs to follow the product's real effect (device-on time, culture negativity, infection-related readmissions), not just the order in the chart. And standardization beats variety: for chronic device care in particular, a consistent kit and agreed-upon cleanser will outperform ad-hoc substitutions. Put simply, the safest hospitals make the right product hard to miss and easy to use in the exact moments where harm tends to start.

Altogether, the literature reinforces a practical view of prevention: the safest hospital is the one with a few well-designed, highly reliable techniques placed at the right moments, supported by local education and light-touch measurement. When those basics are locked in, downstream "rescues" are needed less often.

Altogether, digital technology is changing how prevention is approached in medicine. From smart decision rolls to patient apps and behind-the-scenes analytics, these systems are becoming part of the safety toolkit. The key isn't just making new tools; it's making sure they actually fit into everyday clinical life and support both providers and patients. If we're serious about building safer healthcare, investing in this kind of digital infrastructure should be a priority, not an afterthought.

In summary, integrating technology into treatment and recovery has significantly enhanced patient safety, making healthcare more reliable, innovative, and patient-focused. Devices reduce direct harm, technology-based methods minimize errors and inconsistencies, and digital tools extend support and monitoring beyond the hospital. Continued advances in artificial intelligence, connectivity, and personalized digital solutions will further improve care. Realizing these benefits for all patients will require ongoing collaboration among clinicians, administrators, technology experts, and policymakers. It remains essential to apply these tools thoughtfully and equitably, always prioritizing patient safety and improved health outcomes, especially for children.

Author Contributions/Acknowledgements Conceptualization: Mahesh Shrestha, Allen Terteryan; Writing—original draft preparation: Allen Terteryan(prophylaxis), Ali Baidoun (rest); Review and editing: Mahesh Shrestha, Allen Terteryan, Ali Baidoun; Supervision: Mahesh Shrestha: funding acquisition: none required. Use of AI: in organizing and formatting of content in many sections. All authors have read and agreed to the published version of the chapter.

References

1. Jani YH, Chumbley GM, Furniss D, Blandford A, Franklin B. The potential role of smart infusion devices in preventing or contributing to medication administration errors: a descriptive study of 2 data sets. J Patient Saf. 2021;17(8):e1894–900. https://doi.org/10.1097/PTS.0000000000000751. PMID: 32842073; PMCID: PMC8612907
2. Li E, Clarke J, Ashrafian H, Darzi A, Neves AL. The impact of electronic health record interoperability on safety and quality of care in high-income countries: systematic review. J Med Internet Res. 2022;24(9):e38144. https://doi.org/10.2196/38144. PMID: 36107486; PMCID: PMC9523524
3. VanHorn T, Harris J, Mayes S, Infanti LM, Kennedy A. Evaluation of the effect of smart pump interoperability on infusion errors in the pediatric hospital setting. J Pediatr Pharmacol Ther. 2024;29(3):323–30. https://doi.org/10.5863/1551-6776-29.3.323. Epub 2024 Jun 10. PMID: 38863851; PMCID: PMC11163903
4. Kalata S, Thumma JR, Norton EC, Dimick JB, Sheetz KH. Comparative safety of robotic-assisted vs laparoscopic cholecystectomy. JAMA Surg. 2023;158(12):1303–10. https://doi.org/10.1001/jamasurg.2023.4389. Erratum in: JAMA Surg. 2025;160(5):604. doi:10.1001/jamasurg.2025.0539. PMID: 37728932; PMCID: PMC10512167
5. Rivero-Moreno Y, Echevarria S, Vidal-Valderrama C, Pianetti L, Cordova-Guilarte J, Navarro-Gonzalez J, Acevedo-Rodríguez J, Dorado-Avila G, Osorio-Romero L, Chavez-Campos C, Acero-Alvarracín K. Robotic surgery: a comprehensive review of the literature and current trends. Cureus. 2023;15(7):e42370. https://doi.org/10.7759/cureus.42370. PMID: 37621804; PMCID: PMC10445506
6. Borel AL, Lablanche S, Waterlot C, Joffray E, Barra C, Arnol N, Amougay H, Benhamou PY. Closed-loop insulin therapy for people with type 2 diabetes treated with an insulin pump: a 12-week multicenter, open-label randomized, controlled, crossover trial. Diabetes Care. 2024;47(10):1778–86. https://doi.org/10.2337/dc24-0623. PMID: 39106206; PMCID: PMC11417293
7. Tan SY, Sumner J, Wang Y, Wenjun YA. A systematic review of the impacts of remote patient monitoring (RPM) interventions on safety, adherence, quality-of-life and cost-related outcomes. NPJ Digit Med. 2024;7(1):192. https://doi.org/10.1038/s41746-024-01182-w. PMID: 39025937; PMCID: PMC11258279
8. Ezeamii VC, Okobi OE, Wambai-Sani H, Perera GS, Zaynieva S, Okonkwo CC, Ohaiba MM, William-Enemali PC, Obodo OR, Obiefuna NG. Revolutionizing healthcare: how telemedicine is improving patient outcomes and expanding access to care. Cureus. 2024;16(7):e63881. https://doi.org/10.7759/cureus.63881. PMID: 39099901; PMCID: PMC11298029
9. Grygorian A, Montano D, Shojaa M, Ferencak M, Schmitz N. Digital health interventions and patient safety in abdominal surgery: a systematic review and meta-analysis. JAMA Netw Open. 2024;7(4):e248555. https://doi.org/10.1001/jamanetworkopen.2024.8555. PMID: 38669018; PMCID: PMC11053376

10. Howland K, Edvardsson K, Lees H, Hooker L. Telehealth use in the well-child health setting. A systematic review of acceptability and effectiveness for families and practitioners. Int J Nurs Stud Adv. 2024;8:100277. https://doi.org/10.1016/j.ijnsa.2024.100277. PMID: 39734584; PMCID: PMC11681896
11. Peng Y, Wang H, Fang Q, Xie L, Shu L, Sun W, Liu Q. Effectiveness of mobile applications on medication adherence in adults with chronic diseases: a systematic review and meta-analysis. J Manag Care Spec Pharm. 2020;26(4):550–61. https://doi.org/10.18553/jmcp.2020.26.4.550. PMID: 32223596; PMCID: PMC10391210
12. Park J, Jeon H, Choi EK. Digital health intervention on patient safety for children and parents: a scoping review. J Adv Nurs. 2024;80(5):1750–60. https://doi.org/10.1111/jan.15954. Epub 2023 Nov 10. PMID: 37950382
13. Kirkendall ES, Timmons K, Huth H, Walsh K, Melton K. Human-based errors involving smart infusion pumps: a catalog of error types and prevention strategies. Drug Saf. 2020;43(11):1073–87. https://doi.org/10.1007/s40264-020-00986-5. PMID: 32797355; PMCID: PMC7750013
14. Sowan A, Ha B. Maximizing the impact of smart pump-EHR interoperability in critical care. Intensive Crit Care Nurs. 2024;85:103809. https://doi.org/10.1016/j.iccn.2024.103809. Epub 2024 Aug 24. PMID: 39182391
15. Ouanes K, Farhah N. Effectiveness of Artificial Intelligence (AI) in clinical decision support systems and care delivery. J Med Syst. 2024;48(1):74. https://doi.org/10.1007/s10916-024-02098-4. PMID: 39133332
16. Tennant R, Graham J, Kern J, Mercer K, Ansermino JM, Burns CM. A scoping review on pediatric sepsis prediction technologies in healthcare. NPJ Digit Med. 2024;7(1):353. https://doi.org/10.1038/s41746-024-01361-9. PMID: 39633080; PMCID: PMC11618667
17. Windermere SA, Sconzo D, Askari A, Filippidis A, Binello E. Surgeon-led improvement in compliance with use of sequential compression devices in a neurosurgery patient population. BMJ Open Qual. 2024;13(3):e002807–7.2.
18. Proctor MC, Greenfield LJ, Wakefield TW, Zajkowski PJ. A clinical comparison of pneumatic compression devices: the basis for selection. J Vasc Surg. 2001;34(3):459–64.
19. Murakami M, McDill TL, Cindrick-Pounds L, Loran DB, Woodside KJ, Mileski WJ, et al. Deep venous thrombosis prophylaxis in trauma: improved compliance with a novel miniaturized pneumatic compression device. J Vasc Surg. 2003;38(5):923–927.
20. Shore S, Pienta MJ, Watt TMF, Yost G, Townsend WA, Cabrera L, et al. Non-patient factors associated with infections in LVAD recipients: a scoping review. J Heart Lung Transplant. 2022;41(1):1–16.
21. Johnston J, Stephenson J, Rajgopal A, Bhasin N. "Every patient, every day": a daily ward round tool to improve patient safety and experience. BMJ Open Qual. 2022;11(3):e001829.
22. Pucher PH, Brunt LM, Davies N, Linsk A, Munshi A, Rodriguez HA, et al. Outcome trends and safety measures after 30 years of laparoscopic cholecystectomy: a systematic review and pooled data analysis. Surg Endosc. 2018;32(5):2175–83.
23. Merry AF, Gargiulo DA, Bissett I, Cumin D, English K, Frampton C, et al. The effect of implementing an aseptic practice bundle for anaesthetists to reduce postoperative infections, the Anaesthetists Be Cleaner (ABC) study: protocol for a stepped wedge, cluster randomised, multi-site trial. Trials. 2019;20(1)
24. Alabdulkarim DA, Almohammed OA, Al AMA, Almaklafi NS, Alkathiri MA, Aljohani MA. Venous thromboembolism prophylaxis-prescribing patterns among elderly medical patients in a Saudi tertiary care center: success or failure? J Geriatr Cardiol JGC [Internet]. 2020;17(12):775–81.
25. Chindamo MC, Marques MA. Avaliação do risco de sangramento na profilaxia do tromboembolismo venoso. Jornal Vascular Brasileiro. 2021:20.
26. Huang X, Zhou S, Ma X, Jiang S, Xu Y, You Y, et al. Effectiveness of an artificial intelligence clinical assistant decision support system to improve the incidence of hospital-associated

venous thromboembolism: a prospective, randomised controlled study. BMJ Open Qual [Internet]. 2023;12(4):e002267. [cited 2024 Feb 3]

27. George B, Gonzales S, Patel K, Petit S, Franck AJ, Bovio FJ. Impact of a clinical decision-support tool on venous thromboembolism prophylaxis in acutely ill medical patients. J Pharm Technol. 2020;36(4):141–7.
28. Mohsen A, Kuperman E, McDanel J, Hacker S, Duffy M, Tunning K, et al. Using Electronic Clinical Quality Measures (eCQMs) to perform a venous thromboembolism prophylaxis rapid cycle quality improvement initiative. Joint Comm J Qual Patient Saf. 2019;45(11):750–6.
29. Gibson B, Butler J, Schnock K, Bates D, Classen D. Design of a safety dashboard for patients. Patient Educ Couns. 2020;103(4):741–7.
30. Shaw SJ, Jacobs B, Stockwell DC, Futterman C, Spaeder MC. Effect of a real-time pediatric ICU safety bundle dashboard on quality improvement measures. Joint Comm J Qual Patient Saf. 2015;41(9):414–20.
31. Ansari S, Fung K, MacNeil SD, Nichols AC, Yoo J, Sowerby LJ. The use of standardized order sets to improve adherence to evidence-based postoperative management in major head and neck surgery. Eur Ann Otorhinolaryngol Head Neck Dis [Internet]. 2018;135(5, Supplement):S107–11.
32. Zhou TT, Wang R, Gu SJ, Xie LL, Zhao QH, Xiao MZ, Chen YL. Effectiveness of mobile medical apps in ensuring medication safety among patients with chronic diseases: systematic review and meta-analysis. JMIR Mhealth Uhealth. 2022;10(11):e39819. https://doi.org/10.2196/39819. PMID: 36413386; PMCID: PMC9727690
33. Liu X, Yang G, Xie W, Lu W, Liu G, Xiao W, Li Y. Efficacy of telerehabilitation for total knee arthroplasty: a meta-analysis based on randomized controlled trials combined with a bibliometric study. J Orthop Surg Res. 2024;19(1):874. https://doi.org/10.1186/s13018-024-05381-9. PMID: 39726029; PMCID: PMC11670389
34. Pouliopoulou DV, Macdermid JC, Saunders E, Peters S, Brunton L, Miller E, Quinn KL, Pereira TV, Bobos P. Rehabilitation interventions for physical capacity and quality of life in adults with post-COVID-19 condition: a systematic review and meta-analysis. JAMA Netw Open. 2023;6(9):e2333838. https://doi.org/10.1001/jamanetworkopen.2023.33838. PMID: 37725376; PMCID: PMC10509723
35. Hatef E, Wilson RF, Zhang A, et al. Effectiveness of telehealth versus in-person care during the COVID-19 pandemic: a systematic review. npj Digit Med. 2024;7:157. https://doi.org/10.1038/s41746-024-01152-2.
36. McLean KA, Sgrò A, Brown LR, Buijs LF, Mozolowski K, Daines L, Cresswell K, Potter MA, Bouamrane MM, Harrison EM. Implementation of digital remote postoperative monitoring in routine practice: a qualitative study of barriers and facilitators. BMC Med Inform Decis Mak. 2024;24(1):307. https://doi.org/10.1186/s12911-024-02670-5. PMID: 39434121; PMCID: PMC11492749

Innovation Can Advance Health Equity

Shireen Husami, Nicholas Deleon, Ali Baidoun, and Jocelyn Deleon

Introduction

A. Defining health equity and its significance

Health equity is the condition in which all people have a fair and just opportunity to attain their highest level of health, which entails removing obstacles to health, such as poverty, discrimination, and their consequences [1]. Contemporary syntheses emphasize that equity is not merely a distributive aspiration but an ethical and operational imperative for clinical care and public health: Societies that close unjust gaps achieve better population health, more efficient health systems, and greater social well-being [1].

B. Social determinants of health and structural drivers

A large share of avoidable differences in health arises from the social determinants of health (SDOH), the conditions in which people are born, grow, live, work, and age, structured by the distribution of power, resources, and opportunity [2]. Structural racism operates across housing, education, employment, criminal justice, and health care to produce differential exposure and constrained choices, generating persistent disparities by race and place [3]. Accordingly, equity-oriented strategies must pair clinical improvements with actions targeting upstream drivers and institutional practices.

C. Barriers within the health system: data, design, and diffusion

Even when coverage expands, the features of delivery can entrench inequity. First, the data and algorithms may encode historical disadvantages. A widely used

S. Husami · N. Deleon · A. Baidoun · J. Deleon (✉)
Western Michigan University Homer Styker M.D. School of Medicine, Kalamazoo, MI, USA
e-mail: Shireen.husami@wmed.edu; Nicholas.deleon@wmed.edu; Ali.baidoun@wmed.edu; Jocelyn.deleon@wmed.edu

S. S. Chahin et al. (eds.), *Innovation in Medical Education and Clinical Practice*, https://doi.org/10.1007/978-3-032-19116-8_12

risk stratification algorithm trained to predict healthcare spending systematically underestimated the needs of Black patients; changing the objective reduced racial gaps in referrals for enhanced management [4]. Second, race-based "corrections" embedded in clinical equations have been removed and replaced with race-free formulas (e.g., creatinine–cystatin C and cystatin C-based eGFR), improving diagnostic fairness and accuracy across health systems [5, 6]. Third, the diffusion of new models (e.g., digital health) often favors well-resourced settings, with usability and access hurdles that disproportionately exclude people with limited digital literacy, unstable connectivity, or limited English proficiency. Without explicit gap-closings aims, innovations can widen disparities rather than narrow them [1].

This chapter explores innovation across three interconnected levels of health equity. At the micro-level, we will examine patient-and family-centered approaches, such as culturally tailored education, peer navigation, digital health tools, and community-based support, that improve access and empower individuals. At the meso-level, we will focus on organizational and system redesign, including integrated delivery networks, workforce diversity and retention, hub-and-spoke models, and cross-sector partnerships that align care with community needs. At the macro-level, we discuss broader structural and policy drivers, including payment reform, civil rights protections, infrastructure investment, and accountability frameworks that shape the landscape in which equity efforts succeed. By linking these perspectives, this chapter highlights how coordinated action across levels can drive sustainable and measurable progress towards health equity.

Micro-level Innovations (Individual and Interpersonal Interventions)

Micro-level innovations target individuals, families, and groups to improve health outcomes and reduce disparities, directly engaging with individuals and communities affected by health inequities. Often described as 'grassroots', these strategies lead to changes that are palpable through empowerment, education, and service to the communities and individuals they target. Thus, it is important that they are culturally tailored, community-driven, and rooted in trust-building among the underserved populations. With these principles in mind, micro-level interventions can address barriers to healthcare and build communities.

Community-Based Approach

1. Street Medicine Initiatives—Bringing a Medical Home to the Unhoused
   (a) Street medicine programs are designed to deliver healthcare directly to unhoused and unsheltered individuals in the environments where they reside,

such as in encampments and parks. Unhoused and unsheltered populations often have rates of acute, chronic, and mental illness, which are often comorbid and greater than those of the general population and are exacerbated by being homeless [8]. In fact, some studies have conservatively quoted up to a 2.3-fold difference in mortality between the general public and homeless populations [9]. This approach addresses the critical barriers to equitable healthcare, including transportation challenges, stigma, and lack of documentation, which often prevent this population from accessing traditional healthcare services. Street medicine teams provide a broad spectrum of care, from primary care to behavioral and social services, while utilizing person-centered and harm-reduction strategies [10]. This approach fosters trust and engagement among populations that are often disenfranchised. Trauma-informed and person-centered programs have been shown to improve the quality of life and health outcomes of people experiencing homelessness [11].

2. Community Health Workers

Community health workers (CHWs) play a pivotal role in linking healthcare systems to marginalized communities. These lay individuals deliver health education, facilitate access to care, and navigate social services more cost-effectively than professional healthcare workers do. Additionally, community healthcare workers often share a common language, culture, and socioeconomic status with the individuals they serve, as they are embedded in the communities [12]. This common background enables a peer-to-peer relationship rather than a more traditional provider-client relationship, allowing for more openness. This allows them to serve as valuable, trusted liaisons between individuals and larger healthcare systems.

In Minnesota, Community Health Workers (CHWs) have played a pivotal role in advancing health equity. The state serves as a leading example of how CHWs can be formally integrated into healthcare systems to address health disparities, particularly in racially and ethnically diverse communities. Early on, Minnesota developed infrastructure to support the integration of telehealth into healthcare delivery. This included developing a standardized curriculum and certification process through the Minnesota school systems, enabling CHWs to gain formal recognition in the health workforce [13]. In 2008, the Centers for Medicare and Medicaid Services approved the authorization of hourly payments to CHWs working under the supervision of Medicaid-approved physicians and advanced practice providers, thus establishing a sustainable funding stream [13].

CHWs in Minnesota have been instrumental in serving culturally and linguistically diverse populations, often acting as liaisons between healthcare providers and community members. Because they come from the communities they serve, they have a deep understanding that allows them to address social determinants of health, promote health literacy, and reduce barriers to care. This is especially vital in communities that have historically faced systemic inequities in healthcare access and their outcomes [13].

Additionally, the professionalization of CHWs in Minnesota has provided economic and social benefits to workers. Through training and certification, CHWs gain skills that enhance their employability and earning potential while fostering leadership and empowerment within their communities. This dual benefit of improving population health outcomes and enhancing workforce equity highlights the value of CHWs as both healthcare innovations and investments in underserved communities [13].

Home-Based Healthcare Delivery

1. Home Vaccination Campaigns

Home vaccination programs play a crucial role in addressing disparities in immunization, especially among populations facing mobility limitations, transportation challenges, or medical mistrust. During public health emergencies, such as the COVID-19 pandemic, these challenges can be compounded by the fear of institutional care, further reducing vaccine uptake. As described in the literature, home visits to increase vaccination coverage are among the most resource-intensive strategies but can be particularly impactful in reaching underserved or hesitant populations [14]. Other strategies, such as reminder systems and vaccination programs in schools and community settings, are more cost-effective but may be ineffective in populations with logistical and psychological barriers.

Vaccination programs have emerged as a vital innovation to advance health equity, especially during public health crises, such as the COVID-19 pandemic. An in-home vaccination initiative in Yonkers, NY, found that the program successfully reached older adults who were predominantly female, from racial/ethnic minority groups, and of low socioeconomic status [15]. The inclusion criteria were intentionally broad to avoid excluding vulnerable individuals who may not meet the traditional definitions of disability. The most common motivation for seeking in-home care was being homebound due to disability, especially among those aged 85 and older. Other reasons included transportation barriers, fear of public exposure, and difficulties in navigating digital sign-up systems [15]. For an effective in-home vaccination program, this study emphasizes the need for culturally competent outreach, language translation services, flexible appointment management, and partnerships with local organizations [15]. This emphasizes a key lesson in designing equitable interventions: success depends not only on clinical feasibility but also on reducing administrative barriers and tailoring strategies to meet the needs of the target population.

2. Home Visits for Maternal and Child Wellness

The Mind the Baby initiative demonstrates how culturally competent home-based care can improve maternal and child health outcomes in underserved populations [11]. This program provided regular home visits by nurses and mental health clinicians to medically underserved expectant mothers, beginning in pregnancy and continuing through the child's early years. Through integrated support for parenting, mental health, and infant development, the intervention led to improved outcomes, including a reduction in obesity at age two, especially among Hispanic children, who were initially at elevated risk [11]. These results highlight the impact of embedding culturally and contextually tailored support within the home to effectively reduce disparities, especially in at-risk populations, and promote early life wellness.

Empowering Patients

1. Peer Support Networks

Communities of color and those of lower socioeconomic status often bear a disproportionate burden of chronic disease, yet also share lived experiences that can be harnessed to promote resilience and community. Peer support networks can create spaces where individuals navigate health conditions in the context of their daily lives, while simultaneously building trust, reducing stigma, and enhancing self-efficacy. Evidence from a systematic review demonstrated that across 47 studies, peer support led to significant improvements in health-related outcomes in 94% of cases for a diverse range of conditions, including maternal and child health, diabetes, and other chronic conditions [16]. Critically, these benefits were most pronounced among disadvantaged groups, such as individuals with low health literacy or socioeconomic barriers. In these groups, strategies emphasizing trust and respect were linked to markedly higher retention rates [16]. These findings underscore the adaptability of peer networks across diverse health contexts and their critical role in advancing health equity by engaging and sustaining populations often excluded from conventional healthcare.

2. Culturally Tailored Education

Culturally adapted educational interventions are tools for bridging knowledge gaps and improving health behaviors, particularly within racial and ethnic minority communities that have experienced healthcare inequities and longstanding mistrust of the healthcare system. Effective adaptation involves integrating cultural beliefs, values, and communication styles to enhance the relevance and engagement of the targeted populations. Culturally adapted versions of the Diabetes Prevention Program yielded tangible efficacy and acceptability, as measured by BMI, glucose/insulin levels, and weight loss in their respective target groups [7]. When these cultural factors are deliberately incorporated into educational content and delivery, they foster trust, increase knowledge retention, and promote sustained behavior change. The ability to target interventions is especially important for populations that have historically faced disadvantages. These approaches are essential for equity-driven public health innovation, particularly in the context of increasing population diversity.

3. Health Literacy Interventions

Health literacy, as defined by the CDC, is the degree to which individuals have the capacity to find, understand, and use information and services to inform health-related decisions and actions [17]. Building on this, Liu et al. [18] provided a more complex definition of health literacy. It encompasses skills in processing and gaining new health information, making informed decisions based on that information, and navigating complex healthcare systems to effectively self-manage one's health [18]. In the context of shared decision-making, low health literacy can compromise a patient's ability to advocate for themselves or fully weigh treatment options, making it a crucial component of an effective relationship between a provider and patient. The complexity of health literacy makes it a multifaceted subject that requires multiple levels of intervention, including individual and population-level factors [19].

Health literacy is closely tied to the social determinants of health, such as education, income, language proficiency, and access to care, which shape one's ability to engage effectively with the healthcare system. Individuals with limited health literacy often experience worse health outcomes, not only due to knowledge gaps but also because of structural barriers that inhibit understanding and engagement [20]. In a meta-analysis examining various outcomes, differences in health literacy were associated with increased hospitalization, lower use of preventative and screening services such as mammography and influenza vaccinations, poorer adherence to medications and management of chronic diseases, and in seniors, poorer health and higher mortality [21].

E-health literacy is a vital component of health equity, particularly in an increasingly digitized world. As the use of applications and digital health platforms becomes more ubiquitous, the ability to seek, understand, and use digital health information for informed decision-making becomes increasingly important. Socially disadvantaged groups, often the elderly, those of lower income and education level, and non-English speaking backgrounds, including those with limited reading skills or medical knowledge, are at risk of being marginalized further due to the design of eHealth interventions [22]. A meta-analysis examining the impact of eHealth literacy on eHealth interventions revealed that literacy considerations are often neglected during the development phase [23]. This oversight could pose a significant barrier to care in populations with low eHealth literacy.

To address these gaps, resources such as low-literacy toolkits and decision aids must be designed to be visually engaging, simple and culturally appropriate. The American Heart Association specifically recommends that decision aids and educational materials be simplified and tailored to the literacy level of the target population, using clear language and visual content to enhance understanding and memory retention, thereby supporting equitable participation in shared decision-making and improving care adherence [24]. Routine health literacy screening can identify patients who may benefit from tailored interventions and support the utilization of low-literacy toolkits for effective communication [25]. Additionally, strategies such as teach-back and videos can make information more accessible to patients. The integration of health literacy into school curricula has the potential to improve the health of future generations [24].

Ultimately, advancing health equity through innovation requires a deliberate focus on the eHealth literacy needs of disadvantaged groups, systematic use of low-literacy toolkits, and adoption of health literacy screening to ensure that all patients can meaningfully engage in their care.

4. Targeted Family Programs

Targeted family-based programs, such as Strong African American Families (SAAF) and Familias Unidas, demonstrate the effectiveness of culturally grounded interventions in addressing youth risk behaviors and promoting family resilience. The SAAF program, tailored for rural African American families, strengthens parenting and communication skills to reduce youth conduct problems and substance use [26]. Familias Unidas supports Latinx families through culturally relevant parenting strategies that address the immigrant experience and enhance protective factors [27]. As noted by Boyd et al. [7], these programs are grounded in cultural values and are meant to function within the contexts of their target population's families, schools, and communities, leading to lasting protective outcomes [7]. While these interventions strengthen resilience in the face of many layers of challenges involving individuals and their communities, they do not address the larger systemic and structural stressors that often affect populations. Targeted family programs can play an important role in supporting community initiatives to bolster health equity.

Meso-level Innovations: Community Organizations and Systems of Care

The meso level, including integrated delivery networks, community health centers, public health departments, school-based clinics, and cross-sector coalitions, translates policy into practice and tailors interventions to the local context. This is where redesign directly affects who is reached, how services are offered, and whether innovations close gaps. The following section synthesizes evidence on meso-level strategies with demonstrated or emerging impacts on equity in the United States.

Innovative Care Models

1. Hub-and-Spoke Networks

Regional "hub and spoke" configurations, in which a tertiary or academic hub provides protocols, training, teleconsultation, and quality oversight to community spokes, have been deployed to extend oncology, behavioral health, and other specialty services to rural and underserved communities. Rural residents experience higher cancer mortality and slower gains for several preventable cancers, driven in part by limited access to high-quality care and clinical trials [28, 29]. Reviews highlight hub-and-spoke networks and regionalization, coupled with community partnerships and navigation, as pragmatic levers to improve access and narrow outcome gaps [28]. Evidence from oncology and other domains indicates that when spokes are purposefully sited in high-need areas and supported with telemedicine, workforce development, and shared protocols, access and quality improve for populations historically excluded from specialty care [28, 30].

2. School-Based Health Centers (SBHCs)

Embedding primary and behavioral health services where students already are eliminates common barriers (transportation, time off work, and fragmented care). A national difference-in-differences study (1997–2018) found that county adoption of SBHCs was associated with significant increases in the number of low-income children with a usual source of care and dental visits, alongside large reductions in income-based disparities in insurance coverage and the usual source of care [31]. These population-level gains illustrate how the meso-level placement of services can directly equalize access and utilization, precursors to narrowing outcome gaps.

3. Community-Based Organization (CBO) Partnership

Health systems are increasingly formalizing partnerships with community-based organizations (CBOs) to screen, refer, and follow up on patients' unmet social needs (housing, food, transportation). An implementation science review synthesizing U.S. experience identified multilevel determinants, including payment, cross-sector data exchange, and capacity building in clinics and CBOs, and described five mutually reinforcing activities (awareness, adjustment, assistance, alignment, and advocacy) to integrate social needs care in ways that are sustainable and equitable [32]. Closed-loop referral infrastructures, community care hubs, and shared measurements (that track disparity reduction, not just volume) are meso-level design features that convert screening into resolution.

While these innovative care models reconfigure how and where services are delivered, their impact on equity ultimately depends on how well they resonate with the communities they serve. Expanded access alone does not guarantee meaningful engagement or improved outcomes if programs are not attuned to the cultural contexts, language, and lived experiences. To convert structural innovation into equitable health gains, care models must embed culturally tailored approaches that address barriers and leverage community strength.

Culturally Tailored Chronic-Disease Initiatives

1. Diabetes Prevention and Self-Management

Generic chronic disease programs often underperform in marginalized groups because they do not fit cultural contexts or lived constraints. A 2025 systematic review of culturally tailored Diabetes Self-Management Education and Support (DSMES) for ethnic minority adults found improved uptake and engagement when programs used culturally concordant educators, linguistically appropriate materials, community venues, and social support elements; barriers included language, cost, and fatalism, while local champions and culturally specific strategies facilitated participation [33]. Guidance from the 2025 American Diabetes Association Standards further supports flexible delivery, including telehealth, to expand the reach of DSMES without compromising outcomes in rural and under-resourced settings [34].

2. Retooling Biased Clinical Infrastructure

While community-based tailoring improves individual engagement, system-level reforms are equally critical for sustaining equity. Seemingly technical choices in algorithms and measures can lead to disparities across organizations. The risk stratification example mentioned in the Introduction section demonstrates how measurement objectives can reproduce inequity [4]. Likewise, the adoption of race-free kidney function equations by health systems has been a meso-level infrastructure change that improves diagnostic fairness across populations [5, 6]. Routine governance to audit tools for bias and update them is, therefore, an equity intervention in its own right.

Together, culturally responsive care and equity-oriented infrastructure can address both human and structural dimensions of chronic disease disparities.

Language Access and Workforce Diversity

1. Language-Concordant care and Outcomes

Language barriers impede shared decision-making and adherence to treatment. In a national cohort of adults with hypertension, patient–physician language concordance was associated with a substantially lower risk of major adverse cardiovascular events among allophone speakers compared with language-discordant care [35]. At the meso-level, this translates to staffing, scheduling, and technology policies that prioritize bilingual clinicians, high-quality interpreters across modalities, multilingual portals, and language-concordant outreach.

2. Workforce Representation and Trust

Diversity in the clinical workforce can improve experiences and outcomes via cultural concordance, trust, and advocacy. County-level analyses show that greater Black representation among primary care physicians is associated with higher life expectancy for Black residents and lower Black–White mortality disparities, even after socioeconomic adjustment [36]. Therefore, meso-level strategies, including pipeline programs, targeted recruitment and retention, mentorship, and leadership accountability, are integral components of an equity agenda.

Community-Driven Collaboration and Shared Power

Community-based participatory research (CBPR) offers a durable template for power-sharing in the design, implementation, and evaluation of interventions. Foundational work shows that CBPR enhances the relevance, uptake, and sustainability of programs in marginalized communities by aligning priorities with local knowledge and embedding feedback loops [37]. Recent evaluations in Indigenous communities have demonstrated that co-designed surveillance and case-management systems can reduce suicidal behaviors while increasing the reach of care, underscoring the value of culturally grounded, community-led innovations [38].

Cross-Cutting Meso-level Strategies

Across domains, successful meso-level innovations share common features: [1] explicit gap-closing aims and metrics; [2] place-based delivery that reduces friction for those with the greatest barriers (e.g., school-based SBHCs; hub-and-spoke outreach); [3] culturally and linguistically concordant staffing, tools, and materials; [4] re-engineered data and algorithmic infrastructure to remove encoded bias; and [5] durable partnerships with CBOs, using implementation-science guidance to move from screening to resolution. Together, these strategies translate the aspiration for equity into concrete organizational choices that can be evaluated, scaled, and sustained.

Macro-level Innovations

Structural Reforms

Macro-level innovations that can significantly enhance health equity include solutions targeting specific historical and structural inequalities. These equities are rooted not only in systems of oppression, such as racism and classism, but also in the everyday beliefs that some Americans hold. One specific example of these harmful beliefs is the false belief regarding the biological differences between Black and White people. This belief is not only present in everyday people but also among doctors [43]. This racial bias towards pain perception, which does not have any real basis, results in the African American community being undertreated for their pain symptoms at a systematic level. This bias, along with many other inequities, are all potential targets that could be solved so that marginalized communities can receive equitable healthcare and improve their health outcomes.

One innovative way to target these inequities is at the level of medical education and health care faculty. More specifically, pushing for policies that increase diversity in healthcare teams across the United States. There has been a historical lack of ethnic and racial diversity within medical teams, and adding people who can bridge these cultural gaps will be greatly beneficial to patients in the future. In one study, which examined the diversity of providers across different hospital systems, increased workforce diversity reduced racial health disparities [44]. Improvements were not only seen in the health outcomes of the patients, but improvements were also seen in the overall satisfaction scores of the patients [44].

Furthermore, diversification benefits not only patients but also different industries. For example, studies have shown that diversity in corporate boards improves company productivity and in-company innovation [45]. On a broader level, these findings reveal that diversity has applications beyond just the team treating the patient, but also in non-healthcare-related roles that may still contribute to a person's health, such as urban planning. Therefore, creating and advocating for policies that help create more diversity in the healthcare team is a powerful way to address the many historical and structural inequities that block the achievement of health equity.

Data and Accountability Systems

To ensure that obstacles to health equity are prevented as healthcare continues to develop, data collection is necessary to identify both existing and future disparities that may occur in healthcare. This type of infrastructure allows healthcare workers to immediately see patterns in their respective communities and create solutions that can directly target the problem. For example, during the COVID-19 pandemic, racial minorities were seen to have poorer health outcomes [46]. However, because data infrastructure was not used effectively to track these inequities beforehand, these realizations were only made after the inequities resulted in increased hospitalizations and death from the virus.

Evidently, the infrastructure used in most healthcare systems is not yet up to par with what is necessary to achieve health equity. To achieve this, several changes must be made to the current system. First, it is crucial to have a team with the skills to manipulate data. In general, many existing public health agencies do not have the funding required to maintain a team with these capabilities [47]. Second, many of the current systems used to track health metrics are not optimized for their functions. For example, the CDC operates over 100 surveillance systems that are useful for gathering essential information. However, many of these systems are not properly coordinated with one another and perform redundant tasks, thereby reducing the overall effectiveness of tracking [48]. Moreover, this does not even consider the local and state health tracking departments that operate alongside the CDC's systems, which may also add additional redundancy and wasteful tracking. These problems make it difficult to track and assess problems properly, leading to poorer patient outcomes in communities that would benefit most from this tracking.

For these changes to be realized, more funding is necessary to create a universal system that can track and assess data alongside paying workers who are skilled enough to work with this data. While there have been recent developments in this field due to the challenges faced during the COVID-19 pandemic, it is important that the momentum for these changes is sustained to support the innovations that will create widespread health outcome benefits.

Policy Advocacy for Equity

While equity can be greatly increased at both the micro- and meso-levels of innovation through approaches such as innovative care models and community-based approaches, there are also many benefits to advancing equity through more upstream interventions. For example, policy advocacy can create sustainable change at the systemic level. Once passed, laws and regulations can positively affect millions, especially those in marginalized communities. For example, the Affordable Care Act greatly improved health insurance coverage for both minority groups and people living in poverty [39]. Furthermore, the gaps in adult uninsured rates fell significantly between white and minority communities [40]. Advocating for these policies is therefore vital to creating health equity and better health outcomes for all populations.

However, engaging with local communities is necessary to encourage public advocacy for beneficial policies. Policies are easier to implement when a community understands what the policy is, and the policy itself becomes more effective at addressing the specific challenges that different communities face. Additionally, allowing the community to be active participants has benefits beyond creating and implementing effective policies. Community engagement at this level can also ensure that an implemented policy remains in effect. In one county, opponents of a recently implemented local policy exploited the lack of community knowledge and overturned it within 3 months of implementation [41]. Therefore, it is clear that collective public support and knowledge are necessary to obtain the most benefits. In fact, this approach to involving the community has already been seen to be effective in other areas that are commonly debated, such as environmental protection [42].

However, there does remain some barriers that must be overcome for a community-based approach to be effective in policy implementation. Primarily, framing the actual issue in a way that garners support may prove to be very difficult. Furthermore, communities in which health equity policies will have a significant effect may be environments where systematic oppression has already had a large impact. Despite these potential obstacles, these innovations in policy advocacy will greatly assist in solving the downstream solutions that prevent health equity from being realized in all communities.

Taken together, the innovations described across the micro-, meso-, and macro-levels reveal a clear pattern: structural, community, and clinical strategies can drive equity, but their long-term impact depends on supportive policy environments. Micro-level interventions improve direct care and engagement, meso-level strategies strengthen organizational and community infrastructure, and macro-level innovations address systemic inequities. However, without policy mechanisms to embed, scale, and sustain these changes, their benefits may remain localized and temporary. Therefore, policy advocacy becomes the natural next step, transforming promising innovations into durable, system-wide standards that institutionalize health equity.

Innovation Gaps and Implementation Challenges

Inequitable Access to Innovations

Although there have been many innovations in healthcare over the last several decades, especially in the context of improving health equity, a gap in the accessibility of these advancements continues to exist. Consequently, many communities still face health disparities that exacerbate their health outcomes. Many of these are not even related to healthcare-specific innovations but rather basic community infrastructure. For example, some communities do not have access to clean water and electricity. In Flint, Michigan, for instance, the lead crisis and disease outbreak due to dirty water caused a health crisis that greatly affected the local population [49]. In rural communities, electricity may be difficult to access. This lack of access, paired with hospitals being very far away, makes it clear why these communities have difficulty obtaining all the benefits of healthcare innovations.

In addition to public infrastructure, historical injustices and the marginalization of specific communities continue to negatively affect their respective populations. Race, ethnicity, and socioeconomic status have created disparities despite advancements in civil rights. Consequently, the gap between the less and more marginalized has continued to widen, resulting in poorer health outcomes for those affected [49]. Therefore, policymakers must acknowledge these inequities to ensure that technological and health equity innovations benefit all populations. Although local structures help promote equity in community programs, there is currently no overall system at the federal level that guides larger agencies to consider equity in innovation [49].

Overall, the consequences of inequitable access to healthcare innovations are profound and far-reaching. Innovations can greatly improve health outcomes but will have an even greater impact on the population if they are accessible to all communities.

System Fragmentation

For health equity advancements to be properly distributed, all current systems related to health equity must be interoperable. Currently, a universal platform that can function across all sectors does not exist [48]. This is especially true at the local, state, and federal health department systems levels. There is no cohesion among the different levels of public health agencies. Several groups may have overlapping responsibilities or operate in distinct regions. With over 3000 public health agencies in the country, all of which function independently from one another, optimizing communication and coordination becomes incredibly complex [50]. This can hinder effective responses to public health emergencies, as seen during the COVID-19 pandemic. For instance, there are over 100 surveillance systems that are not properly coordinated and therefore not optimized for providing important information to public health groups [48].

This fragmentation is also true at the level of data sharing. Given the multilayered and complex nature of the health disparity factors a given community may face, it is necessary to have a means to organize that data in a way that allows health departments, research teams, and policymakers to make correct decisions. For example, during the COVID-19 pandemic, data could not be easily exchanged between key stakeholders, which greatly slowed decision-making, thus reducing overall health outcomes [48].

Moreover, public and private healthcare sectors are currently fragmented. Partnerships in this area will allow for more effective data standards that will ease information sharing. Furthermore, public systems need to collaborate more effectively with private departments that deal with community-related problems that may hold new information regarding the social determinants of health.

Finally, the basic infrastructure of electronic data also needs to be improved. Effective responses to public health emergencies require rapid communication of accurate information, which is done electronically. However, as many as 40% of US hospitals are unable to share and receive information through modern electronic reporting systems. These hospitals relied on slower information sharing utilizing fax or phone, which are much more prone to human error [51]. As such, it is crucial for both hospitals and public health agencies to be equipped with the proper infrastructure for rapid and accurate data-sharing. These improvements, along with decreasing the level of fragmentation at all levels of public health, will allow more health innovation benefits to reach the entire population.

Funding and Resource Constraints

Apart from infrastructure and marginalization barriers that prevent the full effects of health equity innovations, there are also large funding gaps that need to be addressed in the future. Improvements at the micro-level, such as telemedicine and community health initiatives, and improvements at the macro-level, such as data infrastructure improvements, require not only massive upfront investment, but also continuous budgeting for operations to sustain them. Despite efforts to address these foundational issues, some analyses report that there continues to be an annual funding gap of $ 4.5 billion [50]. A significant reason for this is the lack of incentives for state and local agencies to match funding. Without federal programs to push for increased investments, the capabilities, benefits, and health equity innovation will continue to be hindered, thus decreasing overall health outcomes.

Future Directions for Innovations and Health Equity

Designing Ecosystemic Frameworks with Emphasis on External Validity

The ecosystemic framework emphasizes that micro-level approaches target individuals and families, meso-level strategies address communities, and macro-level interventions focus on broad policy and structural change, all of which are key to advancing health equity [7]. These layered interventions synergistically prioritize external validity by accounting for the interplay between individual, community, and policy environments. For example, improving outcomes for patients with diabetes can involve ensuring that they understand their treatment regimens through health literacy toolkits, providing community-based support through peer networks, and implementing policies that increase access to insulin and related care.

Boyd et al. argue that scaling health equity interventions entails planning for implementation from the start, requiring adaptable programs [7]. This means designing interventions that function with consideration of variable conditions and can be iteratively adjusted as needs inevitably evolve in dynamic systems. As is commonly seen, macro-level decisions, such as funding or political shifts, can undermine or reinforce micro- and meso-level work. An approach that anticipates such changes prioritizes external validity to bolster function in complex real-world contexts.

Leveraging Community-Based Participatory Research (CBPR) for Comprehensive Impact

To properly assess evolving needs, CBPR should be used to provide a critical foundation for multilevel strategies. While traditional randomized controlled trials maximize internal validity, this often comes at the cost of real-world applicability. CBPR is a model that involves community partners in collaboration with researchers in all stages of the study process to identify problems, set research priorities, design interventions, collect data, and make iterative changes based on outcomes [52]. CBPR ensures that interventions are created with those most affected by inequities, augmenting external validity. It emphasizes engagement with community partners to foster ownership through shared leadership, thus increasing acceptability and supporting sustainability.

Importantly, CBPR informs micro- and meso-level interventions and can catalyze structural change at the macro level. For example, CBPR-informed data and community leadership contributed to policy shifts in Native communities that supported culturally grounded maternal health programs and influenced federal funding priorities in the United States. This case illustrates how community-generated evidence and advocacy can drive policy and resource allocation decisions, bridging local insights with systemic change.

CBPR processes can guide the cultural adaptation of micro-level interventions, inform the prioritization of meso-level structural changes, and strengthen advocacy for macro-level policy reform. By directly linking lived experiences to decision-making processes, CBPR enhances the legitimacy and relevance of policy advocacy efforts. This creates a direct pathway from community-engaged research to systemic transformation, ensuring that health equity gains are not only achieved but also embedded within durable policy and infrastructure frameworks. CBPR facilitates the alignment of local cultural values, community leadership, and evidence-based methods, thus producing measurable health equity gains while critically maintaining cultural integrity and community investment [7, 52].

By directly linking lived experiences to decision-making, CBPR converts community insights into policy and infrastructure changes, creating a clear pathway from engagement to durable, system-level transformation that embeds equity in practice.

Conclusion: A Call to Action

This chapter illustrates how interventions at the micro-, meso-, and macro-levels can augment health equity. Innovation holds transformative potential to reduce health inequities; however, this is only possible if equity is incorporated at every stage, from ideation to implementation. In this chapter, we showed how micro-level strategies (street medicine, CHWs, home-based care, peer networks, health literacy, and culturally adapted education) build trust and improve outcomes for those facing the steepest barriers. At the meso level, delivery-system redesign (hub-and-spoke networks, school-based health centers, CBO partnerships), language access, workforce diversity, and debiased data infrastructure make equity the default in organizations and communities. At the macro-level, structural reforms, interoperable data and accountability systems, and targeted policy advocacy convert local innovations into durable system-wide standards.

However, inequitable access, fragmented systems, and chronic underfunding continue to blunt the impact of these advances and, if unaddressed, can widen existing disparities. The work ahead is therefore ecosystemic: co-designing with communities, operationalizing equity in delivery, and securing it in policy. When these threads are braided together (design, implementation, and institutionalization), innovation moves from promising pilots to measurable and lasting reductions in health inequities.

Ultimately, advancing health equity is not a passive outcome of innovation but must be the central purpose. Innovation achieves its potential when it is co-created with communities, embedded in systems, and secured by policy.

References

1. Prentice KR, Beitelshees M, Hill A, Jones CH. Defining health equity: A modern US perspective. iScience [Internet]. 2024;27(12) [cited 2025 Sep 22]; Available from: https://pubmed.ncbi.nlm.nih.gov/39640575/
2. Marmot M, Allen JJ. Social determinants of health equity. Am J Public Health [Internet]. 2014;104(SUPPL. 4) [cited 2025 Sep 22]; Available from: /doi/pdf/10.2105/AJPH.2014.302200?download=true
3. Bailey ZD, Krieger N, Agénor M, Graves J, Linos N, Bassett MT. Structural racism and health inequities in the USA: evidence and interventions. Lancet [Internet]. 2017;389(10077):1453–63. [cited 2025 Sep 22]; Available from: https://www.thelancet.com/action/showFullText?pii=S014067361730569X
4. Obermeyer Z, Powers B, Vogeli C, Mullainathan S. Dissecting racial bias in an algorithm used to manage the health of populations. Science [Internet]. 1979;366(6464):447–53. [cited 2025 Sep 22]; Available from: /doi/pdf/10.1126/science.aax2342
5. Inker LA, Eneanya ND, Coresh J, Tighiouart H, Wang D, Sang Y, et al. New Creatinine- and Cystatin C–based equations to estimate GFR without race. N Engl J Med [Internet]. 2021;385(19):1737–49. [cited 2025 Sep 22]; Available from: https://www.nejm.org/doi/pdf/10.1056/NEJMoa2102953
6. Pottel H, Björk J, Rule AD, Ebert N, Eriksen BO, Dubourg L, et al. Cystatin C–based equation to estimate GFR without the inclusion of race and sex. N Engl J Med [Internet]. 2023;388(4):333–43. [cited 2025 Sep 22]; Available from: https://www.nejm.org/doi/pdf/10.1056/NEJMoa2203769
7. Boyd RC, Castro FG, Finigan-Carr N, Okamoto SK, Barlow A, Kim BKE, et al. Strategic directions in preventive intervention research to advance health equity. Prev Sci [Internet]. 2023;24(4):577–96. [cited 2025 Apr 21]; Available from: https://pubmed.ncbi.nlm.nih.gov/36469162/
8. Baggett TP, O'Connell JJ, Singer DE, Rigotti NA. The unmet health care needs of homeless adults: a national study. Am J Public Health. 2010;100(7):1326–33.
9. Los Angeles County Department of Public Health C for HIE. Recent trends in mortality rates and causes of death among people experiencing homelessness in Los Angeles County. Br Med J. Los Angeles County. 2019;327
10. Feldman BJ, Kim JS, Mosqueda L, Vongsachang H, Banerjee J, Coffey CE, et al. From the hospital to the streets: bringing care to the unsheltered homeless in Los Angeles. Healthcare. 2021;9(3):100557.
11. Roosa Ordway M, Sadler LS, Holland ML, Slade A, Close N, Mayes LC. A home visiting parenting program and child obesity: a randomized trial. Pediatrics. 2018;141:e20171076.
12. Hill J, Peer N, Oldenburg B, Kengne AP. Roles, responsibilities and characteristics of lay community health workers involved in diabetes prevention programmes: a systematic review. PLoS One. 2017;12:e0189069.

13. Rosenthal EL, Browstein JN. Community health worker- part of the solution.
14. Jacob V, Chattopadhyay SK, Hopkins DP, Murphy Morgan J, Pitan AA, Clymer JM. Increasing coverage of appropriate vaccinations: a community guide systematic economic review. Am J Prev Med. 2016;50:797–808.
15. Jean Struelens M, Castagnoli R, Bhattacharya M, Zhou Meganzhou MS, Copyright fpubh, Zhou MS, et al. OPEN ACCESS EDITED BY Novel in-home COVID-vaccination program for vulnerable populations using public-private collaboration.
16. Sokol R, Fisher E. Peer support for the hardly reached: a systematic review. Am J Public Health. 2016;106:e1–8.
17. US Government CDC Office of Communications. What Is Health Literacy? 2024.
18. Liu C, Wang D, Liu C, Jiang J, Wang X, Chen H, et al. What is the meaning of health literacy? A systematic review and qualitative synthesis. Fam Med Community Health. 2020;8:e000351. BMJ Publishing Group
19. Sørensen K, Van Den Broucke S, Fullam J, Doyle G, Pelikan J, Slonska Z, et al. Health literacy and public health: a systematic review and integration of definitions and models. BMC Public Health. 2012;12:80.
20. Magnani JW, Mujahid MS, Aronow HD, Cené CW, Dickson VV, Havranek E, et al. Health literacy and cardiovascular disease: fundamental relevance to primary and secondary prevention: a scientific statement from the American Heart Association. Circulation. NLM (Medline). 2018;138:e48–74.
21. Berkman ND, Sheridan SL, Donahue KE, Halpern DJ, Crotty K. Low health literacy and health outcomes: an updated systematic review [Internet]. Available from: www.annals.org
22. Kutner, Greenberg, Jin, Paulsen. The health literacy of America's adults: results from the 2003 national assessment of adult literacy. 2003.
23. Cheng C, Beauchamp A, Elsworth GR, Osborne RH. Applying the electronic health literacy lens: systematic review of electronic health interventions targeted at socially disadvantaged groups. J Med Internet Res. 2020;22:e18476. JMIR Publications Inc.
24. White-Williams C, Rossi LP, Bittner VA, Driscoll A, Durant RW, Granger BB, et al. Addressing social determinants of health in the care of patients with heart failure: a scientific statement from the American Heart Association. Circulation. 2020;141(22):e841–63.
25. Olayiwola JN, Magaña C, Kindo B, Soderquist J, Obanua F, Haq F, et al. Screening for health literacy, social determinants, and discrimination in health plans. Am J Manag Care. 2024;30(2):88–94.
26. Brody GH, Chen YF, Kogan SM, Yu T, Molgaard VK, DiClemente RJ, et al. Family-centered program deters substance use, conduct problems, and depressive symptoms in black adolescents. Pediatrics. 2012;129(1):108–15.
27. Pantin H, Prado G, Lopez B, Huang S, Maria IT, Schwartz SJ, Sabillon E, Brown CH, Branchini J. A randomized controlled trial of Familias Unidas for Hispanic Adolescents with behavior problems. Psychosom Med. 2009;71:987–95.
28. Unger JM, McAneny BL, Osarogiagbon RU. Cancer in rural America: improving access to clinical trials and quality of oncologic care. CA Cancer J Clin [Internet]. 2025;75(4):341–61. [cited 2025 Sep 22]; Available from: https://pubmed.ncbi.nlm.nih.gov/40146038/
29. Yabroff KR, Han X, Zhao J, Nogueira L, Jemal A. Rural cancer disparities in the United States: a multilevel framework to improve access to care and patient outcomes. JCO Oncol Pract [Internet]. 2020;16(7):409–13. [cited 2025 Sep 22]; Available from: https://pubmed.ncbi.nlm.nih.gov/32574130/
30. Munhoz R, Sabesan S, Thota R, Merrill J, Hensold JO. Revolutionizing rural oncology: innovative models and global perspectives. Am Soc Clin Oncol Educ Book [Internet]. 2024;44(3):e432078. [cited 2025 Sep 22]; Available from: https://pubmed.ncbi.nlm.nih.gov/38838274/
31. Boudreaux M, Chu J, Lipton BJ. School-based health centers, access to care, and income-based disparities. JAMA Netw Open [Internet]. 2023;6(9):e2334532. [cited 2025 Sep 22]; Available from: https://pubmed.ncbi.nlm.nih.gov/37721750/

32. Kepper M, Walsh-Bailey C, Owens-Jasey C, Gunn R, Gold R. Integrating social needs into health care: an implementation science perspective. Annu Rev Public Health [Internet]. 2025;46(1):151–70. [cited 2025 Sep 22]; Available from: https://pubmed.ncbi.nlm.nih.gov/39476408/
33. Abu S, Llahana S. Factors influencing the uptake of culturally tailored diabetes self-management education and support programmes among ethnic minority patients with type 2 diabetes: a systematic review. Prim Care Diabetes [Internet]. 2025;19(2):103–10. [cited 2025 Sep 22]; Available from: https://pubmed.ncbi.nlm.nih.gov/39894748/
34. Improving Care and Promoting Health in Populations: Standards of Care in Diabetes-2025. Diabetes Care [Internet]. 2025;48(1 Suppl 1):S14–26. [cited 2025 Sep 22]; Available from: https://pubmed.ncbi.nlm.nih.gov/39651974/
35. Reaume M, Labossière MN, Batista R, Van Haute S, Tangri N, Rigatto C, et al. Patient-physician language concordance and cardiovascular outcomes among patients with hypertension. JAMA Netw Open [Internet]. 2025;8(2):e2460551. [cited 2025 Sep 22]; Available from: https://pubmed.ncbi.nlm.nih.gov/39969882/
36. Snyder JE, Upton RD, Hassett TC, Lee H, Nouri Z, Dill M. Black representation in the primary care physician workforce and its association with population life expectancy and mortality rates in the US. JAMA Netw Open [Internet]. 2023;6(4):e236687. [cited 2025 Sep 22]; Available from: https://pubmed.ncbi.nlm.nih.gov/37058307/
37. Wallerstein N, Duran B. Community-based participatory research contributions to intervention research: the intersection of science and practice to improve health equity. Am J Public Health [Internet]. 2010;100((Suppl 1)):S40-6. [cited 2025 Sep 22]; Available from: https://ajph.aphapublications.org/doi/pdf/10.2105/AJPH.2009.184036?download=true
38. Haroz EE, Goklish N, Walsh CG, Cwik M, O'Keefe VM, Larzelere F, et al. Evaluation of the risk identification for suicide and enhanced care model in a native American Community. JAMA Psychiatr [Internet]. 2023;80(7):675–81. [cited 2025 Sep 22]; Available from: https://pubmed.ncbi.nlm.nih.gov/37195713/
39. Lantz PM, Rosenbaum S. The potential and realized impact of the affordable care act on health equity. J Health Polit Policy Law [Internet]. 2020;45(5):831–45. [cited 2025 Sep 22]; Available from: https://openurl-ebsco-com.wmusom.proxy.liblynxgateway.com/contentitem/doi:10.1215/03616878-8543298?sid=ebsco:plink:crawler&id=ebsco:doi:10.1215/03616878-8543298&crl=c
40. Baumgartner J. How ACA narrowed racial ethnic disparities access to health care | Commonwealth Fund [Internet]. 2020 [cited 2025 Sep 22]. Available from: https://www.commonwealthfund.org/publications/2020/jan/how-ACA-narrowed-racial-ethnic-disparities-access.
41. Hossain M. Grassroots innovation: a systematic review of two decades of research. J Clean Prod [Internet]. 2016;137:973–81. [cited 2025 Sep 22]; Available from: https://www.sciencedirect.com/science/article/abs/pii/S0959652616310368?via%3Dihub
42. Calloway EE, Fricke HE, Carpenter LR, Yaroch AL. A qualitative exploration of indicators of health equity embeddedness among public health policy advocacy campaigns. Health Promot Pract [Internet]. 2022;23(3):453–62. [cited 2025 Sep 22]; Available from: https://openurl--ebsco-com.wmusom.proxy.liblynxgateway.com/contentitem/doi:10.1177/1524839920981950?sid=ebsco:plink:crawler&id=ebsco:doi:10.1177/1524839920981950&crl=c
43. Hoffman KM, Trawalter S, Axt JR, Oliver MN. Racial bias in pain assessment and treatment recommendations, and false beliefs about biological differences between blacks and whites. Proc Natl Acad Sci [Internet]. 2016;113(16):4296–301. [cited 2025 Sep 22]; Available from: https://doi.org/10.1073/pnas.1516047113
44. Gomez LE, Bernet P. Diversity improves performance and outcomes. J Natl Med Assoc. 2019;111(4):383–92.
45. Miller T, Del Carmen Triana M. Demographic diversity in the boardroom: mediators of the board diversity–firm performance relationship. J Manage Stud [Internet]. 2009;46(5):755–86. [cited 2025 Sep 22]; Available from: /doi/pdf/10.1111/j.1467-6486.2009.00839.x

46. Mude W, Oguoma VM, Nyanhanda T, Mwanri L, Njue C. Racial disparities in COVID-19 pandemic cases, hospitalisations, and deaths: a systematic review and meta-analysis. J Glob Health [Internet]. 2021;11:05015. [cited 2025 Sep 22]; Available from: https://pmc.ncbi.nlm.nih.gov/articles/PMC8248751/
47. Chandra A, Martin L, Acosta J, Nelson C, Yeung D, Qureshi N, et al. Transforming public health data systems: white papers to inform commission. RAND [Internet]. 2021; [cited 2025 Sep 22]. Available from: https://www.rand.org/pubs/external_publications/EP68744.html
48. Kadakia KT, Desalvo KB. Transforming public health data systems to advance the population's health. Milbank Q [Internet]. 2023;101(Suppl 1):674. [cited 2025 Sep 22]; Available from: https://pmc.ncbi.nlm.nih.gov/articles/PMC10126962/
49. National Academy of Medicine; National Academies of Sciences E and MH and MDB on HSPC on C a F for EST and I in H and M. Taking equity seriously in innovation. Toward equitable innovation in health and medicine: a framework [Internet]. 2023; 1–228. [cited 2025 Sep 22]; Available from: https://www.ncbi.nlm.nih.gov/books/NBK599704/
50. DeSalvo K, Parekh A, William Hoagland G, Dilley A, Kaiman S, Hines M, et al. Developing a financing system to support public health infrastructure. Am J Public Health [Internet]. 2019;109(10):1358. [cited 2025 Sep 22]; Available from: https://pmc.ncbi.nlm.nih.gov/articles/PMC6727291/
51. Holmgren AJ, Apathy NC, Adler-Milstein J. Barriers to hospital electronic public health reporting and implications for the COVID-19 pandemic. J Am Med Inform Assoc [Internet]. 2020;27(8):1306. [cited 2025 Sep 22]; Available from: https://pmc.ncbi.nlm.nih.gov/articles/PMC7313984/
52. Riccardi MT, Valentina P, Marcello DP, Gerardo A, Nurchis MC, Roberta M, et al. Community-based participatory research to engage disadvantaged communities: levels of engagement reached and how to increase it. A systematic review. Health Policy. 2023;137:104905. Elsevier Ireland Ltd

Honing Cultural Humility Can Improve Health Outcomes

Jennifer Lee and Cheryl A. Dickson

Background

The United States of America continues to become more diverse each and every day. The Diversity Index—defined as how likely two people chosen at random will be from different race and ethnicity groups—grew from 54.9% in 2010 to 61.1% in 2020 [1]. Estimates predict that by 2050, approximately 50% of those living in the US will belong to a minority racial or ethnic group [2]. It is only expected that as the US continues to diversify, our health care providers will need to adapt and educate themselves on how to provide sound care to people of many backgrounds.

With this knowledge, increasing awareness has been drawn to evaluating a person's or community's social determinants of health and how they affect their ability to receive adequate and equitable health care. Over the past few decades, attention is being put on the non-financial barriers that impact the patient-physician relationship. This includes mismatches in sociocultural background between patient and provider, lack of provider knowledge of their patient's individual health beliefs and life experiences, and intentional and unintentional acts of bias. The Institute of Medicine had described optimal primary care as having "an understanding of the cultural, nutritional, and beliefs systems of patients and communities that may assist or hinder effective health care delivery" [3]. While taking into consideration a patient's dynamic sociocultural identity is of the utmost importance in primary care, this should be accounted for in all subspecialties in medicine and health care. By the end of this chapter, we will discuss the definition of cultural humility, the clinical history of why this is an important topic to consider in patient care, and how cultural humility impacts the social determinants of health and health outcomes.

J. Lee · C. A. Dickson (✉)
Western Michigan University Homer Stryker M.D. School of Medicine,
Kalamazoo, MI, USA
e-mail: cheryl.dickson@wmed.edu

S. S. Chahin et al. (eds.), *Innovation in Medical Education and Clinical Practice*, https://doi.org/10.1007/978-3-032-19116-8_13

From Cultural Competence to Cultural Humility

Previously, medical training was based in achieving cultural competence. Education was aimed at concretely learning as much as there is to know about a specific cultural subgroup. Essentially, achieving competence meant learning a series of facts and arriving at a pre-defined endpoint through the completion of some form of quantitative assessment of that culture. Even though it is valuable for medical trainees to increase their knowledge of the health beliefs and practices of different cultures and communities, it lends itself to creating a false sense of security in one's training. One may see themselves as a "self-proclaimed expert" because they have learned a slew of facts about a cultural subgroup. However, this can be a harmful model of professional development. It equates having completed a series of training sessions or courses or exams with being culturally competent and negates the lived experiences that each individual has within their own culture.

In the late 1990s, Tervalon and Murray-Garcia shifted the narrative toward the term "cultural humility" [3]. They defined cultural humility as the "commitment and active engagement to the lifelong process of self-reflection as individuals engage with their patients, communities, and themselves". Rather than using the word "competence", the term "humility" allows for more flexibility. It provides individuals the space to admit to themselves and their patients that they do not know the answer when they truly do not know. The ability for health care providers to let go of their ego and express humbleness can strengthen the relationship with their patient at times of unknown.

The lifelong commitment to cultural humility also guides trainees to examine their own patterns of intentional and unintentional acts of bias. It encourages trainees to consciously consider their own multidimensional cultural identities and backgrounds. This includes race, ethnicity, socioeconomic class, religious affiliation, age, sexual orientation, gender identity, language comprehension, and much more. Clinicians can begin to think about how these different facets of sociocultural identity interact with each other. This is a dynamic process where one part of someone's identity may play a larger role depending on the other party they are interacting with. From there, we can examine how the interrelationship of these many facets of identity then shapes an individual's values, beliefs, and behaviors related to health.

Tervalon and Murray-Garcia outlined interventions to implement the principles of cultural humility in patient care. Rather than focusing medical education and professional development on quantitative assessments, they encouraged the use of more qualitative methods. Actions such as journaling, observational learning, interviewing patients, and engaging with community members and organizations, allow trainees the time for self-reflection and critique—both of which are critical to developing skills in cultural humility.

For example, not all of a physician's training should take place in large academic tertiary medical centers. Instead, training should also take place in community clinics and hospitals. The American Academy of Pediatrics, which heavily emphasizes competencies in advocacy, describes medical training in this way to be mutually beneficial. First, by developing a respectful working relationship with the community, clinicians are able to recognize that the focus of expertise is not always within large academic medical centers, but at the heart of the communities they are serving. Second, community members and organizations directly benefit by being able to clearly communicate their health care needs and playing an active role in shaping the way that they receive care.

Clinical History of Cultural Humility

Introduction

Before we explore the progress made in medical education and patient care driven by the principles of cultural humility, it is important to recognize the clinical history of why cultural humility is important to consider. In this section, we will explore different areas of health care, such as mental health, surgical outcomes, and clinical trials, where lack of culturally humility has led to disparities in care.

Call to Action in Pediatrics

In the year 2024, there were approximately 73 million children living in the United States [4] with half being children of color, and 10 million children, or about 14%, living below the poverty threshold. Despite advances in health care research, training, and policy, there are still large disparities in child and adolescent health.

A call to action was made in a 2021 issue of *Pediatrics* [5] for more culturally sensitive interventions in pediatric primary care. It was posited that well-child visits were an excellent starting point to promote health equity. Both vaccine hesitancy and gender and sexual identity are excellent examples where a clinician making space for the patient or family to communicate their unique perspectives and experiences can lend itself to stronger rapport and a more effective clinical plan moving forward.

As an example, there is limited literature on vaccine hesitancy within certain demographics, leading to disparities in rates of vaccine-preventable illnesses within these communities. Rather than health care providers assuming the reason behind a family's hesitancy towards vaccines, needs-based assessments could be conducted with these specific communities to inquire more about their beliefs towards vaccines. By employing principles of cultural humility, clinicians can then provide more personalized counseling geared towards these community-specific questions and concerns. Shared decision-making would allow clinicians and parents to develop plans to help pediatric patients catch up or complete vaccine series, thus decreasing rates of theses vaccine-preventable illnesses.

Other areas that could be explored for more culturally humble care include gender and sexual identity and mental health. Transgender and non-binary youth face significant barriers when seeking sound health care. In individual interviews with young adults aged 18–24 years [6], they identified several key points where physicians could approach care from a humbler perspective. This included "following the lead" of the patient when describing their own anatomy, clearly addressing patient concerns about confidentiality and privacy, and the burden of the patient having to educate their clinician on their identity and needs. Suggestions were made for the development of a rubric on providing culturally humble care, such as starting clinical encounters by asking patients what pronouns they identify with. The balance of clinical competence and cultural humility in these encounters leads to more effective communication and positive patient-provider relationships.

Mental Health Services for Black, Indigenous, and People of Color (BIPOC)

There are many factors that contribute to minority adolescents having less access and lower quality of mental health care compared to their White counterparts [7]. These include but are not limited to systemic discrimination, the history of health care for the BIPOC community, health care organization structures, and financial limitations. Through the lens of cultural humility, more attention is being drawn to how the inherent aspects of the clinical encounter can contribute to disparities in mental health care for BIPOC youth. Such considerations include the demographics of the mental health care provider and their attitude toward the patient. The clinician's expectations and behaviors—both conscious and unconscious—toward the patient can be impacted by the racial and ethnic background of the patient. Similarly, the patient's perception of the clinician and reception to care can also be influenced by the racial and ethnic background of the clinician.

There is evidence that the therapeutic alliance between BIPOC youth and their mental health care provider was improved when their provider adopted elements of cultural humility in their clinical practice [7]. Patients perceived their provider as less likely to commit microaggressions toward them and that if these transgressions were to occur, the health care provider was better able to acknowledge their wrongdoing, recover, and repair the therapeutic alliance they had built. Overall, this led to patient reports of improvement in therapy [7].

Below are a couple of examples of how institutions adopted the principles of cultural humility and drove changes in the way they were providing mental health services to racial and ethnic minority groups. At Mass General Hospital Center for Cross-Cultural Student Emotional Wellness, it was recognized that Asian students, especially those who had grown up outside of the US, had difficulties adjusting to life on campus and were developing maladaptive coping skills [8]. Especially in the wake of the COVID-19 pandemic where Asians in America were facing increases in prejudice and discrimination, more needed to be done to support the mental health of students of Asian background. To accomplish this, didactic teachings and case presentations have been implemented for educators to discuss the mental health of Asian American and Asian international students. Curriculum for faculty also began to focus more on developing cultural humility skills to avoid making overgeneralizations about their students of Asian backgrounds and better support this goal.

After the murder of George Floyd in 2020, New York University's Department of Child and Adolescent Psychiatry bolstered their curriculum to include more training about the principles of cultural humility. The curriculum was focused on faculty reflecting on their own identity. It encouraged White members of their department to explore White privilege and its impact on systemic racism while also empowering BIPOC colleagues to advocate for social justice [9].

Both of these examples in Boston and New York serve as lessons in continuous reflection of our own individual biases as well as the exploration of the lived experiences of others. Both of these processes are increasingly important as clinicians provide care to our ever-diversifying population and in relation to global current events.

Disparities Amongst Surgical Patients

Concepts of cultural humility apply not only to primary care services but to surgical subspecialties as well. There have been noticeable disparities in both surgical outcomes and post-operative care for minority patients compared to White patients [2]. In vascular surgery, Black patients account for 12% of open surgical procedures and 10% of endovascular surgeries for limb salvage, but make up 29% of major lower extremity amputations, leading to higher morbidity and lower quality of life. In pediatric surgery, it is found that non-White neonates with congenital diaphragmatic hernias had approximately 50% increased risk of mortality compared to White neonates when controlling for other pertinent covariables. With regard to trauma surgery and care, Black patients had worse functional outcomes, especially when a traumatic brain injury was present. Cardiac surgery also presents with significant disparities in types of care where Black and Hispanic adults are less likely to receive invasive cardiac procedures, such as angioplasty, bypass surgery, and thrombolytic therapy. Most commonly known amongst physicians is the discrepancy in pain management between racial and ethnic groups. Black patients are often not believed by their physicians in the severity of their pain, and consequently, not provided with adequate multi-modal pain control [10]. This is most highlighted in those undergoing general and orthopedic surgeries.

In addition to disparities in surgical procedures and post-operative outcomes, there is also a significant disparity in the racial and ethnic demographics of surgical providers. While 77% of surgeons are White, only 2% of surgeons are Black and only 3% are Hispanic [2]. As has been discussed above with regard to mental health providers, it is important to consider how the demographics of our surgical providers may affect evaluating patients for types of surgeries, assessing post-operative pain control, and thus, long-term morbidity from these procedures. Additionally, there was interesting data found when surveying surgical providers about these disparities in patient outcomes. Even among those who acknowledged the existence of these discrepancies in care, 91.4% of surgeons believed they were attributed to factors related to the patient only. They did not recognize factors related to the provider, social determinants of health, or power structures within our health care system as possible contributors [2].These findings highlight the need for overhauls in medical education with an emphasis on practicing the principles of cultural humility in all subspecialties of medicine.

Research and Clinical Trials

Just as important as applying the principles of cultural humility is to patient encounters at the clinic and in the hospital is their application in the clinical research trials that guide physicians counseling and therapeutic plans. There are various populations that continue to be underrepresented in clinical research trials, including women as a whole and people of color. Their inclusion—or lack thereof—can play a part in disparities in clinical outcomes because results cannot be as easily generalized to the greater population as a whole.

For example, across the world, BIPOC patients bear the greatest burden of cardiovascular disease but only make up a small portion of those enrolled in randomized controlled trials [11] Even with this knowledge, the percentage of BIPOC participants did not show an increase from 2000 to 2020. The demographics of those participating in cardiovascular health related clinical trials is still made up of a rather homogenous group—North American and European White males. As stated above, this makes results of these trials difficult to generalize to the overall population as race, ethnicity, and gender may influence the efficacies of these treatments. Even biologically, there are discrepancies in the way that different ethnic and racial groups metabolize medications due to minute variations in our genetics. For instance, studies have also shown that angiotensin-converting enzyme (ACE) inhibitors appear less effective in blood pressure reduction in Black adults compared to their White counterparts. Additionally, 86% of Asians carry a genetic variant that is associated with increased warfarin-related bleeding compared to other ethnic groups, and 75% of Pacific Islanders are unable to convert clopidogrel to its active form, resulting in higher risks of adverse outcomes in those at risk of ischemic events [11].

It is also important to consider that racial, ethnic, and gender identities can influence the effects of treatment because of their dynamic relationship with other facets of identity, such as socioeconomic status, transportation access, or the geographic region where they live. Without the inclusion of a diverse population in clinical research trials, it would be difficult to know if these covariables play a part in the efficacy of a treatment. For example, a Black male patient recently diagnosed with hypertension may be given a prescription to start an ACE inhibitor and was counseled by his physician on healthier lifestyle habits. Even without considering how a patient's genetic makeup influences the way they metabolize the medication, healthier lifestyle habits may not be a feasible goal if someone lives in a food desert, a community filled higher air pollutants, or a neighborhood without accessible, safe parks to exercise in.

In addition to not being able to generalize clinical trial results to the overall population, under enrollment of BIPOC in clinical trials deprives them of the benefits of participation. These include closer monitoring, more frequent follow-up appointments, and earlier access to potential beneficial therapies that are often implemented at the end of the trial.

There are multiple strategies that can be implemented to increase cultural humility in randomized controlled trials. Programs can begin by ensuring that research leaders are representative of the diversity of the population that their research is meant to benefit. It should be encouraged that they engage community members and organizations when formulating their research question, designing their methods, and recruiting for and disseminating information about their clinical trial. Protocols should avoid framing exclusion criteria based on language, socioeconomic status, or geographic region. For instance, clinical research trials can provide informational materials tailored to the language and health literacy of the community they are meant to benefit. By integrating the principles of cultural humility into the way that clinical trials enroll participants, results can be made more applicable to the growing diversity of our population and more accurately predict treatment effects in various populations.

Innovation in Medical Education

Training in Cultural Sensitivity

Self-reflection and recognition of our own implicit biases is a key facet in cultural humility. Everyone has implicit bias and it is important to develop skills so it does not affect our future clinical practice behaviors. When implicit biases show themselves during a clinical encounter, it can contribute to health disparities because it can influence the provider's communication practices and potentially their medical decision making [12].

Currently, the Liaison Committee on Medical Education (LCME) has standards listed for structural competence, cultural competence, and health inequities. They have begun to shift from culturally "competent" health care toward evolving frames of thought of cultural humility. Standard 7.6 states that "faculty of a medical school [should] ensure that the medical curriculum provide opportunities for medical students to learn to recognize and appropriately address biases in themselves … and in the health care delivery process" [13]. Even with the medical community having increased awareness of this, the approach to educating medical students and residents is varied and limited. There are also gaps present in faculty training and professional development for health care leadership [14].

Surveys have shown that in order for faculty to help students develops their skills in cultural humility, we should be implementing strategies that are multi-modal and longitudinal [15]. Additionally, suggestions have been made for how to balance creating a safe learning environment, normalizing bias, and reducing self-blame. In this next section, we will discover innovations in medical education, specifically creating virtual and simulation-based learning environments to dive deeper into personal biases and how to communicate with a diverse population of patients in a culturally humble way.

A concrete example of medical education programs putting this philosophy into action can be seen in clinical skills education [16]. Students are taught to begin each clinical encounter with creating a mutual agenda with their patient to ensure that the most pressing medical conditions are worked up and that the patient's concerns are adequately addressed. After taking a careful history, students are also instructed to elicit the patient's perspective of their symptoms and how it has been impacting their day-to-day life. Open-ended questions allow patients to tell their own wellness or illness story without interference from their provider. Practicing clinical encounters in this way eliminates the need for the clinician to completely master every group's health beliefs. The patient is the ideal narrator to tell their own story and can communicate how little or how much their sociocultural identity has to do with each particular symptom or complaint [17]. This then allows for an easy transition to shared decision-making conversations that can lead to more relevant, personalized, and effective preventative care and treatment strategies.

Virtual Simulation Games to Explore Hidden Bias and Racism

Most training in health care professions, such as nursing or medical school, do not directly address issues of racism—whether it is an interaction between patient and provider or provider and provider. One study at the University of Southern Ontario, Canada directly noted that their nursing program curriculums excludes what their students should do if they personally experience racism or witness it [18]. Nursing faculty also reported feeling uncomfortable and unprepared to discuss racism with their students or how to address racist incidents when they occur to students or other colleagues.

To combat this, their program created a didactic presentation and virtual simulation through the A-CHARM nursing project—otherwise named Addressing Culturally based Hidden bias and RacisM. They aimed to examine learner engagement, usability, and effectiveness of the virtual simulation games as an educational intervention for cultural humility and cultural awareness [18].

The simulation experience entitled "Nik's story" showcased Nik, a fourth-year male nursing student of East Indian descent. He arrived at orientation on his final clinical rotation on a medicine unit at the local hospital with two classmates, James and Sarah. They are introduced as Nik's White peers also completing their final rotation on the same unit. During their lunch break, Nik overhears Sarah make a racist comment about the number of immigrant nurses working in the clinical setting. The virtual simulation game then proceeds with nine different decision points with three different choices each on how one might respond to the scenario. Throughout "Nik's story," the Microaggression Triangle Model was introduced, which describes appropriate steps that could be taken by the source, the recipient, and the bystander of the microaggression. After completion of the virtual module paired, learners participated in an accompanying didactic session.

Surveys of participants showed that there was a significant positive change in cultural diversity awareness. Participants rated the learning experience highly in effectiveness, learner engagement, and usability. They reported that virtual simulation games such as "Nik's story" allowed them to think more deeply about racism, how to address it, and cultural humility awareness.

Virtual simulation games provide a safe learning environment to explore sensitive topics, such as hidden bias, racism, and inappropriate comments and actions in the workforce. It is an effective method to foster a perceived sense of a lived experience. The virtual, private setting also allows students to choose between the various decision points without fearing judgement from peers or faculty. This enables exploration of this often-daunting topic in a non-threatening way.

Simulation-Based Education in Pediatric Residencies

The way in which children are brought up and raised varies greatly between families and communities. Sociocultural identities have a large influence over what dietary habits look like, schooling and extracurricular activities, and even the sleeping arrangements within a household. While the American Academy of Pediatrics (AAP) strongly recommends against the practice of co-sleeping or bed-sharing due to risks of accidental suffocation and sudden infant death syndrome, it is a common practice across the world. More than half of mothers born in Asia practice this tradition and it is a practice that is becoming more common in the United States. Pediatricians may face challenges during safe sleep counseling, due to provider's lack of cultural understanding, language barriers, and conflicting opinions within families. This can lead to the inability to develop rapport with patient families, and ultimately broad, distrust in medical advice.

The Department of Pediatrics at Indiana University aimed to use simulation-based education to help residents develop techniques on how to counsel about safe sleep across cultures and to reflect on their own skills in cultural humility [19]. Faculty identified that co-sleeping—a common practice amongst their Burmese patient population—was a point of disagreement often seen between this community and their pediatricians. A simulation was then developed in partnership between a local Burmese refugee organization, the medical director of their newborn unit, and simulation faculty. The scenario involved a 4-week-old male's first well-child visit, played by a trained standardized patient (SP). Residents either asked about the families sleeping situation or were prompted by the SP bringing up worries about the death of a child in her community due to co-sleeping. Directly after completing the simulation, residents were allowed time to debrief, including hearing the perspectives from the SP on their safe sleeping counseling, verbal and written information about safe sleep, and risk mitigation strategies. They were also provided general guidance on how to confidently approach conversations with open-ended questions and a judgement-free tone.

Pre- and post-surveys completed by residents showed they not only felt more confident providing counseling on safe sleep but also felt better prepared to engage in difficult conversations with diverse patient populations. Residents also reported learning valuable skills to improve the care of future patients. Further reflection on the simulation showed that while it was important to learn about proper safe sleep recommendations, they had not received education on risk mitigation for co-sleeping. Cultural humility skills were put into practice by recognizing that it is essential to consider the family's beliefs, perspectives, and environment when engaged in shared-decision making. In topics like safe sleep where strict adherence to AAP recommendations may not be feasible due to cultural traditions or practical reasons, it is important to work with the family to create the safest possible environment for their infant.

Simulation based education like the one described here emphasized the principles of cultural humility both in its development and its facilitation. By conducting a needs-based assessment with the local community, faculty were able to identify a gap in pediatric care. The simulation also utilized a Burmese woman partaking as a standardized patient who could provide her own unique perspective on how this conversation would typically take place at the clinic and provide advice to residents on how to improve communication skills. Overall, simulation-based education allows for a controlled environment where learners can explore how to have difficult conversations prior to having them with real patients in the clinical setting.

Innovation in Diagnostic Testing

There are many factors that cause communities to have unreliable access to adequate health care services. These include economic limitations, geographic regions, transportation limitations, and access to means of communication, such as email or phone. Point-of-care testing enables health care providers to break down some of these barriers. As defined by the International Organization for Standardization, point-of-care (POC) testing is performed near or at the site of a patient with the result leading to possible change in the care of the patient [20]. In this section, we will examine how technological advancements in point-of-care testing have revolutionized diagnostics in low-resource areas and can improve long-term patient outcomes. Because diagnostic testing is able to take place in low-resource settings at immense speeds, patients are able to receive higher quality personalized treatments before needing to be seen in the clinic again.

Point-of-Care Tests Decreasing the Burden of HIV and Other Sexually Transmitted Infections

The European Center for Disease Prevention and Control affirms that POC testing can be a possible solution in reducing health disparities. They state that it can play a "critical role in rapidly diagnosing both infectious and non-infectious diseases and is not only for appropriate and timely treatment but also for the detection of outbreaks and controlling the rapid spread of infectious diseases" [20]. For instance, medical laboratories in Africa often cannot meet the demands of rapidly growing health care delivery. This leads to inadequate diagnostic services, resulting in misdiagnosis and potentially the under or over treatment of a patient's condition. But, POC testing has revolutionized care for individuals living with HIV across Africa. POC viral load testing has a high sensitivity and specificity for the diagnosis of HIV viral load at or above the clinical threshold of 1000 copies/mL, enabling real-time treatment to enhance viral suppression. Additionally, POC lateral flow urine lipoarabinomannan assays have helped to improve tuberculosis detection by lowering diagnostic turn-around times for those living with HIV.

Another application of POC testing is seen in the testing and treatment of sexually transmitted infections (STIs) during pregnancy [21]. STIs are associated with multiple adverse pregnancy and birth outcomes, including miscarriage, pre-term birth, and neonatal eye and respiratory infections. Because of this, the World Health Organization recommends HIV and syphilis testing for all pregnant women attending prenatal clinic visits. Access to STI testing and treatment in low- and middle-income countries can be limited due to multiple socioeconomic, geographic, and cultural barriers. Additionally, there are barriers created in the medical procedures and practices themselves. Previously, these were done by syndromic management or with laboratory-based testing. Syndromic management involved clinicians identifying signs and symptoms associated with various STIs and treating to resolve those symptoms. Laboratory-based testing is dependent on trained personnel, involves waiting up to several days for results, and providing treatment at a later clinic visit. With POC testing becoming more widely available, pregnant patients can receive adequate personalized care at the time of their single prenatal clinic visit and receive treatment to prevent adverse outcomes related to these infections. By meeting patients where they are at and providing real-time diagnostic information, clinicians are able to provide high-quality, equitable, personalized care all in one visit.

Cultural Humility Principles in Action: The Kidney Check Program

Indigenous communities in Canada living in rural and remote geographic areas face various socioeconomic and environmental disparities. This results in limited preventative health services and lack of continuity of care. Because of this, Indigenous populations face higher prevalence of chronic disease diagnosed at younger ages and with higher severity. But, if diagnosed earlier and at lower severity, these conditions can be optimized with lifestyle changes and medications. Otherwise, patients are often faced with sub-optimal management or have to leave their support networks to receiving life-saving treatments, such as dialysis.

In response to these gaps in health equity, the Kidney Check program was launched in 2018 to identify diabetes, hypertension, and chronic kidney disease in Indigenous peoples throughout Canada [22]. Protocols for this program were developed after several years of collaboration between patients, caregivers, community leaders, Indigenous people, researchers, and policy makers. The Indigenous community were included at every level of decision-making and feedback for this program. Community leaders and elders contributed to its success by providing insight on each specific community's cultural practices, how to best engage their people, and how best to use local resources. Health care providers involved are dedicated to approaching each community respectfully to converse about their individual needs, cultures, and practices.

During a Kidney Check screening, patients first watch a video about the purpose and processes involved prior to giving their consent. Each patient has their blood pressure taken to screen for hypertension. Then, finger prick droplet samples are collected and analyzed using an iSTAT Alinity analyzer to evaluate their electrolytes and kidney function. Lastly, DCA Vantage analyzers are used to determine the patient's urine albumin-to-creatinine ratio and Hgb A1c to evaluate patients for diabetes and diabetic nephropathy. With all of the available diagnostic data, an iPad application is used to calculate the patient's estimated glomerular filtration rate (eGFR) and their risk of developing kidney failure in the next 2–5 years using the Kidney Failure Risk Equation. Regardless of risk, patients are given resources about a holistic approach to kidney health—resources that were developed with Indigenous patient partners. Those at high risk for kidney failure are referred for more detailed evaluation by nephrology teams and are given suggestions for pharmacologic management. At the end of each screening, health care providers turn all data that was collected to the local communities to be stored or used how they see fit.

The team involved in the Kidney Check program emphasize promoting cultural safety and principles of self-determination. Providers turned to the expertise of the Indigenous communities to determine how best to care for them. Because their POC testing model allows for minimal to no specimen transport, minimal training needed to perform tests, and tests being performed in front of or near patients, it allowed for health care to be more effective, affordable, and equitable. Faster turn-around times enabled clinicians to make timely, personalized care decisions. The Kidney Check program allowed for effective shared decision-making, empowering Indigenous communities to act on the knowledge they are given by immediate results and create plans to improve their health.

Innovation in Patient Communication

With the advent of mobile technology, there have been numerous innovations in clinical care that align with the principles of cultural humility. Mobile devices make health care information more accessible and understandable to each individual patient. Mobile applications allow patients to access office notes, message their health care provider directly, and view lab results as soon as available. In this section, we will discuss how mobile technology has begun to break down language barriers, especially in areas that may not have access to diverse in-person translation services, thus greatly improving patient-provider communication.

Mobile Technology for Medical Interpretation in Spoken Languages

According to US Census data, approximately 22% of those ages 5 and older speak a language other than English at home and 8.4% classify themselves as speaking English less than "very well", otherwise categorized as Limited English Proficient [23]. Language non-congruence between patients and clinicians poses a significant barrier to accessing equitable health care. This can lead to patients incomplete understanding or complete misunderstanding of their diagnosis and treatment plan, further resulting in missed follow-up appointments, incorrect home medication regimens, and dissatisfaction with care. Language barriers can strain our health care providers system-wide. Misunderstandings can lead to wasteful resource utilization, increased ER visits and longer hospital stays, unnecessary procedures, or inappropriate medications and interventions. Overall, this can lead to increased negative outcomes, such as lower rates of physician visits, lower participation in preventative services, and have decreased quality of care.

Prior to technological advancements in interpretation services, in-person interpreters would need to be consulted. Barriers to in-person interpretation included extended patient wait times and difficulty finding qualified interpreters in less commonly spoken languages for that particular community. It was not uncommon to use family members to help translate between patients and providers. But, without proper training in medical interpretation, it could lead to incorrect translation, misdiagnosis, incorrect treatment plans, and ethical issues with patient confidentiality and privacy.

Systematic reviews have shown that the use of medical interpreters improves clinical care for patients who do not share the same language as their health care provider when compared to the absence of interpreters or the use of ad-hoc interpreters or family members. In an assessment of the portable and shareable devices that can be used during patient encounters for medical interpretation, two major themes of technology use were found [24].

First was the use of mobile technology as a liaison for human interpreters either through audio or video contact. Many hospital and clinic systems throughout the US utilize this type of technology either with a designated phone in the clinic or a tablet rolled that can be brought into each patient room as needed. Both patients and providers showed preference for interpretation modalities that allowed their interpreter to meet face-to-face either in person or over video call. The use of this service also allowed for decreases in overall clinical encounter times and patient wait times. Physicians also noted that face-to-face interpretation made it easier to discern if interpreters were having trouble conveying medical information and needed more clarification from the provider. This method is also ever important when caring for the D/deaf and hard of hearing community whose first language is sign language, which will be discussed further.

Second was the use of interpretation technology as a direct translation tool with both health care and non-health care specific applications that could be easily downloaded on shared mobile devices. Health care-specific applications, such as X-prompt and CALD assist, use voice-over prompts, written pre-set sentences, and pictorial diagrams that are often used in basic history taking or emergency assessments. Non-health care-specific applications, such as Google Translate, are best utilized for common bedside dialogue rather than interpretation of complex medical diagnoses and therapeutic plans.

There are several limitations that must be considered when using this type of technology. Patients with visual and/or hearing deficits may find these applications difficult to use. Additionally, clinicians that may be unfamiliar with using this type of technology will need additional training before it can be implemented. Spatial limitations can also impact the use of medical technology for interpretation. This includes device placement in patient rooms, connectivity to internet, and proper privacy for both patients and interpreters. There are stark differences in the number of qualified interpreters available depending on the language or specific dialect needed. Rarer languages may need to rely solely on non-health care-specific translation that could result decreased quality and accuracy of the translation. Still, evolving technology can play a key role in breaking down language barriers and building rapport through common conversations. Communities that previously had been completely cut off from receiving health care services can begin to access this system through these innovations in interpretation services.

Video Relay Interpretation for the D/deaf and Hard of Hearing Community

As discussed above, communications technology continues to evolve to enable more effective communication for various marginalized communities in health care settings. Persons who are D/deaf—"Deaf" refers to the linguistic minority while "deaf" refers to those with hearing impairment—and hard of hearing (DHH) who use sign language as their first language is one such community. Overall, the DHH community tends to belong to lower socioeconomic statuses. They are more likely to avoid health care providers than those without hearing impairments and also have lower health literacy, possibly due to insufficient knowledge of medical-related vocabulary. This community also has a greater prevalence of obesity, hypertension, and self-reported depression and with less access to health care, these conditions are often under-diagnosed and under-treated.

A systematic review evaluated the use of video remote interpretation (VRI) and assessed whether this technology can enable the DHH community to overcome barriers and improve communication outcomes between them and health care professionals [25]. Early evidence shows that VRI is as equally efficient as in-person interpretation. Prior to these technological advancements, lipreading and note-reading were employed, especially when access to in-person sign language interpretation was limited. But, this assumes that sign language users are proficient in reading and writing in a spoken language, which may not be true. Instead, advantages of VRI include its flexibility, affordability, and ability to override the need for techniques like lipreading and note-reading. It was shown that patient and provider satisfaction has increased with the use of VRI in health care settings and it was recommended that it was best supported with devices with large screens, reliable internet connection, and qualified interpreters.

VRI has the potential to address communication barriers for the DHH community within health care settings, but there are still some limitations. This type of interpretation service is often considered inappropriate for critical care and stressful situations. Sign language interpretation is also dependent on spatial limitations, such as positioning of the tablet or computer, and certain views may make it more difficult for interpreters to identify visual cues for when DHH patients are not fully comprehending their diagnosis or treatment plan instructions. We can apply the principles of cultural humility to further advancing this technology by taking into account the views, beliefs, and perspectives of the patients using it. The D/deaf and hard of hearing community should play a crucial role in its improvement and implementation in various health care services [26].

World Health Organization Be Healthy Be Mobile Initiative

Estimates of 41 million people per year die from noncommunicable diseases each year. This does not include the burden of disease across the world and its negative effect on quality of life from conditions such as cardiovascular disease, cancer, chronic respiratory diseases, and diabetes. To bring more attention to this global crisis, a partnership was formed between the World Health Organization and the International Telecommunication Union to create the Be Healthy Be Mobile initiative [27].

This program aims to change the way that people across the globe access information about their own health. More than 7 billion people globally have mobile telephone subscriptions, with some parts of the world having more reliable access to a phone than to clean water resources. This initiative focuses on using SMS messaging services to educate individuals about noncommunicable diseases and their risk factors. Their program boasts partnerships with private organizations that are focused on this same mission to help create health content and technical support for each health program. For example, over 2 million people in India have enrolled in their mobile health program to quit the use of tobacco products. Over 500,000 people have received education on cervical cancer in Zambia. Several thousands have received education on diabetes management in various low- and middle-income countries. These health programs are built to encourage, reinforce, and sustain the use of health services in the individual's home country while also promoting health and well-being.

Conclusion

Even though the concept of cultural competence was meant to equip health care providers with the knowledge of various cultures in an attempt to provide more directed care to patients, it still had its limitations. Competence training varies widely depending on the medical education curriculum—from yearly video modules to month long integrated curriculums. It can also give trainees a false sense of confidence and mastery and lends itself to creating an unfounded power differential over the patient, as if the provider knew the patient's dynamic identity more than the patient themselves [28]. This can further reinforce stereotypes and lead to care that ignores the patient's insight into their own condition. Additionally, it has been shown that an increase in clinician cultural competency does not equate to consistently improved patient satisfaction, health outcomes, or a decrease in health disparities.

Instead, the concept of cultural humility acknowledges that one's culture is a dynamic state and can be influenced by one facet more at a particular point in time compared to another. By shifting frames of thought to one of a lifelong process of self-reflection, we are able to create a non-judgmental learning and professional environment, and thus, make space for health care providers to humbly admit their lack of knowledge. Health care providers should think critically about this concept long before a clinical encounters take place. They should take stock in their own biases and blind spots. They should acknowledge how social and economic factors shape a patient's diagnosis and treatment prior to them stepping into an exam room [29]. By taking this time to self-reflect, it encourages open communication with patients to provide their unique perspective on their health journey and allow for shared decision making with their clinician.

References

1. Menchaca A, Pratt B, Jensen E, Jones N. United States Census Bureau. 2023. Examining the Racial and Ethnic Diversity of Adults and Children.
2. Smith CB, Purcell LN, Charles A. Cultural competence, safety, humility, and dexterity in surgery. Curr Surg Rep Springer. 2022;10
3. Tervalon M, Murray-García J. Cultural humility versus cultural competence: a critical distinction in defining physician training outcomes in multicultural education. J Health Care Poor Underserved. 1998;9(2):117–25.
4. Children [Internet]. [cited 2025 Oct 29]. Available from: https://www.census.gov/topics/population/children.html
5. Kibakaya EC, Oyeku SO. Cultural humility: a critical step in achieving health equity. Pediatrics. American Academy of Pediatrics. 2022;149
6. Reeves K, Job S, Blackwell C, Sanchez K, Carter S, Taliaferro L. Provider cultural competence and humility in healthcare interactions with transgender and nonbinary young adults. J Nurs Scholarsh. 2024;56(1):18–30.
7. Yan Li AS, Lang Q, Cho J, Nguyen VS, Nandakumar S. Cultural and structural humility and addressing systems of care disparities in Mental Health Services for Black, indigenous, and people of color youth. Child Adolesc Psychiatr Clin N Am. W.B. Saunders. 2022;31:251–9.
8. Lim CT, Chen JA. A novel virtual partnership to promote Asian American and Asian international student mental health. Psychiatr Serv. 2021;72(6):736–9.
9. Lekas HM, Pahl K, Fuller Lewis C. Rethinking cultural competence: shifting to cultural humility. Health Serv Insights. 2020;13
10. Lombardero A, Assemi KS, Jacobs NN, Houmanfar RA, Trejo S, Szarko AJ. An Acceptance and Commitment Training (ACT) framework for teaching cultural humility: a guide for translating ACT from a therapeutic context into a medical education curriculum. J Clin Psychol Med Settings. 2023;30(2):261–73.
11. Zhu JW, D'Angelo F, Miranda JJ, Yancy CW, Cupido B, Zannad F, et al. Incorporating cultural competence and cultural humility in cardiovascular clinical trials to increase diversity among participants. J Am Coll Cardiol. 2022;80(1):89–92.
12. Gonzalez CM, Lypson ML, Sukhera J. Twelve tips for teaching implicit bias recognition and management. Med Teach. 2021;43(12):1368–73.
13. Functions and Structure of a Medical School Standards for Accreditation of Medical Education Programs Leading to the MD Degree. 2025.
14. Robinson D, Masters C, Ansari A. The 5 Rs of cultural humility: a conceptual model for health care leaders. Am J Med. Elsevier Inc. 2021;134:161–3.
15. Binda DD, Harris AC, Tan T, Fischer K, Molina RL, Mehta D. Examining the role of Medical School Faculty in developing students' cultural humility skills: insights from a single-center multimethod study. Glob Adv Integr Med Health. 2024;13:27536130241305090.

16. Wayne Weston W, Belle Brown J, Moira Stewart MA, Weston W. Patient-centred interviewing Part I: understanding patients' experiences.
17. Solchanyk D, Ekeh O, Saffran L, Burnett-Zeigler IE, Doobay-Persaud A. Integrating cultural humility into the medical education curriculum: strategies for educators. Teach Learn Med. 2021;33(5):554–60.
18. Sawhney M, Li JS, Patterson M, Gumapac NP, Sau C, Akbari A. Addressing culturally based hidden bias and RacisM (A-CHARM) using simulation experiences, Nik's story: a quasi-experimental study. Can J Nurs Res. 2025;57(1):47–58.
19. Moore C, Hecht SM, Sui H, Mayer L, Scott EK, Byrne B, et al. Integrating cultural humility into infant safe sleep counseling: a pediatric resident simulation. Cureus. 2021;13(12):e20847.
20. Erasmus RT. Point-of-care testing: connecting communities in Africa and ensuring equity in access to health and diagnostics. Afr J Lab Med. 2022;11(1):2072.
21. Saweri OPM, Batura N, Al Adawiyah R, Causer LM, Pomat WS, Vallely AJ, et al. Economic evaluation of point-of-care testing and treatment for sexually transmitted and genital infections in pregnancy in low- and middle-income countries: a systematic review. PLoS One. 2021;16(6):e0253135.
22. Curtis S, Martin H, DiNella M, Lavallee B, Chartrand C, McLeod L, et al. Kidney check point-of-care testing—furthering patient engagement and patient-centered care in Canada's rural and remote indigenous communities: program report. Can J Kidney Health Dis. 2021;8:20543581211003744.
23. New Data on Detailed Languages Spoken [Internet]. [cited 2025 Oct 29]. Available from: https://www.census.gov/newsroom/press-releases/2025/2017-2021-acs-language-use-tables.html
24. Ji X, Chow E, Abdelhamid K, Naumova D, Mate KKV, Bergeron A, et al. Utility of mobile technology in medical interpretation: a literature review of current practices. Patient Educ Couns. Elsevier Ireland Ltd. 2021;104:2137–45.
25. Velarde MR, Jagoe C, Cuculick J. Video relay interpretation and overcoming barriers in health care for deaf users: scoping review. J Med Internet Res. JMIR Publications Inc. 2022;24:e32439.
26. Grover S, Fitzpatrick A, Azim FT, Ariza-Vega P, Bellwood P, Burns J, et al. Defining and implementing patient-centered care: an umbrella review. Patient Educ Couns. Elsevier Ireland Ltd. 2022;105:1679–88.
27. Be healthy be mobile [Internet]. [cited 2025 Oct 29]. Available from: https://www.who.int/initiatives/behealthy
28. Ogunyemi D, Thind BS, Teixeira A, Sams CM, Ojo M, Dinkins GAE, et al. Integrating cultural humility into medical education using a structured and interactive workshop. Adv Med Educ Pract. 2024;15:575–83.
29. Metzl JM, Hansen H. Structural competency: theorizing a new medical engagement with stigma and inequality. Soc Sci Med. 2014;103:126–33.

Innovation in Medical Decision-Making and Diagnostic Testing

Megan Westphal, Lyndsay Kluge, Allison Harris, and Cheryl A. Dickson

Introduction

Diagnostic medicine is rapidly evolving with innovations that work to expand precision, speed, and accessibility of medicine. Modern diagnostics are transforming how diseases are identified and managed. This includes advancements from genetic testing to point-of-care ultrasound (POCUS) and the use of artificial intelligence (AI). As these tools become more integrated into practice success will depend on consideration of equity, education, and clinical judgement.

Genetic testing has evolved to enable more accurate diagnoses, risk assessment, and treatment planning. A key area of this is preimplantation genetic testing (PGT) which is used in IVF to screen for genetic disorders. This has been useful in identifying a large number of conditions but does raise concerns of embryo viability and ethical implications. Beyond this, use of next-generation sequencing (NGS) and whole exome sequencing (WES) have transformed diagnosis of different neurological, renal, and cardiac disorders. This technology appears to be an excellent tool for advancing personalized medicine but ethical concerns and physiological impacts as well as biological limitations need to be considered.

Additionally, physician experience is being assisted by point-of-care resources and AI in real-time to enhance diagnostics. This includes platforms like UpToDate®, DynaMed®, ClinicalKey®, and BMJ Best Practice which offer quick access to recent guidelines and evidence. New technologies like ClinicalKey® AI and large language models (e.g. ChatGPT) have also become increasingly popular. These all work to synthesize data and support clinical decision-making. This is especially true in resource limited areas. Emerging fields like radiomics work similarly to extract

M. Westphal · L. Kluge · A. Harris · C. A. Dickson (✉)
Western Michigan University Homer Stryker MD School of Medicine, Kalamazoo, MI, USA
e-mail: megan.westphal@wmed.edu; lyndsay.kluge@wmed.edu; allison.harris@wmed.edu; cheryl.dickson@wmed.edu

S. S. Chahin et al. (eds.), *Innovation in Medical Education and Clinical Practice*, https://doi.org/10.1007/978-3-032-19116-8_14

diagnostic information from medical imaging and offer promising insight for the future. However, with this potential these tools have a large risk of bias and misinformation. Rather than replacing physicians, the tools should work to supplement their judgment with adequate ethical considerations and training.

POCUS is also working to enhance more efficient, cost-effective diagnoses. This handheld ultrasound technology is being integrated into multiple specialties including cardiology, nephrology, emergency medicine, family medicine, and primary care. It works to detect various valvular diseases, hydronephrosis, appendicitis, cholecystitis, and more. Adoption of this technology remains low especially in areas with limited resources and training. However, integrating this into medical education could aim to improve diagnostic accuracy as well as benefit the speed, cost, and accessibility of diagnostics.

As medicine continues to evolve tools like genetic testing, AI-powered platforms and POCUS are working to change clinical approach to diagnostics and treatment. They work to enhance accuracy, reduce diagnostic time, and target therapies to conditions. Genetic testing works to enable earlier detection, while AI works to support clinical reasoning and decision making, and POCUS brings these diagnostics to the bedside of the patient. Successful integration, however, will require adequate training, ethical consideration, and continued research to ensure that these diagnostic advancements can improve patient outcomes in all healthcare settings.

Genetic Testing

In the past few decades, genetic testing has evolved from a niche scientific tool to a cornerstone of modern medicine. With the addition of advanced sequencing technologies and an expanding understanding of the human genome, clinicians can now use genetic information to diagnose diseases more accurately, predict individual risk, guide treatment decisions, and even prevent illness before symptoms arise. The goal of this section is to explore the impact of genetic testing across various fields and examine the benefits, highlight its current applications, acknowledge limitations, and expand on considerations that shape its integration into everyday clinical practice.

Preimplantation genetic testing (PGT) appears to be one of the most common uses of modern genetic testing with the goal of reducing genetic disorders. This occurs during in vitro fertilization in order to identify genetic abnormalities in the embryo before they can become implanted in the uterus. The goal of this testing was originally to select the embryos with the greatest likelihood of survival and progression to a healthy infant for implantation. This was theorized to reduce the risk of passing on various genetic disorders. In this process the cells are obtained from developing embryos in a culture and undergo genetic diagnostic testing [1]. With the evolution of technology, a single embryo biopsy can undergo high-quality testing for multiple indications [2]. These include monogenic hereditary disorders, structural chromosomal abnormalities, and numerical abnormalities [3]. This technology is especially useful in cases where the rate of aneuploidies, or an embryo with an abnormal number of chromosomes, is higher such as advanced maternal age, paternal infertility, recurrent pregnancies, or implantation failures [4].

There are a variety of techniques that can be utilized to accomplish PGT. One example is the use of polar body biopsy as polar bodies are produced during meiotic divisions of the oocyte. These only provide maternal information but can be removed without affecting the embryo. Blastomere biopsy is also performed where an embryo is made from six or eight cells which appears to provide better diagnostic efficiency but is only compatible in a very specific time window [4]. It has been noted that with the polar body biopsy only a few cells are analyzed which limits the ability to test for mosaicism and with the blastomere biopsy such a significant portion of cells are drawn that it could affect embryo viability [3]. Trophectoderm biopsy can also be used where the trophectoderm, the precursor to the placenta, is utilized. This procedure appears to be more accurate and, because the trophectoderm is not contributing to fetus formation, appears to be less invasive. There are also non-invasive procedures like blastocentesis which analyzes blastocyst fluid on the opposite side of the inner cell mass and examination of spent culture media. The latter takes cell free DNA found in the media to be examined and unlike the other methods does not require an expert, such as an embryologist, as it does not involve the embryo. Additionally, there are a variety of molecular techniques including Single Nucleotide Polymorphism Array (SNAP), Real Time Quantitative Polymerase Chain Reaction (rtq-PCR), and Next Generation Sequencing (NGS) that can be used to make a similar analysis. The perceived most viable methods are the NGS and trophectodermal biopsy [4].

This technology can be utilized in nearly every field of medicine. It has been useful for conditions such as sickle cell disease, cystic fibrosis, Huntington's disease, Fragile X Syndrome, and myotonic dystrophy. One area that has benefited from PGT is monogenic kidney diseases, specifically autosomal dominant polycystic kidney disease (ADPKD). ADPKD affects nearly 12 million people across the world and is a very prevalent disease. This testing is very specific to couples in which at least one individual has kidney disease. In this case PGT-M, screening to look for a specific mutation, can be conducted to determine the risk of passing this condition on to the embryo [5]. Additionally, it can be used to analyze Fragile X Syndrome. One case analysis was performed on the FMR1 CGG expansion to evaluate its structure. This analyzed those that were mutation carriers and premutation carriers based on the length of the gene expansion. It was found to be more beneficial for premutation carriers and those with ovarian dysfunction to select an unaffected embryo for IVF. There are some associated risks with this type of testing as it can be demanding and reduce the ovarian reserve resulting in fewer oocytes which could make it less appealing [6]. In a similar manner the technology utilized in the detection of ADPKD is associated with the release of hormones that could potentiate kidney and liver tumors which could be a challenge to its utility [5].

While PGT is seemingly a very useful tool in medicine there are a variety of biological limitations. These include conditions in which the genetics cannot be accurately predicted to ensure proper use of this technology like mosaicism, variants, or epigenetic factors [2]. Mosaicism specifically has raised a lot of concerns with this technology as it is a variety of different cell lines in the same embryo. It has been recommended that this technology aim to transfer embryos without, or with as low levels as possible, of mosaicism [4]. Beyond this, there is significant genetic variability to inherited monogenic diseases even without mosaicism. This makes identifying the underlying cause of these disorders very challenging. With respect to structural rearrangements there is a very large range of breakpoints and patterns that can be transmitted which can make it more difficult to assess the genetic alterations accurately [3].

Looking at trophectoderm biopsy specifically, which is believed to have the highest accuracy of the methods used to date, it is not believed that this has accomplished complete diagnostic accuracy. This can be problematic as it can indicate that there is a large amount of missed embryo diagnoses or potentially incorrect diagnoses [7]. Additionally, there is extensive discussion surrounding the safety of these procedures and ethical implications for these patients and future generations [2]. This technology could theoretically prevent a couple from birthing a child with undesirable outcomes which becomes an issue that would require additional professional consults and interventions. Beyond this, genetic screenings can raise more questions and uncertainty than was present initially. These tests have not been proven to be entirely accurate so it can be very difficult for families and caregivers to make drastic decisions based on these results. Sometimes the amount of information alone can overwhelm couples and make it more difficult to go through the IVF process. Different health professionals may need to be recruited in order to work with these couples through issues that they may not be familiar with. Additionally, questions can begin to be raised about where the responsibility to make these decisions lies which can further complicate the use of this technology [8].

To make matters more complicated, there is a specific type of PGT focused on managing the development of aneuploidies, or abnormal number of chromosomes, in the developing embryo for IVF. This specifically uses the previously discussed polar body biopsy method to ensure transfer of embryos with a normal number of chromosomes [9]. There is also use of a single trophectoderm biopsy at specifically the blastocyst stage to determine the number of chromosomes. In a similar manner this would allow for the chromosome number to be checked prior to implantation [10]. There is some suggested evidence that miscarriages are reduced in those undergoing IVF that also undergo PGT-A. However, the clinical support for this remains an area in need of greater development [9].

Initially when this technique was becoming popular, there was simultaneous use of PGT-A with FISH, Fluorescence In Situ Hybridization. Over time it was found that this can be harmful to the developing embryo and is therefore not a viable option for continued investigation [9]. Aside from this, PGT-A is becoming increasingly more popular and more widely demanded by patients. However, there is mixed evidence as to whether or not this reduces the number of miscarriages. Some sources report an increase in miscarriages and decrease in embryo viability after utilization of this technology. This is because the number of embryos is reduced as a result of using some for biopsy. Additionally, these are from such an early stage in development that there are a lot of false positives generated. While it is possible to see chromosomal abnormalities early on, these can occasionally correct themselves later in development. This results in embryos that are not used that could potentially be viable [10].

Similarly, use of PGT-M combined with PGT-A has been attempted to reduce the risk of miscarriage. This however has been not found to be exceptionally effective. As previously stated, the use of PGT-A only potentially reduces the number of miscarriages by a small number, and this is still not clinically proven to be significant. It is theorized that this technology is more useful for those above the age of 35, while PGT-M is more valuable for those that are younger. However, the combination of the two techniques can result in excessive testing and sampling of additional embryos which has only been seen to reduce the number of viable embryos with limited success in scanning for additional abnormalities [11]. Therefore, the combination of these therapies does not appear to prove additional benefit above what is seen with just the PGT-M testing alone. Furthermore, PGT-A remains very controversial as it highlights the desire to obtain embryos without genetic defects, utilizes embryos in testing, and is subject to different ethical considerations and concerns as it advances.

Aside from PGT for monogenic testing, there have been significant advancements in Next Generation Sequencing (NGS) that can aid in disease diagnostics and treatment planning. It was found that a large portion of neuropathy cases were related to five specific genes that were not always identified on previous diagnostic genetic panels. These included: *PMP22*, *MFN2*, *GJB1*, *MPZ*, and *TTR*. This is essential information to aid with earlier diagnostic interventions as peripheral neuropathy is frequently missed due to its nonspecific nature and complex etiology. This can help guide treatment interventions, genetic counseling, and family planning [12]. This identification has also led to use of this technology for more complex diseases. Focusing specifically on epilepsy, this technology has increased knowledge about the causative genetic variants. Epilepsy is very complex and is attributed to multiple different genetic abnormalities. NGS has allowed for the identification of some monogenic genetic abnormalities that can result in this as well as some with polygenic inheritance. The diagnostic accuracy of this testing was found to be somewhere between 20–30% which, although not ideal, can still help guide treatment techniques and therapies [13]. In a similar manner whole exome sequencing, or WES, has been conducted to look at multiple genes related to infantile epileptic syndromes. This has similar accuracy to the NGS at about 25–40%, however it provides the additional benefit of looking at the entire exome to analyze multiple different genes. Through NGS and WES testing SCN1A and SCN2A deficiencies have been demonstrated to be one of the most frequent causes of a rare form of epilepsy common in the first year of life. This precise finding can then allow for development of very directed treatment options. These treatments would aim to restore proper functioning of the gene and avoid treatment options that have been found to exacerbate issues related to loss of function of this specific gene. While these treatments are limited to very specific epileptic etiologies, they demonstrate the utility of this testing as it continues to progress and expand. As the variability of testing expands and costs remain relatively low it appears that this is feasible to incorporate into practice to better understand various diseases and tailor treatments accordingly [14].

Beyond neurological diseases, this technology has become incredibly useful in determining the etiology of different heritable cardiac conditions. These conditions include congenital heart defects as well as specific conditions like Hypertrophic Cardiomyopathy, or HCM. Both conditions contribute significantly to mortality from heart related conditions. HCM has been associated with very specific mutations in MYH7 and MYBPC3 which are myosin proteins related to sarcomere function. More recently, NGS has been utilized to better understand the heterogeneity of this condition. This allowed for sequencing of what were previously considered minor proteins involved in this process. It was found that the number of related genes to this condition was far more extensive than anticipated [15]. In a similar manner, congenital heart defects have been analyzed to better understand underlying mutations. A large portion of these defects are associated with genetic syndromes or extracardiac malformations. However, various genes have been proposed as the underlying cause. With genetic testing, previously suspected genetic mutations can be confirmed, and novel causes can be identified. Additionally, overlapping genetic variants and associated causes can be evaluated to better understand the mechanistic interplay of these genetic factors similar to what is seen in HCM [16].

There is evidence that this genetic testing is underused and could be expanded to assist with cardiac conditions. As discussed, NGS screenings could be used to look for various identified mutations responsible for HCM as it provides a rapid analysis of multiple different causative genes. This permits more directed genetic counseling and therapies for a condition with a lot of phenotypic heterogeneity to hopefully improve long term outcomes [15]. The same can be seen for congenial heart defects as more causes are identified and genetic counseling can be conducted for risk assessment in current and future generations. Additionally, testing can be used as a confirmatory measure when syndromes are suspected. From the results, targeted therapies can be expanded upon to improve outcomes and ultimately reduce mortality. Especially as the technology advances and the cost of testing continues to decline, this appears to be a promising option moving forward [16].

In conclusion, the integration of genetic testing into modern medicine has marked a significant advancement in the ability to diagnose, predict, and manage a wide range of diseases. From reproductive technologies like preimplantation genetic testing (PGT) to advanced sequencing techniques such as next-generation sequencing (NGS) and whole exome sequencing (WES), these tools have enhanced clinical decision-making and personalized care. PGT, particularly, has provided possible avenues for couples at risk of transmitting monogenic disorders or chromosomal abnormalities, and it continues to evolve with increasingly precise and less invasive techniques. However, limitations such as mosaicism, technical variability, reduced embryo viability, and ethical concerns highlight the need for cautious interpretation and multidisciplinary support.

In parallel, NGS and WES have expanded the diagnostic understanding of neurologic, renal, and cardiac conditions. This has offered insights into rare syndromes with novel genetic contributors and guided targeted treatment strategies. Despite notable diagnostic yields, particularly in conditions like epilepsy and cardiomyopathy, these technologies still face challenges in accuracy, clinical interpretation, and equitable access.

Ultimately, while genetic testing is reshaping the future of medicine, its use must be balanced with consideration of its biological, ethical, and psychosocial implications. Continued research, education, and collaboration across specialties will be necessary to ensure these technologies are applied responsibly and effectively. This will hopefully lead to better outcomes for patients and families across the healthcare spectrum.

Point-of-Care Resources and AI

The practice of medicine is shaped by the information available to clinicians. For centuries, physicians relied primarily on their training, experience, and peer consultation to arrive at diagnoses. In the last few decades, there has been a growing use of technology in healthcare diagnostics. This has transformed access to knowledge and reshaped how clinicians approach clinical reasoning. Point-of-care diagnostic tools, such as UpToDate®, DynaMed®, ClinicalKey®, and BMJ Best Practice, are digital platforms that synthesize and deliver evidence in real time. These resources allow a physician to consult the latest guidelines and differential diagnoses within minutes, directly during patient interactions. More recently, artificial intelligence (AI) and machine learning have emerged as a new wave of innovation in diagnostics, raising both hopes for improved care and questions about its risks and challenges.

Among these resources, UpToDate® has grown to play a larger part in medical practice [17]. It provides expert-authored content across almost every specialty, integrates treatment guidelines, and is frequently updated to reflect new evidence [18]. It contains a vast amount of information and is the largest tool of the point-of-care resources. The UpToDate® interface allows for rapid search and clinical applicability, making it a frequently used resource in hospitals. In fact, some studies suggest that the presence of UpToDate® in hospitals is associated with improved patient outcomes, including lower length of stay and mortality for certain conditions, especially in smaller hospitals [19, 20].

Despite its utility, UpToDate® has limitations. The subscription cost can prevent its use, especially for physicians in private practice or those working in under-resourced healthcare systems [21, 22]. While academic centers and teaching hospitals often provide institutional subscriptions, smaller healthcare systems may lack access, creating a knowledge gap between environments. Furthermore, there are concerns about conflicts of interest, since authors are allowed to have financial ties to pharmaceutical industries [21].

Another important critique is the platform's use of racial or ethnic tagging within diagnostic and treatment discussions. When race is linked as a genetic or phenotypic marker rather than understanding social determinants of health or structural inequities, it risks guiding physicians toward inappropriate treatments. Without critical evaluation, clinicians who rely solely on the content in UpToDate® may inadvertently exacerbate disparities [23]. Encouragingly, new initiatives have emerged to build open-access clinical databases that can increase recognition of race-input and eventually be used to work towards eliminating the improper use of race and ethnicity in clinical algorithms. These advancements can hopefully be utilized to make UpToDate® a more reliable tool for physicians [24].

While UpToDate® is dominant, other tools contribute meaningfully to the point-of-care landscape. Many of these resources require paid subscriptions to use, which is a limit to their use since many can only afford to subscribe to one tool. DynaMed® prioritizes frequent updates and emphasizes transparency, with a clear conflict-of-interest policy that is easily accessible to users [21, 25]. ClinicalKey® is another evidence-based point-of-care resource with access to full-text references, and its newer version, ClinicalKey® AI, incorporates generative AI to refine searches and support diagnostic reasoning [26]. BMJ Best Practice stands out for its stepwise guidance and daily updates, offering clinicians structured care pathways that are particularly useful in urgent settings [27]. A more affordable option is Medscape®. Though free to use and widely accessed globally, it depends on advertisement funding and is sometimes criticized for variability in content rigor compared to subscription-based tools [21].

An article from 2017 provides a comparative overview of several of these platforms, highlighting not only their individual strengths and weaknesses to help physicians choose the best tool for them, but also their role in the broader problem of information overload in medicine. The article emphasizes that clinicians should weigh several factors when choosing a tool, such as usability, frequency of updates, and transparency of conflicts of interest when selecting tools [21].

While most of these tools are aimed at physicians, medical students also have the option to subscribe. Exposure early in training allows students to become better at integrating evidence from these resources into their clinical reasoning, preparing them to practice in a rapidly evolving digital environment. Having this experience will help them as physicians, since they already have experience in integrating them into their practice.

As powerful as point-of-care resources have become, the future of diagnostics is likely to be increasingly supplemented by AI. Unlike such platforms, which deliver curated human-authored summaries, AI tools can synthesize raw data, generate new hypotheses, and adapt recommendations in real time. ClinicalKey® AI is one example, embedding generative AI into a familiar point-of-care framework [28]. Beyond this, large language models like ChatGPT are being studied for their ability to generate differential diagnoses, suggest treatment plans, and explain medical concepts to patients. While generative AI has potential, it is something that must be implemented properly with a focus on "human wellbeing" over technology to improve patient outcomes [29]. Using it as an aid rather than a replacement for physicians is critical to its success.

A potential merit of AI is that it can be useful in medical settings with fewer resources. This can help to reduce diagnostic errors, counteract human biases, and aid in decision making in such settings where expertise may be scarce. For example, in rural or low-resource hospitals, an AI tool could provide immediate access to diagnostic reasoning that might otherwise require referral to an outside party. If used in such ways, AI has the potential to narrow disparities in access to specialized knowledge.

Emerging fields such as radiomics push this field even further. Radiomics involves extracting high-dimensional data from standard imaging modalities such as CT, MRI, or PET scans, and applying pattern recognition algorithms that can be used for diagnosis [30]. Applications in oncology are particularly promising, with studies suggesting radiomics can help classify tumors and predict survival [30]. This represents a shift from imaging as purely visual to one enhanced by quantitative, AI-driven biomarkers.

ChatGPT is another area of research as an emerging diagnostic support tool. One study provided ChatGPT with several standardized clinical vignettes. Measuring accuracy and performance, it was found that ChatGPT achieved an overall accuracy of 71.7% but inferior performance for differential diagnosis and clinical management. It was concluded that ChatGPT is best to be used for final diagnoses. ChatGPT does need to be used with caution, as model hallucinations and improper model training can skew data [31]. These findings suggest that AI may be best deployed as a confirmatory tool helping clinicians test hypotheses rather than as a primary diagnostic engine.

Still, AI carries risks. Models are only as representative as the data on which they are trained. If minority populations are underrepresented in datasets, AI outputs may be less accurate for these groups, reproducing and even amplifying inequities. Similarly, issues with AI transparency can decrease clinician trust in these tools if clinicians cannot understand or explain how an algorithm reached its conclusion or if its output is "hallucinated". In clinical settings, this could have dangerous consequences, making cross-referencing critical.

The rapid expansion of diagnostic tools raises many questions about the future of medicine. For instance, it is important to consider how clinicians should integrate technology without losing the humanistic core of medicine. While these tools can improve efficiency, they cannot replace the human aspect of care, such as thorough patient histories and cultural awareness. Clinicians need to acknowledge the limits of both their own knowledge and the tools they use and remain open to the patient's lived experience as a vital piece of diagnostic data.

Many patients have several identities and social determinants of health that play a role in their care. AI models are not advanced enough to take all of these factors into account when creating diagnostic suggestions, making a physician's lens vital to capturing the nuances in their care. Because of this, diagnostic tools should be seen as supports to help enhance care rather than something to replace a human physician.

With the growing use of technological tools, new governing and ethical practices must be put in place to keep their use effective and keep the physicians in check to prevent inappropriate use. Institutions that implement AI into their practices need to create guidelines for oversight, bias detection, and frequent education. This includes ensuring the AI tools they use have diverse datasets with explainable outputs, and that physicians understand both the merits and risks of such tools. This will help to improve trust on all ends, including physician trust in the tools and patient trust in the physicians.

Diagnostic decision-making is entering a new era, with technology at the forefront. Tools such as UpToDate® have already revolutionized how clinicians access evidence at the point of care, while AI-enabled platforms are the future to further transform the diagnostic process by analyzing patterns, generating hypotheses, and extending expertise to underserved regions. Yet, innovation must be paired with equity and humility. Without attention to issues of cost, access, and algorithmic bias, these tools risk reinforcing the very disparities they seek to resolve.

The future of diagnostics will not be determined solely by the sophistication of algorithms, but by the values with which they are deployed. A hybrid model where clinician judgment is augmented by evidence-based resources and AI but grounded in cultural humility offers the best path forward. Using this approach, point-of-care diagnostics and AI are not the sole decision-makers, but tools to provide in-depth care.

POCUS

As technology has developed, physicians have added more tools to their repertoire to aid in accurate, efficient, and cost effective diagnosis of patients. Point-of-care ultrasound (POCUS) is one tool that is becoming more widely used with the development of hand-held ultrasound systems accessible to physicians in many disciplines. Due to the recent advancements to POCUS, it has been suggested that in the future this tool could be an addition to the four pillars of clinical bedside physical examination (observation, palpation, percussion, osculation) as a way to enhance medical diagnosis and care [32]. As knowledge and research is expanding there have been many applications identified for POCUS in clinical practice, medical education, telemedicine, and under-resourced areas.

POCUS is used in a variety of medical disciplines, with one of the major disciplines being cardiology. It is frequently compared in studies to standard transthoracic echocardiography (sTTE) to assess utilization in clinical practice. POCUS was shown to be able to diagnose mitral regurgitation, aortic regurgitation, aortic stenosis, and prosthetic valvular abnormality with high sensitivity and specificity [33]. It was also used to assess for early signs of infective endocarditis in patients with bacteremia and candidemia. Valvular regurgitation, valvular vegetation, hepatomegaly, and splenomegaly were detected with POCUS [34]. Acute aortic syndromes, which present with very general symptoms, have a potential to be missed on diagnosis. POCUS being used on assessment decreased the time to diagnosis of this rare syndrome compared to using clinical score, and successfully ruled out this diagnosis in patients where this was unlikely [35]. Thoracic aortic aneurysm was specifically demonstrated to be detected using POCUS with high positive predictive value [36].

The current gold standard for valvular heart disease assessment is standard transthoracic echocardiography (sTTE). A study in 2013 compared the use of portable transthoracic echocardiography (pTTE), a type of POCUS, to standard transthoracic echocardiography (sTTE). It was found that there was significant agreement between the results of pTTE and sTTE. When comparing sensitivity of pTTE to low-risk and high-risk groups unsurprisingly pTTE was found to be more sensitive with detection of abnormalities in the high-risk group of patients compared to detection in the low-risk group. Additionally, when compared to sTTE, pTTE was also shown to be quicker than sTTE which could aid in initial emergency department assessments of patients [37]. With this evidence, cardiac pathology could be more readily assessed for in patients. Cardiology, emergency medicine, internal medicine, and family practice physicians have the capabilities to assess, diagnose, and begin treatment. This will decrease the time patients spend waiting for a diagnosis or treatment and has the potential to decrease the cost of seeing many different providers to get a diagnosis.

In nephrology, there is a slow incorporation of POCUS into clinical practice. Many of the providers need more training to better utilize POCUS in clinical practice [38]. In a study of infants with hydronephrosis, POCUS was shown to be as effective as conventional ultrasound when performed by providers who had undergone training in POCUS [39]. It was suggested that POCUS also can be used to detect hydronephrosis in patients with acute kidney injury, where POCUS was compared to CT and traditional ultrasound and shown to be as effective [40]. In patients with renal colic, POCUS was suggested to be useful as an initial tool in determining patient diagnosis and future steps in treatment [41]. Renal colic is a common presentation in patients presenting to primary care, urgent care, and the emergency department. It is described as excruciating pain, therefore the ability to assess this immediately at presentation allows providers to begin treatment sooner bringing patients faster relief of their pain.

There are many indications for use of standard ultrasound in diagnosis of abdominal pathology. Currently, there is research into how POCUS could be used for diagnosis. POCUS was demonstrated to effectively diagnose routine acute gallbladder pathology, specifically acute cholecystitis and assessment of the common bile duct compared to other radiological studies [42]. There have also been suggested approaches for different techniques to use POCUS for the biliary system, liver, free fluid, appendix, and renal system [43]. Many of these diagnoses are urgent or emergent requiring nearly immediate treatment. Continuing to research the uses of POCUS and expanding the use for abdominal pathology has the potential to increase the diagnostic information quickly, and at the bedside, for patients.

There have been many identified uses for POCUS in family practice, specifically in rural medicine, however currently it was discovered that less than 10% of family practice physicians utilize POCUS in their care [44]. Increasing the training and usage of POCUS in primary care would give physicians a stronger differential diagnosis for patients, preventing unnecessary visits to the emergency department and proper referrals to specialists when it is determined to be necessary. Being able to understand more about the patient in primary care can help confirm that each patient is immediately getting necessary care that is specific to their diagnosis. Additionally, there is no radiation exposure with POCUS which is beneficial for patients in circumstances where POCUS can glean at least as much information as Computed Tomography (CT) about a potential diagnosis.

The implementation of POCUS has sparked discussion of when it should be introduced to medical students and residents and what POCUS training looks like for students. A study performed in 2012 suggested that use of POCUS by fourth year medical students improved diagnostic specificity from 84.9% to 93.6% and sensitivity from 25.9% to 74.1% [45]. Recently, Kameda described experience with instructing students on POCUS. Based on observation, the student's best understanding of POCUS was after identifying an abnormality during another part of the physical exam and using POCUS for more information and confirmation of the findings [46]. This provides evidence that even during training POCUS can be a useful tool for both learning and diagnostics. There has been significant encouragement to incorporate POCUS training from many fields including neonatology, emergency medicine, cardiology, and anesthesia [45, 47–49]. Aside from using POCUS as a tool to improve clinical reasoning in medical education, this tool was also demonstrated to improve anatomical knowledge in the undergraduate medical education curriculum. POCUS lessons were incorporated into the anatomy curriculum in addition to the other avenues of anatomical study. These additional POCUS sessions resulted in students feeling more confident in both ultrasound technique and anatomical knowledge [50]. As technology advances in clinical practice, it is pertinent that medical education evolves with the advancements. Use of POCUS in medical education improves both the educational experience and development of clinical understanding in medical students and residents throughout their training.

Over the last few years, there have been advancements in telemedicine and ways care can be provided without requiring patients to come in-person for an office visit. Interestingly, POCUS was investigated for patient use in home-based imaging. In the prospective study, patients with no previous training received a slideshow with background information about POCUS and instructions on proper technique. The scans taken by patients were compared to the same scans taken by emergency medicine faculty who received fellowship training in emergency ultrasound. Surprisingly, the quality and interpretability of the scans did not differ between groups [51]. This provides evidence that there are applications for POCUS outside of clinic and hospital settings. Additional studies on patient use could provide more data with the potential to improve care via telemedicine. Furthermore, this could improve healthcare access by increasing the information obtained from a telemedicine call creating more avenues for patients to use for access to care.

One major benefit to POCUS is that devices are compact and affordable, making it possible for this tool to advance care in under-resourced areas. A study using POCUS to aid in diagnosis of patients in rural Uganda showed that in 50% of patients diagnostic findings were confirmed and in 23% of patients diagnosis was changed based on the POCUS findings [52]. A different study from rural Germany showed that POCUS findings in a primary care office impacted future management of 80.4% of cases and a survey of emergency medicine physicians in rural Canada showed that almost all of the physicians used POCUS in their clinical practice [53, 54]. This could increase the knowledge a physician gains from initial assessment of the patient under circumstances where there is limited access to labs or other imaging modalities. It has been commonly used for trauma, heart, and lung visualization, aiding in rapid diagnosis. In one example, a handheld POCUS device was used to detect a pleural effusion in a child in Chad, Africa when no x-ray was available. During this same expedition it was identified that POCUS was used in direct management of 75% of patients [55]. Overall, POCUS was demonstrated to positively aid in rapid diagnosis by confirming or providing evidence to change the diagnosis which positively impacted future management of these patients.

In addition to the diagnostic benefits of POCUS, there have also been cost benefits to POCUS. A cost analysis of pTTE compared to sTTE, which were both used to diagnose valvular heart disease, determined there would be a 31% cost reduction using POCUS compared to sTTE [37]. The cost of POCUS is less than $10,000 whereas the cost of a CT machine is around 10x greater, more evidence supporting use of POCUS in under-resourced areas. Medical costs continue to increase, making the most modern solutions to care inaccessible for many patients. Additionally, alternative options for medical imaging can be very expensive for patients. This is an opportunity to lower medical costs without sacrificing proper diagnosis.

Although POCUS has been proven to have significant benefits, there are also drawbacks to widespread implementation. This is not unusual for new medical technology, as at one point the stethoscope, blood pressure cuff, and electrocardiogram were all considered to have extensive drawbacks [32]. Since POCUS is a newer technology, many of the studies do not contain sample sizes large enough to draw concrete conclusions. However, the current research provides a strong foundation for future research. More data can suggest concrete conclusions on where POCUS is most beneficial and where implementation efforts should be directed. POCUS training is another aspect requiring future development. Many disciplines have identified uses for POCUS in practice, however time for and access to training can be difficult for physicians. As this technology develops there are progressively more suggestions on ways to incorporate POCUS into physician training, to further implement use in clinical practice [45–49]. The training barrier is specifically prevalent in under-resourced communities with one suggested solution being to train a small group of physicians who can then continue to train others in their community [55]. Additionally, although POCUS is affordable compared to other imaging modalities, there are still many costs associated with implementation along with the $4000 device cost. This purchase is not always feasible for many low-resource clinics [55], expanding the barriers to access in under-resourced communities.

POCUS has been shown to be useful in many settings including clinical care, clinical education, telemedicine, and under-resourced areas. There are many ways where POCUS is demonstrated to be as effective as other imaging modalities in making diagnoses, while being accessible and cost-effective. It also can provide more information where imagining is not traditionally used. Furthermore, POCUS often decreases the time to diagnosis while simultaneously increasing the clarity of the clinical picture of a patient. It is essential to continue research to define more ways to utilize POCUS. In the future, POCUS has the potential to expand diagnostic ability for providers which will allow them to provide better, more accessible care for all patients.

Conclusion

The use of medical technology in diagnostics and decision making is rapidly advancing, specifically with the expansion of tools such as genetic testing, AI-powered platforms, and POCUS. Although the future of these advancements appears promising, there are a number of factors to consider prior to the widespread implementation of these technologies. Implementing genetic testing has the potential to make diagnostics earlier, allowing treatment to start earlier, however the ability to prevent miscarriages and accurately prevent chromosomal abnormalities is still up for debate. Ethical considerations and cost also contribute to the hesitation towards widespread implementation. Similarly, there are a number of ethical considerations for incorporating AI usage into diagnosis and patient care. The potential for bias with AI usage requires critical examination of the platform and data being used prior to applying the output information to the patient. There are many discussions for POCUS on the ways training can be done to best reach physicians practicing in clinic and under-resourced settings, not only hospital usage. Additionally, since the many applications of POCUS are still being discovered, more research is required to confirm the findings. Furthermore, as technology continues to advance, it is pertinent that physicians continue to prioritize the patient-physician relationship as to not lose the humanistic side of medicine. Together, with continuing advancements and research, these tools show potential for earlier diagnostics with more information gained directly at the bedside of the patient.

References

1. Brezina PR, Kutteh WH. Clinical applications of preimplantation genetic testing. BMJ. 2015;350:g7611.
2. Kakourou G, Sofocleous C, Mamas T, Vrettou C, Traeger-Synodinos J. The current clinical applications of preimplantation genetic testing (PGT): acknowledging the limitations of biology and technology. Expert Rev Mol Diagn. 2024;24(9):767–75.
3. Giuliano R, Maione A, Vallefuoco A, Sorrentino U, Zuccarello D. Preimplantation genetic testing for genetic diseases: limits and review of current literature. Genes. 2023;14(11):2095.
4. Greco E, Litwicka K, Minasi MG, Cursio E, Greco PF, Barillari P. Preimplantation genetic testing: where we are today. Int J Mol Sci. 2020;21(12):1–29.

5. Knoers NVAM. Prenatal and preimplantation genetic testing for monogenic kidney disorders. Kidney Int. 2025;107(2):255–61.
6. Persico T, Tranquillo ML, Seracchioli R, Zuccarello D, Sorrentino U. PGT-M for premature ovarian failure related to CGG repeat expansion of the FMR1 gene. Genes. 2023;15(1):6.
7. Chen K, Hu Z, Lian Y, Han Y, Zhou X, Li Y, et al. The diagnostic accuracy of preimplantation genetic testing (PGT) in assessing the genetic status of embryos: a systematic review and meta-analysis. Reprod Biol Endocrinol. 2025;23(1):1–18.
8. Kaye DK. Addressing ethical issues related to prenatal diagnostic procedures. Matern Health Neonatol Perinatol. 2023;9(1):1.
9. Cornelisse S, Zagers M, Kostova E, Fleischer K, van Wely M, Mastenbroek S. Preimplantation genetic testing for aneuploidies (abnormal number of chromosomes) in in vitro fertilisation. Cochrane Database Syst Rev. 2020;9(9):CD005291.
10. Gleicher N, Patrizio P, Brivanlou A. Preimplantation genetic testing for aneuploidy—a castle built on sand. Trends Mol Med. 2021;27(8):731–42.
11. Scriven PN. Combining PGT-A with PGT-M risks trying to do too much. J Assist Reprod Genet. 2022;39(9):2015–8.
12. Roggenbuck J, Morales A, Ellis CA, Dratch L, Stetler M, Tan CA, et al. Diagnostic and clinical utility of comprehensive multigene panel testing for patients with neuropathy. J Peripher Nerv Syst. 2024;29(3):363–7.
13. Møller RS, Dahl HA, Helbig I. The contribution of next generation sequencing to epilepsy genetics. Expert Rev Mol Diagn. 2015;15(12):1531–8.
14. Bayat A, Bayat M, Rubboli G, Møller RS. Epilepsy syndromes in the first year of life and usefulness of genetic testing for precision therapy. Genes. 2021;12(7):1051.
15. Cecconi M, Parodi MI, Formisano F, Spirito P, Autore C, Musumeci MB, et al. Targeted next-generation sequencing helps to decipher the genetic and phenotypic heterogeneity of hypertrophic cardiomyopathy. Int J Mol Med. 2016;38(4):1111–24.
16. Cowan JR, Ware SM. Genetics and genetic testing in congenital heart disease. Clin Perinatol. 2015;42(2):373–93.
17. Kinengyere AA, Rosenberg J, Pickard O, Kamya M. Utilization and uptake of the UpToDate clinical decision support tool at the Makerere University College of Health Sciences (MakCHS), Uganda. Afr Health Sci. 2021;21(2):904.
18. Evidence-based Clinical Solutions for Healthcare | UpToDate | Wolters Kluwer [Internet]. Available from: https://www.wolterskluwer.com/en/solutions/uptodate
19. Isaac T, Zheng J, Jha A. Use of UpToDate and outcomes in US hospitals. J Hosp Med. 2012;7(2):85–90.
20. UpToDate Research Studies | Wolters Kluwer [Internet]. Available from: https://www.wolterskluwer.com/en/solutions/uptodate/about/research
21. Andrews R, Mehta N, Maypole J, Martin SA. Staying afloat in a sea of information: point-of-care resources. Cleve Clin J Med. 2017;84(3):225–35.
22. Baxter SL, Lander L, Clay B, Bell J, Hansen K, Walker A, et al. Comparing the use of DynaMed and UpToDate by physician trainees in clinical decision-making: a randomized crossover trial. Appl Clin Inform. 2022;13(1):139.
23. Cerdeña JP, Asabor EN, Plaisime MV, Hardeman RR. Race-based medicine in the point-of-care clinical resource UpToDate: a systematic content analysis. EClinicalMedicine. 2022;52:101581.
24. Visweswaran S, Sadhu EM, Morris MM, Vis AR, Samayamuthu MJ. Online database of clinical algorithms with race and ethnicity. Sci Rep [Internet]. 2025;15(1) Available from: https://pubmed.ncbi.nlm.nih.gov/40157976/
25. DynaMed | Point of Care | Clinical Decision Support | Evidence Based | EBSCO [Internet]. Available from: https://about.ebsco.com/clinical-decisions/dynamed-solutions/dynamed
26. ClinicalKey | Elsevier [Internet]. Available from: https://www.elsevier.com/products/clinicalkey

27. Homepage | BMJ Best Practice [Internet]. Available from: https://bestpractice.bmj.com/info/us/
28. Trusted content. Powered by responsible AI | ClinicalKey AI [Internet]. Available from: https://www.elsevier.com/products/clinicalkey/clinicalkey-ai
29. Reddy S. Generative AI in healthcare: an implementation science informed translational path on application, integration and governance. Implement Sci IS. 2024;19(1):27.
30. Mayerhoefer ME, Materka A, Langs G, Häggström I, Szczypiński P, Gibbs P, et al. Introduction to Radiomics. J Nucl Med. 2020;61(4):488.
31. Rao A, Pang M, Kim J, Kamineni M, Lie W, Prasad AK, et al. Assessing the utility of ChatGPT throughout the entire clinical workflow: development and usability study. J Med Internet Res. 2023;25:e48659.
32. Narula J, Chandrashekhar Y, Braunwald E. Time to add a fifth pillar to bedside physical examination: inspection, palpation, percussion, auscultation, and Insonation. JAMA Cardiol. 2018;3(4):346–50.
33. Wen S, Naqvi TZ. Point-of-care ultrasound in detection, severity and mechanism of significant Valvular heart disease and clinical management. J Clin Med. 2023;12(20):6474.
34. Palmero SL, Zúñiga MAL, Martínez VR, Parrilla RR, Muñoz AMA, Romera WSY, et al. Point-of-Care Ultrasound (POCUS) as an extension of the physical examination in patients with bacteremia or Candidemia. J Clin Med. 2022;11(13):3636.
35. Morello F, Bima P, Castelli M, Capretti E, Soeiro A d M, Cipriano A, et al. Diagnosis of acute aortic syndromes with ultrasound and d-dimer: the PROFUNDUS study. Eur J Intern Med. 2024;128:94–103.
36. Hesami M, Denkewicz R, Boivin Z, Bhalodkar S, Li JJ, Moore C. Association of dilated aortic root on point-of-care ultrasound with aortic aneurysm and dissection. Am J Emerg Med. 2025;95:89–94.
37. Kitada R, Fukuda S, Watanabe H, Oe H, Abe Y, Yoshiyama M, et al. Diagnostic accuracy and cost-effectiveness of a pocket-sized transthoracic echocardiographic imaging device. Clin Cardiol. 2013;36(10):603–10.
38. Cook DL, Patel S, Nee R, Little DJ, Cohen SD, Yuan CM. Point-of-care ultrasound use in nephrology: a survey of nephrology program directors, fellows, and fellowship graduates. Kidney Med. 2023;5(4):100601.
39. Cheon EJ, Yoon JM. Reliability of renal point-of-care ultrasound (POCUS) performed by pediatric postgraduates to diagnose hydronephrosis in infants. Front Pediatr. 2024;12:1361223.
40. Nepal S, Dachsel M, Smallwood N. Point-of-care ultrasound rapidly and reliably diagnoses renal tract obstruction in patients admitted with acute kidney injury. Clin Med. 2020;20(6):541–4.
41. Bourcier JE, Gallard E, Redonnet JP, Abillard M, Billaut Q, Fauque L, et al. Ultrasound at the patient's bedside for the diagnosis and prognostication of a renal colic. Ultrasound J. 2021;13:45.
42. Dumbrava BD, Bass GA, Jumean A, Birido N, Corbally M, Pereira J, et al. The accuracy of Point-of-Care Ultrasound (POCUS) in acute gallbladder disease. Diagnostics. 2023;13(7):1248.
43. Boling B, Solis A. Point-of-care ultrasonography in the critical care setting: abdominal POCUS. AACN Adv Crit Care. 2023;34(3):216–27.
44. Niblock F, Byun H, Jabbarpour Y. Point-of-care ultrasound use by primary care physicians. J Am Board Fam Med. 2021;34(4):859–60.
45. Panoulas VF, Daigeler AL, Malaweera ASN, Lota AS, Baskaran D, Rahman S, et al. Pocket-size hand-held cardiac ultrasound as an adjunct to clinical examination in the hands of medical students and junior doctors. Eur Heart J Cardiovasc Imaging. 2013;14(4):323–30.
46. Kameda T. The combination of physical examination and point-of-care ultrasonography in undergraduate medical education. J Med Ultrason. 2023;50(3):273–4.
47. Kurepa D, Boyar V, Zaghloul N, Beachy J, Zaytseva A, Teng D, et al. Structured neonatal point-of-care ultrasound training program. Am J Perinatol. 2021;38(S 01):e284–91.

48. Kalagara H, Manson W, Townsley MM. Point-of-Care Ultrasound (POCUS) training for anesthesiologists: is it time to embrace and attain competency? J Cardiothorac Vasc Anesth. 2022;36(1):30–2.
49. Lazarow F, Deal AK, Shaves SC, Knapp B, Byars D, Goodmurphy CW, et al. Evaluation of a point-of-care ultrasound curriculum and ocular phantom in residency training. J Ultrasound. 2021;25(2):259–63.
50. Olivares-Perez ME, Graglia S, Harmon DJ, Klein BA. Virtual anatomy and point-of-care ultrasonography integration pilot for medical students. Anat Sci Educ. 2022;15(3):464–75.
51. Duggan NM, Jowkar N, Ma IWY, Schulwolf S, Selame LA, Fischetti CE, et al. Novice-performed point-of-care ultrasound for home-based imaging. Sci Rep. 2022;12(1):20461.
52. Baker DE, Nolting L, Brown HA. Impact of point-of-care ultrasound on the diagnosis and treatment of patients in rural Uganda. Trop Dr. 2021;51(3):291–6.
53. Lo H, Frauendorf V, Wischke S, Schimmath-Deutrich C, Kersten M, Nuernberg M, et al. Ambulatory use of handheld point-of-care ultrasound (HH-POCUS) in rural Brandenburg—a pilot study. Ultraschall Med – Eur J Ultrasound. 2021;43:584–91.
54. Andani R, Jacques Q, Yi Y, Jelic T, Micks T, Bradbury-Squires D, et al. Rural Canadian emergency physician experiences using point-of-care ultrasound. Can J Emerg Med. 2025;27(3):191–7.
55. Dana E, Nour ADM, Kpa'Hanba GA, Khan JS. Point-of-Care Ultrasound (PoCUS) and its potential to advance patient care in low-resource settings and conflict zones. Disaster Med Public Health Prep. 2023;17(5)

Innovations in the Delivery of Optimized Care

Mary Haddad, Adam Haddad, Juanita Moses, and Summer Chahin

Introduction

Population Change and the Need for Healthcare Modifications

The United States is an ever-evolving community. According to recent census data over the last 10 years, the United States population has increased 7.4% to over 330,000,000 people [1]. In 2023, 1 in 6 people in the United States were 65 years old or older, and the Census Bureau predicts this subset of the population will exceed that of children and adolescents by 2040 [1]. Additionally, the number of people being 18–64 years of age will be near 230 million by 2060 [1]. Reflecting on these demographic indicators, one can infer there is a shift happening in the United States which will require changes in current pathways of providing patient care. More emphasis, resources, and providers will likely be needed to direct their attention to geriatric care and chronic disease management, among other topics.

Due to the changes in the population, adjustments to how healthcare delivery is provided to an aging population will need to be made. There are many reasons for this. Firstly, an aging population, such as in the United States, will require more healthcare services than a younger population [1]. The older an individual becomes, the more prone they become to severe infections and chronic diseases like hypertension, diabetes, and chronic obstructive pulmonary disease. With advancements in modern medicine, patients are living longer and thus require longer management of

M. Haddad · A. Haddad
Michigan State University College of Human Medicine, Grand Rapids, MI, USA
e-mail: Haddad12@msu.edu; Haddada5@msu.edu

J. Moses · S. Chahin (✉)
Western Michigan University Homer Stryker M.D. School of Medicine, Kalamazoo, MI, USA
e-mail: Juanita.moses@wmed.edu; Summer.chahin@wmed.edu

S. S. Chahin et al. (eds.), *Innovation in Medical Education and Clinical Practice*, https://doi.org/10.1007/978-3-032-19116-8_15

their medical conditions than ever before. Likewise, due to their weaker immune systems, senior citizens require closer monitoring than younger individuals. With increasing life expectancy and improved treatments for acute and chronic conditions, individuals are living longer but often with complex, long term care needs. This requires sustained, coordinated management rather than episodic or reactive care. Due to this population's risk factors and likelihood of developing chronic diseases, the design and implementation of healthcare services directed to geriatric patients should be a priority. Chronic diseases have been known to complicate a person's quality of life. To help prevent compounding disability from these diseases, more resources should be allocated to research topics such as early disease prevention and management [1].

Throughout my year of core rotations, I have had the privilege of serving as an active member of the multidisciplinary care teams responsible for many geriatric patients. Reflecting on these experiences, a common theme stands out. Patients, their caregivers, and their loved ones consistently would ask what specialty I was interested in. I would share that I was undecided to which they would urge me to become a geriatrician. This deficiency in geriatric providers is not only evident to members of the healthcare community but also the patients themselves.

In summary, population aging and demographic shifts necessitate comprehensive modifications in how healthcare is delivered. Innovation must focus on scalability, sustainability, and personalization to meet the needs of a changing society—one that is older, more diverse, and living longer than ever before.

Optimized Care and Its Importance

According to Merriam-Webster, "to optimize" means to make something more effective and perfect [2]. Thus, delivering optimized care to patients means providing effective, efficient, and patient-focused healthcare. While this may seem like a challenging task, the long-term benefits in the individual and national healthcare system will be significant.

Healthcare plays a major role in our lives. From our first breath to our last, the utilization of medical services is intertwined. Finding a way to personalize the care provided to a specific patient should always be a priority. Working in the healthcare field allows you to meet a patient in their most vulnerable state and lending a listening ear may make all the difference. As one patient once said, "All I want when I come to a hospital is for someone to be nice to me" [3]. For this patient, showing kindness and empathy may be all she needs to feel her care being optimized. For others, it may be cost-efficiency, time-efficiency, improved data collection, etc. The list can go on and on.

Changing the methods in which we provide healthcare in the United States is essential because of our dynamic population. Outdated approaches will no longer work to provide adequate care for individuals in our evolving communities. Each person has their own expectations, biases, and experiences with the healthcare system which need to be taken into account. "Nothing about us, without us" is a phrase used for hundreds of years signifying the importance of the involvement of people affected by the change in the process of developing the described change [4]. To deliver optimized care to our patients, new innovations are required to keep up with the times and bring light to a system that has been neglected for too long.

Drivers in Innovation

The reform of the healthcare system in the United States has been a challenging and ongoing process. From providers to patients to conglomerates and insurance companies, it is no secret that the majority of those involved in healthcare are unsatisfied with their current state. To effectively assess the changes necessary for optimizing healthcare delivery in the United States, the various obstacles currently facing the healthcare system need to be examined.

Resources and finances are major stressors for many industries in the world. Looking more specifically at healthcare, this fact still holds true. In 2018, over $3.5 trillion was spent on healthcare, which accounts for over 17% of the United States' Gross Domestic Product [5]. Although a significant amount of cash goes towards healthcare, 25% of said spending is considered "wasted" [5]. Why is that? Well, different medical services or diagnostic tests can be overutilized, while others are underutilized [6]. For example, many patients in the emergency department receive CT scan orders. Imaging studies get billed and added to the overall cost of the hospital visit. The question that needs to be asked is "Is this study necessary for this patient?" A study found that the more recent a physician graduated from medical school or completed allopathic training, the less "lower-valued" services they used while providing patient care [5]. A community having many providers can lead to overuse, while having too few primary care providers can lead to underuse [6]. As healthcare prices rise, ensuring the value of said care must be a priority [5].

Although this is not newfound information, recent years have shed more light on healthcare disparities in the United States which have been catalysts for innovation in the field. In 2003, the Institute of Medicine Report: Unequal Treatment Confronting Racial and Ethnic Disparities in Health Care found that not much has improved when addressing the disparities facing Black Americans in this country [3]. Even with adjustment for potential confounding factors such as social determinants of health, Black individuals had worse outcomes when compared to White Americans [3]. In more recent years, Black Americans had 3.3 times more COVID-19-related hospitalizations than White Americans [3].

Additionally, healthcare providers' feelings and opinions are drivers of innovation. It is no secret that physicians and other healthcare team members have a lot on their plate. With the state of the current healthcare system, physician burnout is at an all-time high, further worsened by the COVID-19 pandemic. Globally, whether from emotional exhaustion, horrible work-life balance, or feelings of detachment and loss of purpose, providers are dissatisfied with the current system [7]. At least

40% of physicians in America have felt at least one symptom of burnout, which in turn has been shown to lead to ineffective care practices, more self-reported errors, and less professionalism [7]. One can infer burnout leads to physicians leaving the field, especially during the COVID-19 pandemic. The attrition of providers just adds to the problems already facing a falling healthcare system. Imagine putting over a decade into what was once a dream of yours and waking up to a life in a broken system that does not appreciate both the medical and social services you aim to provide. A system that lacks the resources, support, and empathy needed to deliver optimized care, not only for the patients, but for the healthcare team as well.

When we look at today's world, it is strikingly different from 100, let alone 50 years ago. With the advancements in technology, many Americans have access to information at their fingertips. This access does not stop for healthcare. For example, long ago, a patient would visit their physician, get a diagnosis, start treatment, and come back in 'X' days to months to see how it was working or to ask any follow-up questions. Nowadays, patients may do a quick internet search before even considering scheduling an appointment with a healthcare provider. Patients now have the ability to research the diagnosis, imaging, or treatment options in the comfort of their own home [8]. This improved access to information is a driver for innovation in many fields, including healthcare.

As we've often heard before, knowledge is power. However, what happens when one does not know how to apply that knowledge, or if one doesn't know how to critically analyze the information? In such cases, our society's increasing access to information, health-related or not, may at times be detrimental. From children to elders, practically everyone has access to search engines and social media. From scrolling through your "For You" page on TikTok to the various ads that populate on Facebook to the random questions searched on Google, information is always being presented to us. It is easy to believe individuals online who speak confidently about a topic they claim expertise in. With terms such as "doctor", "specialist", and "expert" frequently used to imply credibility, it becomes increasingly difficult for the average person to differentiate truth from falsehood.

One way to overcome this obstacle is building strong patient-physician relationships. During these encounters, physicians can encourage patients to improve their health literacy. As healthcare providers, explaining to patients their diagnoses in plain language and tailoring your encounters to best fit the individual in front of you is one method. Additionally, making room for patients to ask questions and using the teach-back method, as we are taught in our training, also improves health literacy.

As mentioned above, patients have been known to input their symptoms or medical questions into their chosen search engine. Today, OpenEvidence, an online AI search engine used by healthcare professionals, has been running full steam ahead. I have seen internists, obstetricians, and pediatricians utilizing this evidence-backed resource. Healthcare providers can input their clinical questions, and the AI will look through evidence-based, published research to formulate a concise answer while providing links to the research articles used as evidence. Imagine an evidence-based version for patients where explanations are provided in layman's terms and the best next steps are addressed. This may be a tool to help decrease the burden on the emergency departments nationwide, helping patients differentiate between going to their primary care provider's office, urgent care, or emergency room.

Advancements in Optimized Care

A Brief Look at Past Innovations

Healthcare innovations have been around for centuries. From the creation of the first medical school to the creation of antibiotics, the field has never ceased evolving. To start off the main section of this chapter, a look at some of the history of advancements in optimized care will help paint a clearer picture for the current and future evolution of healthcare delivery.

First, a brief history lesson. In 1795, the first American medical school was created. Within the next coming years, many medical schools opened, but after rules and regulations were put in place, many shut down, leaving just 66 [9]. It was only in the 1800s that handwashing was found to be important in patient care by Ignaz Semmelweis. Florence Nightingale helped discover the connection between living conditions and death rates among soldiers. Ernest Codman, a surgeon, advocated for the standardization of hospital [10]. These individuals, like many others, helped pioneer the healthcare system we see today. Of course, no history lesson about healthcare is complete without discussing antibiotics. The first antibiotic, penicillin, was discovered in 1928 by Alexander Fleming.

Additionally, governments have gotten involved in healthcare. In 1965, the United States government created Medicare and Medicaid programs [10]. This was done in efforts to increase access to healthcare services to underserved communities. These programs are still around today and continue to improve the delivery of optimized care.

Technology has also found its way into healthcare delivery. The electronic health records (EHRs) have become intertwined in medicine since the 1990s [11]. Never before was there a "one-stop-shop" for every medical aspect of a patient. Rather than having paper charts and having to communicate through fax machines and endless "on hold" phone calls, providers and patients have access to the majority of patient information in one entity. With a few clicks of the mouse or taps on a smartphone screen, physicians can send prescriptions, update specialists, or upload media into the patient's chart, while patients can view labs and upcoming appointments, and direct message their providers.

Recent Advancements in the Delivery of Optimized Care

Wearable Technology

In the twenty-first century, there have been drastic improvements in technology, profoundly impacting industries like healthcare [12]. These advancements have provided opportunities to improve health outcomes, patient empowerment, and efficiency [13]. Some of the innovations include incorporating wearable technology in medicine, the widespread adoption of electronic health records (EHR), the increasing use of telemedicine, and the revolutionary use of artificial intelligence (AI) [14].

The evolution of medical devices into wearable forms has integrated healthcare into daily life. These devices can have various functions, including remote patient monitoring and activity tracking. They are also capable of providing real-time monitoring of various physiological parameters, such as blood pressure, respiratory activity, body temperature, stress levels, sleep patterns, and adherence to medications [15, 16]. Wearable devices, like activity monitors and smartwatches, promote greater patient autonomy in health management, advancing the shift towards patient-centered care. With their advanced technology, these devices can provide personalized ideas for improvement [16].

Due to physical inactivity being the "fourth most significant contributor to global mortality," there is a growing emphasis among society on improving physical fitness and maintaining an active way of life [16]. Physical inactivity has also been shown to be linked to an increased likelihood of developing chronic conditions. This has brought more attention to wearable activity trackers as they encourage and improve our push towards a healthier lifestyle. In fact, the use of these devices has recently seen a drastic increase, "with a staggering 1444% rise in global shipping from 2014 to 2020" [16]. For tracking physical activity, these wearables enable the monitoring of physical activity-related indicators, such as step count, distance moved, cardiac output, and heart rate. They support behavior change strategies like goal setting, self-monitoring, and feedback provision to improve physical therapy activities. Additionally, wearables give users insight into their long-term performance, allowing for informed changes to their exercise regimens. The use of wearable technology is correlated with improved physiological results, decreased BMI, and reduced blood pressure. Since physical activity has been shown to have antidepressant effects, wearables can help alleviate anxiety and depression [16].

When an individual is stressed, their body releases hormones like adrenocorticoids, glucocorticoids, catecholamines, growth hormones, and others. These hormones can have significant effects on the body, such as increased heart rate, elevated blood pressure, increased breathing frequency, and heightened muscle tension. This gives wearable devices the ability to identify elevated stress levels by monitoring heart rate and suggesting relaxation, mindfulness, breathing exercises, and meditation to promote mental well-being by managing stress [16].

Wearable devices can also use skin temperature, motion sensors, and optical photoplethysmography (PPG) sensors to more accurately identify sleep stages. PPG is a non-invasive and cost-effective technique to monitor heart rate and changes in blood flow volume. Daily, non-intrusive tracking of sleep plays a vital role in assessing sleep's impact on health and disease. The use of wearable technology has given us the opportunity to enhance our understanding of sleep health [16].

In addition to these features, the ability of wearable devices to provide continuous, real-time physiological data has allowed them to be utilized for the treatment and management of various chronic diseases. They allow physicians to precisely customize treatment regimens and can lead to reduced costs and improved patient outcomes by adopting a patient-centered approach [17]. Continuously monitoring vital signs and physiological parameters allows them to detect trends across a wide range of medical specialties and improve outcomes for various patient demographics [17, 18].

In cardiology, wearable devices can be beneficial for monitoring hypertension and detecting arrhythmias. Ambulatory and home blood pressure (BP) monitoring have been recommended for hypertension management by many physicians. A wrist-worn, watch-like, BP monitor called the HeartGuide was found to provide reliable and reproducible measurements. A study found that the differences between wearable BP monitors and ambulatory BP monitoring were acceptable. Therefore, wearable BP monitors like the HeartGuide can improve hypertension management [18]. Also, wearables patients are able to receive immediate feedback on the effects of their physical activity and diet. This can further encourage patients to make healthier choices to improve their health [17].

Additionally, wearable devices, like smartwatches, can detect atrial fibrillation and atrial flutter due to their ability to measure pulse rates. For example, the Apple Watch uses an algorithm to identify events that suggest atrial fibrillation. In the Apple Heart Study, among the participants wearing an ECG patch and Apple Watch, 84% of irregular pulse notifications corresponded with atrial fibrillation detected on ECG patch monitoring at the same time. Other devices like the Fitbit, CardioTracker, and AT-Patch have also been shown to effectively detect atrial fibrillation. These wearables provide the ability for noninvasive monitoring to enhance patient care [18].

For respiratory health, wearable devices can continuously monitor respiratory rate and oxygen saturation allowing them to help diagnose and treat respiratory diseases like asthma, COPD, and sleep apnea. Fitbit activity tracking and smartphone applications can assist patients with COPD to increase physical activity after pulmonary rehabilitation and improve self-management of COPD [18]. Fitness trackers can also efficiently track sleep disorders in asthma patients. Fitbit measurements showed improved sleep quality can improve asthma impact in pediatric patients, suggesting that wearable devices can increase asthma self-management. Additionally, wearable devices can increase patient engagement and management of obesity-related respiratory diseases [18].

Wearables have also been utilized in neurology for seizure detection and monitoring Parkinson's disease. They can detect, track, and manage seizures and are often used for managing epilepsy. Also, they can "distinguish between convulsive psychogenic non-epileptic seizures and convulsive epileptic seizures" [18]; These devices are best used to detect tonic-clonic seizures and further enhancements are needed to detect all types of seizures [18].

Patients with Parkinson's disease have symptoms that increase the risk of falls and balance loss like bradykinesia, posture, and rigidity. Wearable devices like smartwatches can monitor motor impairments and movements for early detection of symptoms like tremors. Gyroscopes and accelerometers have been shown to effectively monitor bradykinesia and assess gait. Additionally, devices can monitor Parkinson's long-term, assess disease severity, and identify the type of tremor. Wearables have also been shown to have a role in neurologic rehabilitation for patients with stroke, neurodegenerative ataxias, and multiple sclerosis [18].

Another specialty wearable devices have a significant role in is endocrinology. Wearables can assist patients with thyroid dysfunction monitoring, fertility tracking, and diabetes management. Wearables are used to monitor thyroid function and can predict thyroid dysfunction using heart rate data. Heart rate data can also be used to predict changes in T4 enabling timely changes to treatment plans for those with thyroid dysfunction [18]. For women, wearable devices can track their fertility window. They use biomarkers like basal body temperature, hormone levels, and other parameters to accurately detect six-day fertility windows [18].

Various devices like smartwatches and fitness trackers can manage diabetes by providing real-time monitoring of blood glucose levels, physical activity, and other parameters. The Dexcom G6 and FreeStyle Libre can measure glucose levels in interstitial fluid without fingerstick calibration, significantly improving glycemic control and patient adherence. Also, fitness trackers can also improve glycemic control in type 1 diabetes patients by integrating activity levels, heart rate, and caloric data with insulin delivery. Other devices like the iGLU 2.0 can also accurately monitor glucose levels noninvasively [18]. Machine learning models in wearables analyze the glucose data and can optimize insulin therapy by changing doses in real time. Wearables can also prevent complications like hypoglycemia and hyperglycemia, thus improving patients' quality of life [17].

Wearable devices have been shown to have positive impacts on patient health outcomes across a variety of specialties. They can optimize the delivery of care by promoting data-driven personalized care and adherence to treatment regimens. Additionally, their potential extends to broader public health policies by reducing disease complications and hospitalization [17]. Aggregating their data can give insights into public health issues and outbreaks [18]. The ability to consistently monitor data by using wearable devices improves care by decreasing hospitalization, emergency interventions, and improving patient quality of life. The integration of artificial intelligence (AI) into healthcare is projected to advance real-time data analysis and patient monitoring by predicting disease exacerbations and enabling timely interventions that could reduce hospitalization rates [17].

Artificial Intelligence (AI)

Recently, artificial intelligence has been integrated into medicine and has drastically impacted various aspects of healthcare. AI tools have been able to assist with disease detection, precise diagnoses, and treatment planning. Additionally, AI has increased efficiency in the medical field, assisted with drug discovery, and further expanded access to remote monitoring and telemedicine. AI has also been used for medical imaging. It has been very efficient and quick in detecting abnormalities in images like X-rays. AI can assist radiologists with interpreting images and making the process more accurate and efficient by detecting minor abnormalities and disease detection [19]. Some have even speculated whether AI could step in and take jobs away from radiologists.

AI can be used as a tool to analyze and process large amounts of data quickly. This can be used to predict health outcomes and determine a patient's risk of developing certain conditions. Some Apollo Hospitals use "AI-powered predictive analytics models to analyze patient data and medical records, enabling early detection and proactive management of chronic diseases" [19]. Additionally, AI can be utilized for data analysis in research. This can speed up the process of writing manuscripts, giving researchers more time to focus on other projects. AI's speed and efficiency can thus lead to more research projects being completed, and more clinical information being available for physicians to determine how to best treat their patients. For example, deep learning AI has been increasingly used in pharmaceutical research and drug discovery [19].

Artificial Intelligence in the form of robots has assisted with processes like patient registration, billing, and data entry. They have been used to speed up tasks and free up healthcare staff to spend more time with patients or work on other tasks. Robots have also assisted with surgeries. Robot-assisted surgery provides surgeons with greater precision, control, and dexterity during surgical procedures. It has enabled minimally invasive procedures that improve surgical outcomes in various fields, like Interventional Radiology [19].

Virtual assistants and chatbots like ChatGPT provide personalized support, answer medical questions, provide support for medication management and guidance, and can even assess symptoms. Many patients are using chatbots to ask specific questions about their health to provide them with more information. Even though AI can provide data backed medical advice, it is important to complement, not replace, medical professionals. Utilizing AI in medicine has some challenges including data privacy and security, and skepticism from physicians. Despite these challenges, AI is being increasingly adopted in healthcare. As more improvements are made in AI, some of the challenges will be addressed and new features will be added [20].

Communication

Telemedicine gives physicians the ability to provide healthcare services without needing an in-person visit. Recent technological advancements in telemedicine have revolutionized how medical services are provided by addressing challenges in accessibility. This has had a major impact on rural and underserved areas by allowing providers to extend their range into further regions. Patients who are far from physicians, or those who lack access to transport, are able to use telemedicine to receive care from their providers. Additionally, for patients with chronic conditions that require regular visits with their providers, telemedicine can be an efficient way to reduce travel time and improve efficiency while still maintaining regular monitoring. Also, telemedicine allows providers in rural areas to refer their patients to specialists that may be far from their clinic, ensuring their patients are receiving the best care possible [21]. Overall, telemedicine has had a drastic effect on the efficiency of and access to medicine, especially for patients in underserved and rural areas.

The widespread adoption of electronic health records has been a major positive in the healthcare industry. EHRs have improved accuracy of documentation by reducing their errors. This has been able to improve patient safety by making it easier for physicians to monitor patient information like medications and allergies. Additionally, EHRs are critical for improving care coordination across different specialties, clinics, and hospitals. They allow for the quick and easy transfer of patient information, providing physicians with a vast amount of information on the patient's prior medical visits. This allows physicians to understand the context of their patient's past medical history, which can prevent negative drug interactions [22].

Electronic health records also give the patient the ability to track their progress and view the documentation of their past medical visits on their own. This provides patients with all of the information on what happened on their visits. If a patient forgets something their physician told them, like medication instructions and wound care, they could just check their EHR without having to call or go to the clinic. EHRs have had a positive effect on physicians by providing them with all of their patients' information, and on patients by allowing easy access to their medical information.

Possible Future Advancements in Optimized Care

With a lot of attention in today's media being directed towards personal health and wellness alongside endless technological advancements, the possible future advancements to optimize patient care are vast.

Research-Supported Patient AI Search Engine

We have all seen an uproar in the use of AI. It has been incorporated into education, healthcare, businesses, and more. While rotating through different services in the hospital during medical school, it was noted that attending and resident physicians were utilizing research-based AI. such as OpenEvidence, to help answer medical questions that come up. Similarly, we have all run to our preferred search engine to self-diagnose ourselves when new symptoms develop. The answers we find are usually worse-case scenarios and leave us with heightened anxiety until we are able to schedule an appointment with our primary care provider (PCP) or visit the nearest urgent care or emergency department. Additionally, a quick scroll through practically any social media platform will show you non-medical professionals providing medical advice online. Social media users flock to the comment sections and interact with these posts. The more interactions it gets, the more people are exposed to the post and potentially doing something harmful or nonbeneficial to their bodies rather than seeking the assistance of a medical professional.

Due to this, a tool I believe our society would benefit from would be an OpenEvidence for patients. This could be a site where patients could input their chief complaint, set of symptoms they are experiencing, or medical questions they have and get a science-backed answer. It would be linked to published research articles and summarize the findings in layman's terms while encouraging follow up with a medical provider. Minimizing the false information available to patients and providing them with free access to medically backed information could improve health outcomes and patient-physician relationships.

Similarly, I could also see this being utilized as an online triage tool where it could tell patients where they should go to receive care, like a primary care provider's office, urgent care, or emergency room, based on the level of urgency. One major issue plaguing our healthcare system is emergency department overcrowding. In recent years, this problem has only worsened and has led to poorer patient care and satisfaction, quality of care, and increased mortality and morbidity [23]. Utilizing an online triage tool could be a massive win for the American healthcare system. The main purpose of an emergency department is to treat emergency and urgent cases that need immediate attention. By finding a way to limit overcrowding and overuse, we may improve patient outcomes and emergency department employee satisfaction [23].

Remembering Your "Why?"

The research that went into creating this chapter not only shed light on the delivery of optimized care, but also an even more significant one. Yes, efficiency, accuracy, productivity, improved access to care and information, as discussed in this chapter, are important for providing optimized care, but there is one important detail missing- the knowledge and wellbeing of the individual providing the care.

Filling Your Cup

It is common knowledge that one cannot pour from an empty cup. To become a physician in the United States, one must complete a bachelor's degree and pass various prerequisites, succeed on the MCAT, and go through a medical school application cycle. If you are lucky, one cycle will be all you need, but unfortunately, this is not the case for many. Once you matriculate into medical school, you will need to pass courses, semesters, and most importantly at least two licensing exams on top of all the extracurriculars to be a competitive applicant into the specialty of your choice. The road is not over here. Many letters of recommendation, personal statement edits, rotations, and sub-internships later; you match into a program and start June/July of your application cycle. The schedule for residency, no matter the specialty, is known to be rigorous. You will not have control over your schedule during this at least 7-year period of your life, and there will always be something you will be working towards.

You successfully complete the aforementioned journey of becoming a physician, and many individuals are drained. They are tired, overworked, and the light that brought them into this field has been dimmed. A survey was conducted on trainee physicians and found that 50% experienced burnout, while 80% of them shared experiences of high stress levels [24]. The expectations of yourself, the program, the fellowship you may be aspiring to be a successful applicant in, and most importantly, your patients fall on that resident physician's shoulders. These symptoms of burnout have had a pivotal effect on physician well-being, relationships, and potentially patient care [24].

By reconnecting and filling your own cup, you ensure you have something to pour from when supporting others. In medicine, this holds even more significance as the field revolves around improving the health and wellbeing of patients. Starting a patient encounter from a burnt out, tired, or angry outlook does not help cultivate an environment where you can foster a strong patient-physician relationship. The USA's Physician Foundation found 58% of physicians experienced burnout in 2020 compared to 40% just two years prior [25]. With physician mistrust already being problematic today, making sure these interactions are impactful, compassionate, and restorative is more important than ever.

Nowadays, information is very accessible, and it is no secret that a lot of physicians are unhappy. Social media allows people to share their experiences. In healthcare, sharing experiences of burnout and dissatisfaction within the career may be a deterrent to some from pursuing this career path in the future, thus worsening the physician shortage in this country and blocking the delivery of optimized care to patients. Additionally, they are more likely to struggle with depression, substance dependence, and cardiovascular disease [25].

On top of the personal struggles these physicians may be experiencing; the stigma regarding this subject matter worsens the situation. In medicine, the physician's mental and physical health can be seen as an indicator of their medical competence. Thus, confessing your struggles or seeking treatment for burnout-related symptoms can be seen as weakness by the physician's colleagues. This perceived stigma has contributed to the lack of seeking assistance [25]. More work needs to be done to better understand and decrease the stigma associated with physician burnout both to improve work life satisfaction, patient care, and attract students to the profession.

Conclusion

The United States of America's population is changing. With the increase in life expectancy and chronic diseases, patient care modifications are necessary. In this chapter, we discussed the delivery of optimized care in relation to current and future innovations. With the increased financial burden and resource scarcity in the healthcare system, finding ways to mitigate these stressors and other disparities can improve the quality of patient care from a systematic standpoint.

From the first medical school to the standardization of hospitals to the creation of antibiotics, medicine and healthcare has been an ever-evolving sector. Systems have been created to address disparities such as Medicaid and Medicare. Recent advancements in technology have had a major impact on the medical field with EHRs. Wearable devices have integrated healthcare into daily life by allowing remote patient monitoring and activity tracking. Their ability to provide real-time monitoring of physiological parameters allows them to be used in the treatment of various chronic conditions. Some of these devices have been integrated with artificial intelligence. Although new and improving, AI has already increased efficiency in the medical field by assisting patients and processing vast amounts of information quickly. Telemedicine and electronic health records have improved communication between patients and providers by improving access to medicine and medical information. These recent technological advancements have ultimately led to improved health outcomes, patient empowerment, and autonomy, and improved efficiency. Future advancements include a new triage system and an "OpenEvidence"-inspired patient search engine.

Addressing the problems in medical education, alongside patient care, is also important. Creating resources to remove the stigma on medical students and provider burnout should have resources allocated. After all, you cannot pour from an empty cup. In the end, the United States healthcare system necessitates a system overhaul. There is dissatisfaction from every angle you look at. With the advancements in technology and the vast realization of the problems plaguing the healthcare system, adjustments addressing the various problems can improve job satisfaction, patient care, and cost.

References

1. Portrait of American Healthcare [Internet]. www.ncbi.nlm.nih.gov. Agency for Healthcare Research and Quality (US); 2023. Available from: https://www.ncbi.nlm.nih.gov/books/NBK600454/
2. Definition of OPTIMIZE [Internet]. Merriam-webster.com. 2019. Available from: https://www.merriam-webster.com/dictionary/optimize
3. Beverley M, Holson DA, Hewlett D. Patient engagement and cultural sensitivity as a strategy to improve health inequities: the solutions are as simple as they are complex. J Natl Med Assoc [Internet]. 2022;114(6):578–583. Available from: https://www.ncbi.nlm.nih.gov/pmc/articles/PMC9525216/
4. Dember LM. What patients teach us about patient engagement in research. Clin J Am Soc Nephrol. 2022;17(2):176–8.
5. Landon SN, Padikkala J, Horwitz LI. Identifying drivers of health care value: a scoping review of the literature. BMC Health Serv Res. 2022;22(1)
6. Saini V, Garcia-Armesto S, Klemperer D, Paris V, Elshaug AG, Brownlee S, et al. Drivers of poor medical care. Lancet [Internet]. 2017;390(10090):178–190. Available from: https://www.sciencedirect.com/science/article/pii/S0140673616309473
7. Hodkinson A, Zhou, A, Johnson J, Geraghty K, Riley R, Zhou A, et al. Associations of physician burnout with career engagement and quality of patient care: systematic review and meta-analysis. BMJ [Internet]. 2022;378(8352):e070442. Available from: https://www.bmj.com/content/378/bmj-2022-070442
8. Towbin AJ, O'Connor T, Perry LA, Moskovitz JA, Miñano GG, Regan J, et al. Using informatics to engage patients. Pediatr Radiol. 2020;50(11):1514–24.
9. Sheingold BH, Hahn JA. The history of healthcare quality: the first 100 years 1860–1960. Int J Africa Nurs Sci [Internet]. 2014;1(1):18–22. Available from: https://www.sciencedirect.com/science/article/pii/S2214139114000043
10. Marjoua Y, Bozic KJ. Brief history of quality movement in US healthcare. Curr Rev Musculoskelet Med [Internet]. 2012;5(4):265–273. Available from: https://www.ncbi.nlm.nih.gov/pmc/articles/PMC3702754/
11. Rampton V, Böhmer M, Winkler A. Medical technologies past and present: how history helps to understand the digital era. J Med Humanit. 2021;43(2)
12. Ibanga IJ. Human and technology in the 21st century. Bincang Sains dan Teknologi. 2024;3(02):40–3.
13. Alhur A. Impact of technological innovations on healthcare delivery: a literature review of efficiency, patient care, and operational challenges. World J Biol Pharm Health Sci. 2024;18(2):216–9.
14. Matcha A. Innovations in healthcare: transforming patient care through technology, personalized medicine, and Global Health crises. Int J Sci Res. 2023;12(12):1668–72.
15. Vishwakarma AK, Ranjan R, Verma K, Kumar R. Exploring the potential impacts of wearable technology in reshaping healthcare. 2024 15th International Conference on Computing Communication and Networking Technologies (ICCCNT) [Internet]. 2024 Jun 24 [cited 2024 Dec 22];1–7. Available from: https://www.semanticscholar.org/paper/Exploring-the-Potential-Impacts-of-Wearable-in-Vishwakarma-Ranjan/2a4db835ea03c71e56001c7ebb8a032ab5f42e57
16. Sieniawska J, Proszowska P, Madoń M, Kotowicz Z, Orzeł A, Pich-Czekierda A, et al. Measuring health: wearables in fitness tracking, stress relief, and sleep management. J Educ Health Sport [Internet]. 2024;67:50673. Available from: https://apcz.umk.pl/JEHS/article/view/50673
17. Oni O, Awofala TB. Utilization of wearable technology data in chronic disease management. World J Adv Res Rev. 2022;16(3):1189–95.

18. Jafleh EA, Alnaqbi FA, Almaeeni HA, Faqeeh S, Alzaabi MA, Al Zaman K. The role of wearable devices in chronic disease monitoring and patient care: a comprehensive review. Cureus [Internet] 2024;16(9). Available from: https://pubmed.ncbi.nlm.nih.gov/39381470/
19. Valdya R, Kulkarni SM, Galkwad T, Jadhav S. Advancing healthcare through artificial intelligence: opportunities, challenges and future directions. Int Res J Adv Eng Manag. 2024;2(05):1302–8.
20. Weerarathna IN. Artificial intelligence in healthcare. 2024;346–62.
21. Alqahtany AS, Khrami SA, Alsharari AS, Alsharari SF, Alshamari MR, Alsharari AS, et al. Advancements in telemedicine: transforming healthcare delivery and enhancing access for providers and patients alike. Int J Health Sci [Internet]. 2022;6(S10):1771–85. Available from: https://www.neliti.com/publications/580858/advancements-in-telemedicine-transforming-healthcare-delivery-and-enhancing-acce
22. Razzano AV. A scoping review on the impacts of electronic health record systems on healthcare delivery. Int J Health Sci Res [Internet]. 2024;14(7):276–282. Available from: https://www.ijhsr.org/IJHSR_Vol.14_Issue.7_July2024/IJHSR37.pdf
23. Sartini M, Carbone A, Demartini A, Giribone L, Oliva M, Spagnolo AM, et al. Overcrowding in emergency department: causes, consequences, and solutions—a narrative review. Healthcare [Internet]. 2022;10(9):1625. Available from: https://www.ncbi.nlm.nih.gov/pmc/articles/PMC9498666/
24. Zhou AY, Panagioti M, Esmail A, Agius R, Van Tongeren M, Bower P. Factors associated with burnout and stress in trainee physicians. JAMA Netw Open. 2020;3(8):e2013761.
25. Favre S, Bajwa NM, Dominicé Dao M, Audétat Voirol MC ., Nendaz M, Junod Perron N, et al. Association between burnout and stigma in physicians. Gascón S, editor. PLoS One 2023;18(4):e0283556.

New and Innovative Ideas in Medical Specialties and Subspecialties

From Crisis Innovation to Lasting Reform: The Role of Telehealth in Equitable and Sustainable Healthcare

Lauren Herschelman and Cheryl A. Dickson

Introduction

The COVID-19 pandemic catalyzed a dramatic transformation in the delivery of medical care across the United States and beyond. What began out of necessity as an urgent and temporary adaptation in response to an unforeseen and unprecedented crisis has evolved into a lasting paradigm shift in which elements have proved to provide benefit to patients and the practice of medicine broadly. The demonstrable benefits of these changes to the healthcare system have given them longevity and transformed the way we practice medicine today. One of these shifts was the adoption of telemedicine into standard medical practice which has rapidly become a critical tool to maintain access to essential health services while minimizing infection risk and accommodating public health restrictions [1, 2]. Despite a relative decrease in total primary care encounters by over 20% in 2020, telemedicine utilization expanded at an unprecedented rate. Prior to the pandemic, virtual visits accounted for just 1.1% of all encounters during Q2 2018–2019. By Q2 of 2020, that proportion had risen to 35.3%, representing approximately 35 million primary care visits compared to an average of 1.4 million quarterly visits pre-pandemic [3]. Extending beyond primary care, across all specialties approximately half of all visits were via virtual visits during the height of the viral pandemic in April of 2020 [4]. This rapid shift reflects not only the healthcare system's ability to scale digital

L. Herschelman
Western Michigan University Homer Stryker M.D. School of Medicine, Kalamazoo, MI, USA
e-mail: Lauren.Herschelman@wmed.edu

C. A. Dickson (✉)
Department of Pediatric and Adolescent Medicine, Western Michigan University Homer Stryker M.D. School of Medicine, Kalamazoo, MI, USA
e-mail: Cheryl.Dickson@wmed.edu

S. S. Chahin et al. (eds.), *Innovation in Medical Education and Clinical Practice*, https://doi.org/10.1007/978-3-032-19116-8_16

infrastructure under pressure but also the willingness of patients and providers to adapt to new models of care delivery.

Post- pandemic utilization rates have declined, but have stabilized at levels much higher than those pre-pandemic. A study of adult patients published in JAMA concluded that in 2022, 43% of patients have at least one telehealth visit annually with a positive association between use of telemedicine and female sex as well as those with chronic medical conditions or participating in multiple visits within a 12 month period [4]. This transition was particularly pronounced in women's health, primary care including pediatrics, behavioral health, where virtual care has filled longstanding gaps in access as well as select subspecialties particularly in underserved populations and minority groups within the United States. Telemedicine proved indispensable in preserving continuity of care for time-sensitive medical needs across diverse settings: it enabled uninterrupted access to family planning and contraception services, facilitated timely follow-up for pediatric patients with developmental delays, and allowed for behavioral health evaluation and management despite geographic, logistical, and regulatory hurdles [5–10]. These examples illustrate how telemedicine has evolved from an emergency stopgap into a durable supplement to in-person care. By bridging geographic barriers, reducing time and transportation burdens, and mitigating infection risk, it has extended life-saving and time-sensitive interventions to populations that might otherwise face critical barriers to access. In doing so, the pandemic not only accelerated a long-discussed but slow-moving innovation, it reset expectations for what accessible, patient-centered care can and should look like in the future [1, 2].

The History of Virtual Healthcare and Its Access

Historically, early applications of telehealth were developed to serve populations with limited access to in-person care, such as members of the military, incarcerated individuals, and residents of rural communities. Among the most influential early models was the "telestroke" program, first implemented in 1999. This initiative emerged in the wake of the pivotal NINDS rt-PA Stroke Trial, which demonstrated that timely administration of tissue plasminogen activator (tPA) within 3 hours of symptom onset could significantly reduce stroke-related morbidity and mortality [11]. Because many hospitals lacked on-site neurologists, telestroke networks leveraged videoconferencing to allow remote stroke specialists to evaluate patients, review neuroimaging, and guide local clinicians in real time. This innovation enabled hospitals without in-house expertise to deliver reperfusion therapies promptly. The model was not only revolutionary in its capacity to democratize access to specialized stroke care, but also became one of the first large-scale demonstrations of telemedicine's ability to directly improve patient outcomes. Subsequent evaluations of telestroke programs confirm that hospitals participating in these networks achieve higher rates of reperfusion therapy and lower 30-day mortality compared to hospitals without such access, underscoring the model's lifesaving potential [12]. Meta-analysis of modern virtual cardiovascular disease monitoring using telephone support programs have shown a reduction in rehospitalization rates of up to 25% [13]. In many ways, telestroke became the prototype for future telehealth models, proving that virtual care could not only supplement in-person medicine but also extend lifesaving interventions to patients who would otherwise be excluded by structural barriers.

Despite such promising examples, telemedicine adoption remained limited in the decades preceding COVID-19 due to significant regulatory, logistical, and cultural barriers. One major factor was the lack of robust, large-scale data proving that telemedicine provided clear, reproducible benefits across specialties. Without compelling evidence, enthusiasm among health systems and clinicians was tempered. Financial barriers also played a central role. Even as regulatory changes, such as the Interstate Medical Licensure Compact, created pathways for physicians to practice across state lines, reimbursement policies remained restrictive and inconsistent. Prior to the pandemic, many payers limited coverage for telehealth services. This fragmented approach discouraged adoption and left both clinicians and patients facing uncertainty about the financial sustainability of telemedicine [14]. Medicare, in particular, lagged behind Medicaid and many commercial insurers, covering telehealth services only for patients in designated rural areas and only when visits occurred at approved "originating sites" which explicitly excluding patients' homes. This sharply limited access for most beneficiaries and further contributed to low utilization rates. These restrictions were strict and had very little exceptions, only including chronic conditions such as hemodialysis requirements or substance use disorder treatment, though even within these exceptions ambulatory presentation to a clinic or a hospital site was required in fixed time intervals [15, 16]. These constraints sharply curtailed access, particularly in urban and suburban populations. Reflecting these barriers, telemedicine utilization prior to 2020 was negligible. For example, in a large national commercial insurance database, only 0.12% of outpatient visits were conducted via telemedicine, with notable disparities based on age, comorbidity burden, income level, and rurality [17].

During the global COVID-19 pandemic, the urgent need to reduce in-person contact, preserve resources, and increase availability of quality healthcare triggered widespread implementation of remote care models. In March of 2020, the Centers for Medicare and Medicaid Services updated the previously enforced restriction on reimbursement for telehealth services. These new guidelines lifted restrictions of geographic barrier related reimbursement for virtual services and allowed for a rapid adoption of these services [18]. Telehealth utilization increased by 20- to 70-fold in key specialties during this timeframe, with the many dramatic and sustained changes in pediatrics, women's health, behavioral health, and selected medical subspecialties [19–23]. In adult populations, this shift to remote care was associated with improved follow-up. One study found that no-show rate disparities in follow-up previously associated with high social vulnerability index (SVI) scores were no longer present after telemedicine expansion [24].

This finding demonstrates the capacity of rapid deployment of telehealth to reduce access disparities and improve retention in care for underserved adult populations, mitigating structural barriers that have historically limited engagement for socially and economically vulnerable groups. With realization of these very tangible benefits, the Society of General Internal Medicine has released a position statement emphasizing the long-term importance of telemedicine beyond the temporary pandemic waivers. Telehealth services, specifically audio-video and audio-only encounters, were shown to expand dramatically during the pandemic and demonstrated potential to advance the quintuple aim of healthcare: patient experience, health outcomes, cost, clinician well-being, and equity. Their policy priorities include ending outdated geographic and originating site restrictions, expanding coverage to include audio-only services, establishing telemedicine-specific service codes, and ensuring equitable broadband access. Clinical recommendations stress that telemedicine should be integrated intentionally to strengthen longitudinal care and that modality selection should occur through patient-clinician shared decision-making [25].

Medical Subspecialties and Telemedicine

Pediatrics

In pediatrics, similar gains were observed and appreciated. Telehealth visits with subspecialists surged from 1 per 1000 child enrollees in 2019 to 68 per 1000 in 2020, a staggering 68-fold increase. While this expansion in virtual encounters did not fully offset the steep decline in in-person visits during the height of the pandemic, it highlighted telehealth's ability to preserve continuity of care in the face of massive disruption [26]. For children, particularly those with special health care needs and those facing systemic barriers to access, the stakes of disrupted care are especially high. Disruptions in care for these children can result in delayed diagnoses, gaps in treatment, and widening health disparities that may have long-term consequences on the patient and the family navigating complex healthcare needs. Telehealth has become foundational to implementing the medical home model which allows for high-value, coordinated, and family-centered pediatric care. The American Academy of Pediatrics (AAP) has been outspoken about telehealth becoming a critical tool for maintaining access to quality acute, chronic, and preventive care. This is especially important for under-resourced populations and in times of health care disruption, such as during the COVID-19 pandemic. The group has warned that rollback of these gains threatens the creation of dangerous gaps in care for young patients in critical need [19]. Data from a large academic center exemplify this trend: Pediatric subspecialty telehealth visits increased by over 5000%, from 150 in March–June 2019 to 7675 in the same period of 2020, while in-person visits fell by more than half [27]. The AAP cautions that dismantling the systems and investments that enabled this transformation would erode not only children's access to "the right care at the right place at the right time" but also the preventive infrastructure that helps reduce costly hospitalizations and long-term morbidity. Stripping this investment would have a rippling effect on all stakeholders in the medical home and ultimately undermine patients, families, and the broader healthcare system alike [19].

This need becomes magnified further for conditions requiring close follow-up and high-intensity intervention. Developmental delay, affecting roughly 13% of young children, represents a prime example [6]. Children with developmental delay require frequent and closely coordinated visits to monitor developmental milestones, adjust individualized therapies, and ensure timely referrals to specialists. These needs are best met through integrated multidisciplinary care teams which include speech therapists, occupational and physical therapists, developmental-behavioral pediatricians, and educators. Evidence is clear that consistent follow-up translates to improved outcomes for children with developmental delay. One study, a systematic review of extremely preterm infants, found that for every 1% decrease in follow-up rate, there was a 1.1% increase in the reported rate of neurodevelopmental impairment at 18 to 24 months of age [28]. This relationship demonstrates that higher rates of follow-up are associated with lower rates of neurodevelopmental impairment at a further timepoint, supporting the importance of close and persistent follow-up care for maximizing the potential for improved developmental outcomes in this population. Additionally, independent of follow up rates, the difficulty to receive follow-up can also play a major role in the outcomes of these patients. Factors such as missed appointments or the need to travel to alternative sites prove strikingly worse long-term outcomes. A study found that despite a near-identical follow up rate of 87%, children of school age who were more difficult to follow-up with had over double the rate of neurodevelopmental disability at school age compared to their peers who did not demonstrate these barriers, 42% vs. 20%, respectively. These difficulties included multiple broken appointments, the need for patient assessment at an alternate location to the clinic, and parental inability to present the child for assessment [29].

These findings underscore the critical role of consistent follow-up in improving neurodevelopmental outcomes for children with developmental delay. Telehealth offers the opportunity for consistent follow-up and a reduction in gaps of care that could otherwise delay intervention and compromise long-term outcomes. By removing barriers such as transportation challenges, time off work for caregivers, and long wait times for appointments, telemedicine provides an opportunity to sustain the intensity of care needed to support developmental progress. These barriers were only magnified during the pandemic which disrupted this high-intensity and continual process, providing a prime opportunity to utilize telehealth visits for this patient population. Data from a large developmental-behavior pediatric clinic showed that retention for telehealth was greatly increased when compared to in-person visits in 2019 and 2020 with 75.3% vs. 64.4% completed visits for telehealth vs in-person respectively [8]. In addition to improving access and continuity, telehealth has demonstrated measurable clinical benefits for children with developmental delay. A randomized clinical trial evaluating internet-delivered parent-child interaction therapy (iPCIT) for young children with developmental delay and externalizing behavior problems showed significantly improved behavioral outcomes compared to usual referrals. Children receiving the virtual care option demonstrated greater reductions in externalizing behaviors and higher compliance with caregiver direction at 6- and 12-months post-treatment. Importantly, the benefits extended beyond the patient to encompass the caregiving environment. Caregivers who engaged in virtual sessions reported a steeper decreased reliance on harsh or inconsistent discipline strategies and, on structured observation, demonstrated a more consistent use of positive parenting techniques than non-iPCIT families. These improvements in parenting behaviors are particularly significant, as caregiver practices are among the most powerful predictors of long-term child developmental and behavioral outcomes. By equipping caregivers with effective, evidence-based tools and reinforcing them through consistent virtual contact, telehealth interventions can strengthen the parent-child relationship, foster healthier family dynamics, and build caregiver confidence. In this way, virtual care extends its impact beyond the immediate therapeutic encounter, creating a ripple effect that supports resilience and growth in both the child and the family system [6]. Notably, this trial included primarily low-income and racially minoritized families, highlighting the capacity of telehealth to address persistent disparities in access to high-quality behavioral interventions. By reducing barriers such as transportation challenges, limited availability of local specialists, and caregiver work constraints, telehealth creates more equitable opportunities for consistent engagement in care. These findings underscore the promise of telehealth platforms in extending the reach of effective interventions to underserved populations, supporting both the child and caregiver in achieving better long-term developmental outcomes while fostering stronger family dynamics, caregiver confidence, and resilience.

Women's Health

In women's health, including maternal care, telehealth was rapidly adopted for prenatal, postpartum, and mental health visits, transforming how care was delivered during the pandemic. A rapid review of 44,894 patients found that supplementing or replacing in-person maternity care with telehealth resulted in similar or better clinical and patient-reported outcomes, with high patient satisfaction [30]. This shift occurred not only nationally, but across the globe, even in countries previously labelled as high telehealth adopters in 2018. International survey data show that before the pandemic, 57.6% of women had never used telemedicine, but use increased substantially during the pandemic, especially for audio-based and chat-based services. The expansion of telehealth adoption in women's healthcare was especially significant for women from racial and ethnic minority groups, those experiencing financial hardship, and sexual minority populations, groups historically marginalized and underserved within healthcare systems. These populations often face structural barriers including limited access to transportation, inflexible work schedules, childcare constraints, and geographic or systemic scarcity of culturally competent providers. Telehealth mitigates many of these obstacles by allowing patients to engage in care from home or other convenient locations, reducing the burden of travel and time off work, and increasing access to providers who understand and respect their specific needs.

Analysis from international data shows that women who identified as lower-income or as sexual minorities were significantly more likely to switch to telehealth services, suggesting that these platforms may play a critical role in reducing inequities in access and improving continuity of care for those most vulnerable. By offering flexible, accessible, and patient-centered care, telehealth not only preserves essential women's health services during crises but also has the potential to fundamentally enhance equity in healthcare delivery. While the pandemic prompted a surge in telemedicine adoption, especially among women from marginalized and minority groups, many users who were new to the technology reported mixed or poor experiences [21]. This reflects broader challenges in digital literacy, infrastructure, and accessibility that must be addressed to ensure equitable care. As telemedicine becomes a more permanent fixture in healthcare, it is critical for policymakers and healthcare providers to identify and eliminate barriers, improve patient experience, and ensure that telehealth systems are adaptable across diverse social and economic contexts.

While telehealth helped bridge gaps in maternal and preventive care during the pandemic, its role extended beyond routine visits. One critical area where telemedicine became a lifeline was reproductive health, particularly abortion care. Direct-to-patient telemedicine for medication abortion emerged as an essential resource during clinic closures and travel restrictions, offering a safe and accessible alternative when in-person services were disrupted [1, 2]. The need for this service is evidenced by data showing its cascading impact on reducing delays, complications, and inequities in access to abortion care during the COVID-19 pandemic. The pandemic significantly disrupted access to women's healthcare services worldwide, particularly in reproductive health including abortion services. Unsafe or delayed abortion is associated with increased rates of maternal morbidity and mortality, including higher risks of hemorrhage, infection, and complications from unsafe procedures. The American College of Obstetricians and Gynecologists (ACOG) estimates that globally, unsafe abortions account for up to 15% of maternal deaths, with major causes including hemorrhage, sepsis, and injury from unskilled procedures. This is striking because ACOG also notes that the risk of death from childbirth is fourteen times that of an abortion procedure performed with safe and modern practices [31]. Disruptions in access to abortion services led to measurable negative health outcomes. In Louisiana, for example, clinic closures and service reductions resulted in a 31% decrease in abortions with a resulting significant increase in the odds of second-trimester abortions, which are associated with higher complication rates compared to first-trimester procedures. Importantly this policy change cannot be corrected with patient travel to surrounding states without these regulations as the decrease was not measurably offset with an increase in out-of-state abortions [32]. Globally, where abortion services were postponed or restricted, there was a documented rise in second-trimester abortions and an increased risk of unsafe abortion, particularly in low and middle income countries [32–34].

Nationally representative data show that the number and type of barriers to reproductive health care increased between 2017 and 2021, with the largest increases observed among individuals from historically disadvantaged populations, including those with lower educational attainment, lower income, and non-English speakers [35]. In addition to access-related barriers which included decreased use of public transportation and reduction in childcare workforce, pandemic-specific factors such as the classification of reproductive health services as nonessential lead to clinic closures and reduced service availability [7, 21, 35, 36]. The reduction in Title X family planning clinics in 2019 further limited access, with a documented decrease in family planning visits from 2019 to 2020 [35].

As family planning visits declined, telemedicine women's health and abortion services filled a critical gap when in-person services were severely disrupted, preventing increases in unsafe abortion and resultant maternal morbidity and mortality [37]. In Canada and several other high-resource settings, the removal of restrictive regulations facilitated a robust transition to telemedicine, ensuring that women's health services, including induced pregnancy termination, remained accessible as an essential service [1, 9]. Qualitative data from interviews with women in Canada who obtained abortion care during the pandemic reveal that virtual visits provided relief and gratitude for access to remote abortion services. Several interviewees explicitly stated that without telemedicine they would have faced significant distress, prolonged uncertainty, and potentially been unable to obtain care at all. Similar findings were reported in Scotland, where women emphasized that telemedicine abortion services provided critical flexibility and privacy and that lack of access would have resulted in significant hardship as well as had a negative psychosocial impacts long term [38, 39]. During the pandemic, telemedicine models for medication abortion demonstrated safety and effectiveness equivalent to in-person care, with complete abortion rates exceeding 97% and serious adverse events below 0.5% [40]. Telehealth directly addressed barriers such as travel, cost, and fear of COVID-19 exposure, enabling earlier access to care and reducing the risk of complications associated with delayed or denied abortion. The rapid expansion and high patient satisfaction with telehealth abortion care during this period underscore its essential role in safeguarding women's health and saving lives when traditional healthcare infrastructure was inaccessible.

Mental Health

Just as telehealth mitigated critical barriers to reproductive care, it has similarly emerged as a vital tool for expanding the reach of mental health services. Limited and inconsistent access to mental health care in the United States contributes to significant psychological, clinical, and social burdens. Adults with unmet psychiatric needs experience higher levels of distress, greater severity of depression and anxiety, and worse long-term outcomes. This patient population demonstrates lower adherence to treatment plans and reduced follow-up engagement [41, 42]. This is critical to address as 9% of American adults annually are affected by Major Depressive Disorder alone with a 30% lifetime prevalence for women. Depression is not only linked to an eightfold increase in suicide risk but also contributes to higher all-cause mortality and billions of dollars in lost workplace productivity. Even among those who do initiate treatment, outcomes are often suboptimal with only about 18% achieve a 50% or greater reduction in symptoms within six months, underscoring the need for consistent monitoring and accessible, high-quality care [43]. What is frightening is fewer than half of U.S. adults with any diagnosable mental disorder receive any treatment at all [41]. Financial barriers, medical debt, and lack of insurance drive this gap in care, especially for low-income groups [41, 42]. Insufficient access to mental health services is not merely a matter of inconvenience, rather it is a driver of preventable suffering, chronic illness, and economic burden at the population level. Expanding access to timely, affordable, and sustained psychiatric and psychological services is therefore crucial for improving both individual and public health as well as health equity broadly.

Before the COVID-19 pandemic, the use of telehealth for mental health care in the United States was negligible, accounting for less than 0.2% of all mental health visits among commercially insured patients, with slightly higher uptake among younger adults and residents of western United States [44]. Many argued that virtual mental health services were underutilized in medicine as the most critical aspects of evaluation, the mental status examination and a detailed history, are effectively obtained verbally. Telepsychiatry data at that time demonstrated that virtual and in-person encounters produced equivalent outcomes in patient satisfaction, treatment adherence, and symptom reduction across a multitude of mental health diagnoses. Despite these early calls for the expansion of telehealth in the psychiatry and psychology spaces, most psychotherapy and psychiatric care was delivered in person, with telehealth hindered by strict regulations, lack of reimbursement parity, and limited technological infrastructure [44, 45].

The onset of the pandemic prompted a transformation of the delivery of healthcare which was particularly lucrative in the mental health space at this time as the World Health Organization estimated that global prevalence of psychiatric conditions such as depression and anxiety saw an uptick of 25% within the first year of global viral spread [46]. Following the Centers for Medicare & Medicaid Services' removal of geographic and site restrictions, which allowed telehealth services to be delivered to patients in any location and reimbursed at rates equivalent to in-person care, telehealth use for mental health surged as outpatient encounters transitioned from in-person to virtual. In the United States, nearly half of monthly outpatient mental health visits in 2020 were conducted via telehealth, while in-person visits dropped by half during the early months of the pandemic [46–48]. It is reported that this increase in virtual mental health encounters was able to completely offset the decline in in-person visits. Interestingly, virtual uptake varied by psychiatric diagnosis, with patients with psychotic disorders representing 2% or less of telehealth visits, compared with roughly 25% among those with anxiety or panic disorders

[47]. Psychologists reported similar shifts in practice. Prior to the pandemic, only 7% of their clinical work was virtual, but this rose to over 85% at the height of the pandemic, with over two-thirds operating their practice entirely online [49].

Among Medicare beneficiaries, telehealth visits for mental health reached 55% of all outpatient encounters from January–February of 2020 [50]. Consistent and accessible care, such as through telehealth, improves follow-up and treatment adherence. For example, the transition to telehealth among low-income, racially and ethnically minoritized patients was associated with a significant reduction in missed appointments and improved depressive symptoms [51]. These rapid shifts and expansion in mental health service accessibility were enabled by federal and state policy changes, including reimbursement parity and temporary relaxation of privacy regulations, which data shows many providers hope will remain available for at least a portion of their patients [52]. The data outlines the critical role of telehealth in sustaining access to mental health care during the pandemic and raised the question of whether such elevated levels of virtual utilization could be maintained once emergency policies were lifted, especially given massive support behind the continuance.

After the initial surge, virtual mental health service use declined but did not revert to pre-pandemic levels. By late 2021, between 18–35% of outpatient mental health visits continued to be delivered virtually, depending on population and geography [46, 47, 50]. Providers report sustained intentions to use telehealth, often in hybrid models that combine in-person and virtual visits to maximize patient benefit and preference [47, 53, 54]. Utilization remains higher among younger adults, urban residents, and those with anxiety or depressive disorders, whereas uptake is lower among older adults, rural residents, and patients with substance use disorders [47, 50, 55]. These patterns suggest that while telehealth has expanded access for many, it may also widen disparities for populations less likely to use virtual care. Addressing these gaps will be essential to ensure telehealth strengthens, rather than fragments, equitable access to mental health services if the widespread use remains so high and continues to account for almost a quarter of all mental healthcare visits.

Beyond changes in utilization, robust evidence demonstrates that telehealth for mental health is effective and clinically comparable to in-person care while enhancing patient engagement and follow-up adherence. Systematic reviews and meta-analyses consistently show that telehealth interventions for depression, anxiety, and PTSD achieve equivalent, if not superior, outcomes in symptom reduction, quality of life, and therapeutic alliance compared with traditional face-to-face therapy [10, 43, 56–61]. For example, a meta-analysis of randomized controlled trials found no difference in depressive symptom reduction between video-based psychotherapy and in-person therapy, with attrition rates that were similar [60]. Another meta-analysis found no difference in depression severity post-treatment between telehealth and in-person care [59]. Importantly the therapeutic alliance, a cornerstone of psychotherapy, appears to be preserved in the virtual setting. Patients and providers report high levels of satisfaction with telehealth, and concerns about diminished therapeutic connection have not been elucidated in empirical data [10, 56]. Working alliance and patient satisfaction remain strong in telehealth cognitive behavioral therapy (CBT), mirroring in-person experiences [62]. Patients using telehealth are more likely to attend scheduled psychotherapy sessions and less likely to cancel or miss appointments compared to those receiving in-person care. One large cohort study found a 26% increase in the total number of psychotherapy sessions attended, and patients were five times more likely to complete all scheduled visits via telehealth than in-person [63]. Similarly, among low-income, racial and ethnic minority populations, telehealth adoption during the pandemic was associated with significantly fewer missed appointments and clinically meaningful reductions in depressive symptoms [51]. Remote delivery eliminates barriers related to geography, transportation, and scheduling, and enables dissemination of structured, evidence-based psycho- and pharmacotherapy to underserved populations. These findings suggest that telehealth can improve continuity of care and treatment adherence, particularly for populations facing structural barriers to in-person attendance.

Current Achievements and Ongoing Challenges in Telehealth

Telehealth has advanced from a marginal service to a central component of modern care in an extraordinarily short period of time. The rapid scaling during the pandemic proved that patients and providers alike are not only willing to adapt, but that virtual care can maintain, and in many cases improve, outcomes across mental health, women's health, and pediatrics. Evidence consistently demonstrates that patients engaging in telehealth psychotherapy, psychiatric care, or routine follow-up experience comparable symptom improvement, treatment adherence, and satisfaction as those seen in person. Telehealth also preserved continuity for children with developmental delays, provided safe access to reproductive health services, and reduced missed visits among historically underserved populations. Virtual care reduces traditional access barriers such as transportation, childcare, and time away from work, all of which disproportionately affect low-income, rural, and minoritized populations.

During the pandemic, several studies found that telehealth significantly improved attendance and engagement among Black, Hispanic, and low-income patients, who historically face higher dropout rates in in-person therapy [47, 51]. In these respects, the transformation has been a resounding success. However there remains inherent clinical limitations including gaps in digital infrastructure, governing policy, and healthcare equity within this digital space. Uneven access to broadband, language services, private space, and reimbursement can blunt its impact. For every family who avoided missed visits thanks to a virtual option, another was unable to log on because of an outdated device or insufficient internet. For every woman who accessed contraception or counseling more conveniently, another struggled with privacy in a crowded home. For every child with developmental delays who benefited from consistent telehealth follow-up, another faced diagnostic uncertainty because nuanced physical or behavioral assessments could not be conducted remotely.

Structural Barriers to Equitable Telehealth

The next stage of virtual health care is to ensure reliability, accountability, safety, and fairness. This requires confronting the persistent barriers that limit access and quality. These challenges include structural access gaps such as the digital divide, inconsistent reimbursement and licensure policies, clinical limitations where in-person evaluation is still necessary, and the risk of inequities widening if telehealth is not deliberately designed to meet the needs of vulnerable populations. Addressing these issues will determine whether telehealth remains a supplement to care for some or evolves into a truly transformative model that expands access to all, strengthens continuity, and promotes equity across the healthcare system.

One of the most significant barriers that remains is the structural access gap, often referred to as the "digital divide." Telehealth depends on reliable broadband, high-speed internet that allows for smooth video and audio transmission, as well as functioning devices and affordable data plans. Over one-quarter of the US population lacks broadband in their homes, with this deficit concentrated among individuals with annual incomes less than $30,000 [64]. Additionally, only 49% of adults above the age of 65 own smartphones and only a quarter of this demographic use the internet at all [65]. In the rural United States, nonmetropolitan households are nearly twice as likely to lack any digital access compared to metropolitan households [66]. Many under resourced families, rural communities, and older adults continue to lack these basic prerequisites for video care. When payment policies prioritize video over audio-only encounters, patients in phone-only households are unintentionally excluded. Even for those with internet access, many individuals, particularly those with limited English proficiency, low health literacy, or disabilities, struggle with the digital navigation required to log in, download applications, or troubleshoot connectivity problems in real time. Adult patients with limited English proficiency had a 20% lower odds of telehealth use compared to English-proficient adults [67].

Compounding this finding is the significantly lower active portal function usage of digital patient portals among non-English-speaking families [68]. Non-English-speaking families with lower active portal use miss out on critical features like secure messaging with providers, access to test results, medication refills, and appointment scheduling, which can reduce their engagement in care and delay treatment. Their lower usage may stem from language barriers or lack of culturally tailored portal design, nonetheless this discrepancy may limit the patient's ability to engage as a stakeholder in their own healthcare. Without targeted support, such as device-lending programs, technical help lines, or dedicated digital navigator roles, telehealth risks widening disparities it was originally intended to reduce.

Clinical and Policy Limitations of Telehealth Today

Privacy adds another layer of complexity: patients who cannot secure a quiet or safe space at home for sensitive conversations, such as those related to contraception, intimate partner violence, or trauma, may be unable to engage openly, undermining both candor and clinical quality [69, 70]. This limitation highlights the reality that access is not defined only by broadband or devices but also by the conditions and environments that allow patients to safely participate. Without safeguards to ensure privacy, such as discreet screening protocols, alternate communication channels, or audio-only options, telehealth risks excluding some of the very patients it was designed to help. These challenges also underscore that the pandemic-era improvements in access and attendance among low-income and minoritized patients remain fragile. If connectivity gaps, lack of affordable devices, and limited coverage for audio-only services are not addressed, the advances made during this period could erode, leaving behind communities that already shoulder disproportionate barriers to in-person.

Even as telehealth has proven its clinical value, policy, payment, and regulatory frictions continue to undermine its long-term stability. Coverage and reimbursement remain inconsistent across payers, leaving clinics uncertain about whether telehealth visits will be compensated at the same rate as in-person care. While reimbursement parity laws expanded rapidly during the pandemic, gaps persist, particularly for audio-only encounters, which remain essential for patients without broadband access or reliable devices [5, 19]. Without guaranteed parity, safety-net clinics and small practices serving vulnerable populations face ongoing disincentives to sustain telehealth infrastructure, as the administrative burden of navigating variable codes and coverage policies can outweigh the potential benefits.

Licensure adds another layer of complexity. Patients who move across state lines, such as college students or migrant families, often face disruptions in care because many providers are not licensed to practice outside their home state. While regional licensure compacts and temporary waivers have begun to address this barrier, they remain incomplete and unevenly implemented, limiting continuity of care for patients who are among the most mobile and at risk [5, 19]. Program sustainability poses an additional challenge. Many health systems scaled up telehealth capacity during COVID with the aid of short-term grants and emergency funding, which allowed them to hire digital support staff, purchase equipment, and expand remote monitoring. Now, however, as these temporary funds expire, clinics are confronting budget cliffs, forcing difficult decisions about whether they can maintain technical support teams or replace outdated devices. Without stable financing mechanisms, the very programs that enabled telehealth to demonstrate its value risk being dismantled, leaving patients with fewer options and threatening the progress made in expanding access to equitable virtual care [26].

Together, these barriers do not diminish the progress that has been made but highlight where future work must focus. Broadband must be treated as health infrastructure, interpreter and culturally responsive services need to be integrated directly into telehealth platforms, reimbursement parity should be secured for both video and audio-only encounters, and clinicians must be supported with training and clear guidelines on when virtual care is appropriate and when in-person evaluation is necessary.

Future Directions for Telemedicine in a Post-COVID19 Landscape

Immediate, evidence-based action is needed to ensure telehealth fulfills its potential for equitable, high-quality care. The Society of General Internal Medicine calls for the elimination of geographic and site restrictions, expansion of telemedicine definitions to include audio-only services, and universal broadband access to address disparities in digital infrastructure and access [25]. The American Heart Association urges policymakers to invest in broadband infrastructure, particularly in rural and underserved areas, and to harmonize reimbursement policies to achieve payment parity for both video and audio-only visits, thereby supporting care for patients with limited digital resources [65, 71]. Health systems and regulatory bodies should also prioritize the development and implementation of standardized telehealth quality metrics. The American Academy of Pediatrics recommends rigorous, equity-focused frameworks to ensure that telehealth is evaluated consistently across populations, settings, and conditions [5, 19]. Such quality measures should inform institutional accountability, payer decisions, and system-wide improvement efforts. Expanding awareness and digital literacy, alongside targeted training for both clinicians and patients, is another consideration for telehealth is to reach its full potential. Many individuals, both patients and providers, remain uncertain about how to navigate virtual platforms or are skeptical of their value compared to in-person care. By investing in public education campaigns, incorporating digital literacy into community health programs, and providing hands-on training for the clinical workforce, we can ensure that both patients and providers are equipped to confidently and effectively engage in virtual care [72].

A strength of telehealth is an accessible direct and consistent connection between provider and patient. A key direction is deeper integration of telehealth with digital health technologies as they have become so widely used. Remote patient monitoring tools, such as continuous glucose monitoring systems for diabetes management, can transmit real-time data to electronic health records, allowing physicians to assess trends, adjust therapy, and intervene earlier during virtual visits. These integrations can improve chronic disease management from a primary care approach, reduce hospitalizations, and create a more complete picture of a patient's health status outside clinic walls [73]. Advocacy at local, regional, and national levels remains essential to drive governmental policy changes, secure reimbursement parity, and establish durable regulatory frameworks. The North American Society for Pediatric Gastroenterology, Hepatology and Nutrition emphasizes that such advocacy is necessary for sustainable telehealth integration into routine care [74]. Telehealth platforms must be codesigned with patients, caregivers, and clinicians to address usability, accessibility, and health literacy barriers [71]. Inclusive design can strengthen engagement, ensure cultural responsiveness, and reduce disparities in digital navigation and utilization. Finally, research funding for studies evaluating virtual medicine must be increased to support an extensive body of data to support the creation of digital quality metrics that reflect real-world outcomes and address disparities [5, 19]. By aligning research priorities with practice and policy, health systems can ensure that telehealth evolves as a patient-centered, evidence-driven model of care.

Taken together-, priorities such as policy reform, equitable infrastructure investment, rigorous quality measurement, coordinated advocacy, inclusive design, integration of remote health data, and robust research will secure telehealth's role in modern medicine.

Conclusion

Telehealth has evolved from an emergency response into a durable pillar of modern healthcare, proven to deliver high-quality care across a broad spectrum of conditions and populations, often with greater convenience and equal or better outcomes compared to traditional visits. Its future, however, will not be defined by how many visits take place virtually, but by whether those visits are delivered fairly, effectively, and sustainably. Progress to date shows what is possible: improved follow-up, reduced missed appointments, expanded access for underserved groups, and preserved therapeutic quality. But realizing telehealth's full promise will require addressing the remaining barriers with the same urgency and creativity that drove its rapid expansion. If broadband access, reimbursement equity, and culturally responsive implementation can be secured, telehealth will not only maintain the gains of the past several years but extend them further. Telehealth will redefine what it means to provide accessible, patient-centered care in the twenty-first century.

References

1. Ennis M, Wahl K, Jeong D, Knight K, Renner R, Munro S, et al. The perspective of Canadian health care professionals on abortion service during the COVID-19 pandemic. Fam Pract. 2021;38(Supplement_1):i30–6.
2. Cohen MA, Powell AM, Coleman JS, Keller JM, Livingston A, Anderson JR. Special ambulatory gynecologic considerations in the era of coronavirus disease 2019 (COVID-19) and implications for future practice. Am J Obstet Gynecol. 2020;223(3):372–8.
3. Alexander GC, Tajanlangit M, Heyward J, Mansour O, Qato DM, Stafford RS. Use and content of primary care office-based vs telemedicine care visits during the COVID-19 pandemic in the US. JAMA Netw Open. 2020;3(10):e2021476.

4. Chang E, Penfold RB, Berkman ND. Patient characteristics and telemedicine use in the US, 2022. JAMA Netw Open. 2024;7(3):e243354.
5. Curfman A, Hackell JM, Herendeen NE, Alexander J, Marcin JP, Moskowitz WB, et al. Telehealth: opportunities to improve access, quality, and cost in pediatric care. Pediatrics. 2022;149(3):e2021056035.
6. Bagner DM, Berkovits MD, Coxe S, Frech N, Garcia D, Golik A, et al. Telehealth treatment of behavior problems in young children with developmental delay: a randomized clinical trial. JAMA Pediatr. 2023;177(3):231.
7. Turner K, Brownstein NC, Whiting J, Arevalo M, Islam JY, Vadaparampil ST, et al. Impact of the COVID-19 pandemic on women's health care access: a cross-sectional study. J Women's Health. 2022;31(12):1690–702.
8. Ripp A, Steinway C, Katzow MW, Jan S, Chen J, Chen V. Telehealth utilization and follow-up visits in developmental-behavioral pediatrics during the COVID-19 pandemic in 2020. J Dev Behav Pediatr. 2022;43(5):297–302.
9. Pearlman Shapiro M, Myo M, Chen T, Nathan A, Raidoo S. Remote provision of medication abortion and contraception through telemedicine. Obstet Gynecol. 2023;141(6):1056–61.
10. Bellanti DM, Kelber MS, Workman DE, Beech EH, Belsher BE. Rapid review on the effectiveness of telehealth interventions for the treatment of behavioral health disorders. Mil Med. 2022;187(5–6):e577–88.
11. Levine SR, Gorman M. "Telestroke": the application of telemedicine for stroke. Stroke. 1999;30(2):464–9.
12. Wilcock AD, Schwamm LH, Zubizarreta JR, Zachrison KS, Uscher-Pines L, Richard JV, et al. Reperfusion treatment and stroke outcomes in hospitals with Telestroke capacity. JAMA Neurol. 2021;78(5):527–35.
13. Schwamm LH, Chumbler N, Brown E, Fonarow GC, Berube D, Nystrom K, et al. Recommendations for the implementation of telehealth in cardiovascular and stroke care: a policy statement from the American Heart Association. Circulation [Internet]. 2017 [cited 2025 Sept 30];135(7). Available from: https://www.ahajournals.org/doi/10.1161/CIR.0000000000000475
14. Barbosa W, Zhou K, Waddell E, Myers T, Dorsey ER. Improving access to care: telemedicine across medical domains. Annu Rev Public Health. 2021;42(1):463–81.
15. Brotman JJ, Kotloff RM. Providing outpatient telehealth services in the United States. Chest. 2021;159(4):1548–58.
16. Barnett ML, Huskamp HA, Busch AB, Uscher-Pines L, Chaiyachati KH, Mehrotra A. Trends in outpatient telemedicine utilization among rural Medicare beneficiaries, 2010 to 2019. JAMA Health Forum. 2021;2(10):e213282.
17. Poeran J, Cho LD, Wilson L, Zhong H, Mazumdar M, Liu J, et al. Pre-existing disparities and potential implications for the rapid expansion of telemedicine in response to the coronavirus disease 2019 pandemic. Med Care. 2021;59(8):694–8.
18. Demeke HB, Pao LZ, Clark H, Romero L, Neri A, Shah R, et al. Telehealth practice among health centers during the COVID-19 pandemic — United States, July 11–17, 2020. MMWR Morb Mortal Wkly Rep. 2020;69(50):1902–5.
19. Curfman AL, Hackell JM, Herendeen NE, Alexander JJ, Marcin JP, Moskowitz WB, et al. Telehealth: improving access to and quality of pediatric health care. Pediatrics. 2021;148(3):e2021053129.
20. Patel SY, Mehrotra A, Huskamp HA, Uscher-Pines L, Ganguli I, Barnett ML. Variation in telemedicine use and outpatient care during the COVID-19 pandemic in the United States: study examines variation in total US outpatient visits and telemedicine use across patient demographics, specialties, and conditions during the COVID-19 pandemic. Health Aff Millwood. 2021;40(2):349–58.
21. Tan RKJ, Hensel D, Ivanova O, Bravo RG, Olumide A, Adebayo E, et al. Telemedicine use during the COVID-19 pandemic in 8 countries from the international sexual health and

reproductive health consortium: web-based cross-sectional survey study. J Med Internet Res. 2025;27:e60369.
22. Witkowska-Zimny M. Telemedicine in emergency medicine in the COVID-19 pandemic—experiences and prospects—a narrative review. Int J Environ Res Public Health. 2022;19(13):8216.
23. Mosenia A, Li P, Seefeldt R, Seitzman GD, Sun CQ, Kim TN. Longitudinal use of telehealth during the COVID-19 pandemic and utility of asynchronous testing for subspecialty-level ophthalmic care. JAMA Ophthalmol. 2023;141(1):56.
24. Dekker PK, Bhardwaj P, Singh T, Bekeny JC, Kim KG, Steinberg JS, et al. Telemedicine in the wake of the COVID-19 pandemic: increasing access to surgical care. Plast Reconstr Surg – Glob Open. 2021;9(1):e3228.
25. Chen A, Ayub MH, Mishuris RG, Rodriguez JA, Gwynn K, Lo MC, et al. Telehealth policy, practice, and education: a position statement of the Society of General Internal Medicine. J Gen Intern Med. 2023;38(11):2613–20.
26. Uscher-Pines L, McCullough C, Dworsky MS, Sousa J, Predmore Z, Ray K, et al. Use of telehealth across pediatric subspecialties before and during the COVID-19 pandemic. JAMA Netw Open. 2022;5(3):e224759.
27. Cahan EM, Maturi J, Bailey P, Fernandes S, Addala A, Kibrom S, et al. The impact of telehealth adoption during COVID-19 pandemic on patterns of pediatric subspecialty care utilization. Acad Pediatr. 2022;22(8):1375–83.
28. Guillén Ú. Relationship between attrition and neurodevelopmental impairment rates in extremely preterm infants at 18 to 24 months: a systematic review. Arch Pediatr Adolesc Med. 2012;166(2):178.
29. Doyle LW, Anderson PJ, Burnett A, Callanan C, McDonald M, Hayes M, et al. Developmental disability at school age and difficulty obtaining follow-up data. Pediatrics. 2018;141(2):e20173102.
30. Cantor AG, Jungbauer RM, Totten AM, Tilden EL, Holmes R, Ahmed A, et al. Telehealth strategies for the delivery of maternal health care: a rapid review. Ann Intern Med. 2022;175(9):1285–97.
31. Increasing Access to Abortion: ACOG committee opinion, number 815. Obstet Gynecol. 2020;136(6):e107–15.
32. Roberts SCM, Berglas NF, Schroeder R, Lingwall M, Grossman D, White K. Disruptions to abortion care in Louisiana during early months of the COVID-19 pandemic. Am J Public Health. 2021;111(8):1504–12.
33. Ong I, Zulkarnain ADM, Lim KZQ, Teh DBL, Tam W, Huang Z. The global impact of COVID-19 on abortion care. Heliyon. 2023;9(5):e16094.
34. Pilecco FB, McCallum CA, Almeida MDCCD, Alves FJO, Rocha ADS, Ortelan N, et al. Abortion and the COVID-19 pandemic: insights for Latin America. Cad Saude Publica. 2021;37(6):e00322320.
35. Adler A, Biggs MA, Kaller S, Schroeder R, Ralph L. Changes in the frequency and type of barriers to reproductive health care between 2017 and 2021. JAMA Netw Open. 2023;6(4):e237461.
36. Tam MW, Davis VH, Ahluwalia M, Lee RS, Ross LE. Impact of COVID-19 on access to and delivery of sexual and reproductive healthcare services in countries with universal healthcare systems: a systematic review. Ortega JA, editor. PLoS One. 2024;19(2):e0294744.
37. Aiken ARA, Wells ES, Gomperts R, Scott JG. Provision of medications for self-managed abortion before and after the *Dobbs v Jackson women's health organization* decision. JAMA. 2024;331(18):1558.
38. Boydell N, Reynolds-Wright J, Cameron S, Harden J. Women's experiences of a telemedicine abortion service (up to 12 weeks) implemented during the coronavirus (COVID-19) pandemic: a qualitative evaluation. BJOG Int J Obstet Gynaecol. 2021;128(11):1752–61.

39. Hukku S, Ménard A, Kemzang J, Hastings E, Foster AM. "I just was really scared, because it's already such an uncertain time": exploring women's abortion experiences during the COVID-19 pandemic in Canada. Contraception. 2022;110:48–55.
40. Upadhyay UD, Koenig LR, Meckstroth K, Ko J, Valladares ES, Biggs MA. Effectiveness and safety of telehealth medication abortion in the USA. Nat Med. 2024;30(4):1191–8.
41. Moon KJ, Linton SL, Mojtabai R. Medical debt and the mental health treatment gap among US adults. JAMA Psychiatry. 2024;81(10):985.
42. Olfson M, McClellan C, Zuvekas SH, Wall M, Blanco C. Trends in psychological distress and outpatient mental health care of adults during the COVID-19 era. Ann Intern Med. 2024;177(3):353–62.
43. Simon GE, Moise N, Mohr DC. Management of depression in adults: a review. JAMA. 2024;332(2):141.
44. Arifkhanova A, Elhabr A, Murray C, Khushalani J, Neri A, Kaminski J, et al. Telemental health utilization in commercial health insurance plans in the United States from 2010 through 2019. J Clin Psychiatry [Internet] 2023 [cited 2025 Aug 25];85(1). Available from: https://www.psychiatrist.com/jcp/telemental-health-in-the-us-2010-2019/
45. Saunders NR, Kurdyak P, Stukel TA, Strauss R, Fu L, Guan J, et al. Utilization of physician-based mental health care services among children and adolescents before and during the COVID-19 pandemic in Ontario, Canada. JAMA Pediatr. 2022;176(4):e216298.
46. Rossom RC, Yeh HH, Ma L, Penfold RB, Hooker SA, Miller-Matero LR, et al. Changes in utilization of in-person and virtual outpatient mental health visits before and during the COVID-19 pandemic: an observational cohort study. Medicine (Baltimore). 2025;104(17):e42305.
47. Zhu JM, Myers R, McConnell KJ, Levander X, Lin SC. Trends in outpatient mental health services use before and during the COVID-19 pandemic: study examines trends in outpatient mental health service using before and during the COVID-19 pandemic. Health Aff Millwood 2022;41(4):573–580.
48. McBain RK, Cantor J, Pera MF, Breslau J, Bravata DM, Whaley CM. Mental health service utilization rates among commercially insured adults in the US during the first year of the COVID-19 pandemic. JAMA Health Forum. 2023;4(1):e224936.
49. Pierce BS, Perrin PB, Tyler CM, McKee GB, Watson JD. The COVID-19 telepsychology revolution: a national study of pandemic-based changes in U.S. mental health care delivery. Am Psychol. 2021;76(1):14–25.
50. Hayek MA, Kum HC, Park S, Ohsfeldt R, Lawley MA, Bovin MJ. Utilization of outpatient mental health services during and 2 years after the COVID-19 pandemic. Telemed E-Health. 2025:tmj.2024.0581.
51. Gamoran J, Xu Y, Buinewicz SAP, Liu J, Mowrey W, Goldentyer G, et al. An examination of depression severity and treatment adherence among racially and ethnically minoritized, low-income individuals during the COVID-19 transition to telehealth. Psychiatry Res. 2024;342:116221.
52. Kisicki A, Becker S, Chaple M, Gustafson DH, Hartzler BJ, Jacobson N, et al. Behavioral healthcare organizations' experiences related to use of telehealth as a result of the COVID-19 pandemic: an exploratory study. BMC Health Serv Res. 2022;22(1):775.
53. Molfenter T, Heitkamp T, Murphy AA, Tapscott S, Behlman S, Cody OJ. Use of telehealth in mental health (MH) services during and after COVID-19. Community Ment Health J. 2021;57(7):1244–51.
54. Appleton R, Williams J, Vera San Juan N, Needle JJ, Schlief M, Jordan H, et al. Implementation, adoption, and perceptions of Telemental health during the COVID-19 pandemic: systematic review. J Med Internet Res. 2021;23(12):e31746.
55. Provision of Telemental health before and after COVID-19 onset. Am J Manag Care. 2023;29(3):118–23.
56. Hagi K, Kurokawa S, Takamiya A, Fujikawa M, Kinoshita S, Iizuka M, et al. Telepsychiatry versus face-to-face treatment: systematic review and meta-analysis of randomised controlled trials. Br J Psychiatry. 2023;223(3):407–14.

57. Nowrouzi-Kia B, Bani-Fatemi A, Jackson TD, Li AKC, Chattu VK, Lytvyak E, et al. Evaluating the efficacy of telehealth-based treatments for depression in adults: a rapid review and meta-analysis. J Occup Rehabil [Internet]. 2024 [cited 2025 Aug 26]; Available from: https://link.springer.com/10.1007/s10926-024-10246-3
58. Crowe M, Inder M, Manuel J, Carlyle D. Characteristics of effective teletherapy for major depression: a systematic review. J Affect Disord. 2023;327:175–82.
59. Scott AM, Clark J, Greenwood H, Krzyzaniak N, Cardona M, Peiris R, et al. Telehealth *v.* face-to-face provision of care to patients with depression: a systematic review and meta-analysis. Psychol Med. 2022;52(14):2852–60.
60. Giovanetti AK, Punt SEW, Nelson EL, Ilardi SS. Teletherapy versus in-person psychotherapy for depression: a meta-analysis of randomized controlled trials. Telemed E-Health. 2022;28(8):1077–89.
61. Kelber MS, Smolenski DJ, Boyd C, Shank LM, Bellanti DM, Milligan T, et al. Evidence-based telehealth interventions for post-traumatic stress disorder, depression, and anxiety: a systematic review and meta-analysis. J Telemed Telecare. 2025;31(6):757–67.
62. Swartz HA, Bylsma LM, Fournier JC, Girard JM, Spotts C, Cohn JF, et al. Randomized trial of brief interpersonal psychotherapy and cognitive behavioral therapy for depression delivered both in-person and by telehealth. J Affect Disord. 2023;333:543–52.
63. Connolly Gibbons MB, Duong L, Chiu RY, Crits-Christoph P, Gallop R, Mandell D, et al. A cohort study of engagement in telehealth psychotherapy versus in-person services. Psychother Res. 2025;35(6):990–1000.
64. Tilhou AS, Jain A, DeLeire T. Telehealth expansion, internet speed, and primary care access before and during COVID-19. JAMA Netw Open. 2024;7(1):e2347686.
65. Masterson Creber R, Dodson JA, Bidwell J, Breathett K, Lyles C, Harmon Still C, et al. Telehealth and health equity in older adults with heart failure: a scientific statement from the American Heart Association. Circ Cardiovasc Qual Outcomes [Internet]. 2023 [cited 2025 Sept 2];16(11). Available from: https://www.ahajournals.org/doi/10.1161/HCQ.0000000000000123
66. Curtis ME, Clingan SE, Guo H, Zhu Y, Mooney LJ, Hser Y. Disparities in digital access among American rural and urban households and implications for telemedicine-based services. J Rural Health. 2022;38(3):512–8.
67. Chang E, Davis TL, Berkman ND. Differences in telemedicine, emergency department, and hospital utilization among nonelderly adults with limited English proficiency post-COVID-19 pandemic: a cross-sectional analysis. J Gen Intern Med. 2023;38(16):3490–8.
68. Casillas A, Abhat A, Vassar SD, Huang DYC, Mahajan AP, Simmons S, et al. Not speaking the same language—lower portal use for limited English proficient patients in the Los Angeles safety net. J Health Care Poor Underserved. 2021;32(4):2055–70.
69. Cantor AG, Nelson HD, Pappas M, Atchison C, Hatch B, Huguet N, et al. Telehealth for women's preventive Services for Reproductive Health and Intimate Partner Violence: a comparative effectiveness review. J Gen Intern Med. 2023;38(7):1735–43.
70. Goldstein KM, Rushton S, Lewinski AA, Shapiro A, Lanford-Davey T, Coleman JN, et al. Experiences receiving and delivering virtual health care for women: qualitative evidence synthesis. J Med Internet Res. 2025;27:e68314.
71. Takahashi EA, Schwamm LH, Adeoye OM, Alabi O, Jahangir E, Misra S, et al. An overview of telehealth in the management of cardiovascular disease: a scientific statement from the American Heart Association. Circulation [Internet]. 2022 [cited 2025 Sept 27];146(25). Available from: https://www.ahajournals.org/doi/10.1161/CIR.0000000000001107
72. Li X, Huang L, Zhang H, Liang Z. Enabling telemedicine from the system-level perspective: scoping review. J Med Internet Res. 2025;27:e65932.
73. Ferguson T, Olds T, Curtis R, Blake H, Crozier AJ, Dankiw K, et al. Effectiveness of wearable activity trackers to increase physical activity and improve health: a systematic review of systematic reviews and meta-analyses. Lancet Digit Health. 2022;4(8):e615–26.
74. Franciosi JP, Berg EA, Rosen JM, Lee JA, Sandberg KC, Srinath A, et al. North American Society for Pediatric Gastroenterology, Hepatology, and Nutrition Position Statement for Telehealth. J Pediatr Gastroenterol Nutr. 2023;76(5):684–94.

Implementation of 3D Modeling in Medical Care

Channing Pezet and Adil Akkouch

Introduction

Three-dimensional (3D) modeling has rapidly become an important tool in contemporary medical care. When medical images are converted into detailed digital or physical models, clinicians, trainees, and patients can better visualize complex anatomy and pathology in ways that are not possible with two-dimensional (2D) images alone. In medical education, 3D models enhance anatomical understanding, improve procedural training, and allow repeated practice. In clinical care, they facilitate surgical planning, guide prosthetic design, and enhance patient counseling through patient specific models. As 3D modeling technologies continue to integrate with virtual and augmented reality, computer aided design, and advanced 3D printing platforms, their role is expanding from an auxiliary teaching aid to an essential component of precision medicine. This chapter reviews the current applications of 3D modeling across medical education and clinical care, outlines technical workflows from imaging to printed models, and highlights opportunities and limitations that affect adoption.

C. Pezet
Western Michigan University Homer Stryker M.D. School of Medicine, Kalamazoo, MI, USA

A. Akkouch (✉)
Department of Surgical Sciences, Division of Orthopaedic Surgery and Division of Biomedical Engineering, Western Michigan University Homer Stryker M.D. School of Medicine, Kalamazoo, MI, USA
e-mail: adil.akkouch@wmed.edu

S. S. Chahin et al. (eds.), *Innovation in Medical Education and Clinical Practice*, https://doi.org/10.1007/978-3-032-19116-8_17

Medical Education

3D modeling provides new ways for learners to understand human anatomy and various pathologies. Traditional medical education relies on textbooks and 2D images to introduce anatomical structures and functions, followed by exposure to cadaveric dissection. The shift from the textbook to a real human body can be overwhelming, especially for early learners who are still developing spatial reasoning. High-quality 3D models can bridge this gap and allow students to rotate, enlarge, and selectively hide structures so they can study anatomy at their own pace and in the manner that matches the curriculum.

Cadavers have traditionally been at the forefront of anatomy education, and for good reason: they provide learners with direct visualization of structures as they would be seen in surgery. However, embalming alters tissue color and texture, some architectural distortion can occur in organs like the kidneys, though other organs like the liver and spleen remain well-preserved. Aging embalmed cadavers undergo changes to the vascular structures making them less realistic. Some structures, such as the cardiac conduction system of the heart or parts of the lymphatic system, are nearly impossible to visualize. There is also considerable anatomic variation between cadavers, which can confuse early learners. 3D models can compensate for these limitations by presenting a high-resolution variations of the same structure and by permitting repeated dissections without damaging the specimen.

3D-Printed Models

Plastination techniques, which replace water and fat in a cadaver with plastic, were an important step toward durable anatomic teaching tools. 3D-printed models extend this idea and provide a long-lasting alternative to cadavers. They can be produced at true scale or enlarged for better visualization of small or deep structures, such as the spinal cord, inner ear, or neck. Components of the 3D-printed models can be made removable to expose internal anatomy. Unlike a cadaveric heart that must be cut open to visualize the valves and cannot be restored, a 3D-printed heart model, as seen in Fig. 1, can be opened and closed repeatedly for demonstration.

3D printing is also reshaping procedural skills training. For decades, students practiced suturing on synthetic pads or animal tissue. These options are useful for learning instrument handling, but they rarely match the viscoelastic properties of human skin, and they can raise cost or ethical concerns when many repetitions are needed. Custom 3D-printed suture trainers can be engineered to mimic multilayer closure, variable skin tensions, or challenging locations such as the face or hand. Learners have reported higher realism and preference for these models compared to porcine feet and sponge-based trainers because they better approximate clinical tasks [2].

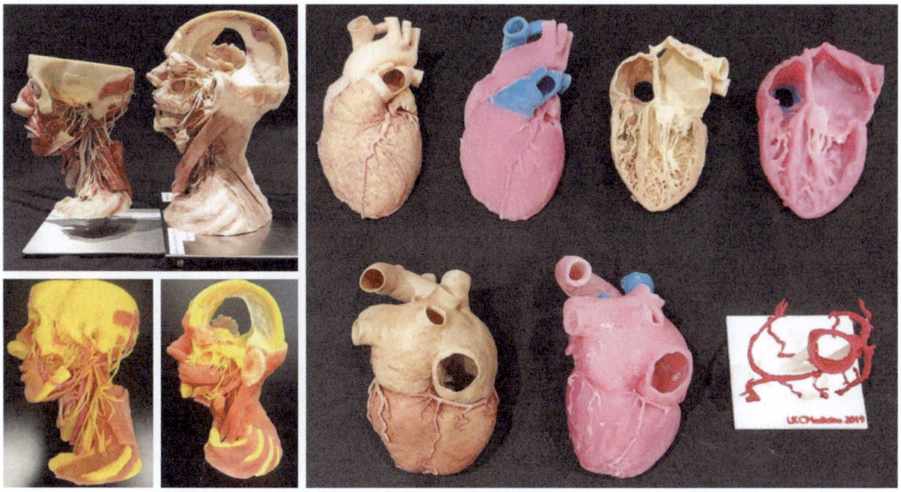

Fig. 1 Plastinated (upper left) and 3D-printed models of neck (lower left) and heart (right) [1]

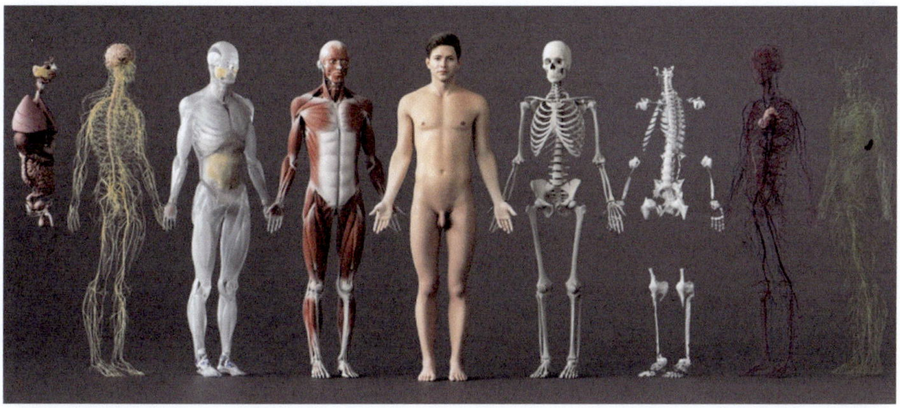

Fig. 2 3D anatomy model from Atomedge showing digestive, nervous, musculoskeletal, cardiovascular and lymphatic systems [3]

Digital 3D Models

Digital 3D models provide an additional layer of interaction. On a computer, tablet or smart phone, students can isolate a single system, such as the musculoskeletal or vascular system, remove fascia and adipose tissue, as demonstrated in Fig. 2. This manipulability supports spatial cognition and can help close achievement gaps for learners who struggle with 3D visualization. Several medical schools have adopted a cadaver free or cadaver light curricula, in which digital and printed 3D models are the primary tools for anatomy instruction, with some studies reporting higher post test performance compared to cadaver only teaching [4].

The advantages of 3D modeling in medical education are not limited to physician training. Nursing students use vascular arm models connected to pumps to practice venipuncture before performing procedures on patients (Fig. 3a). Paramedic and anesthesia trainees use 3D airway heads to rehearse intubation in a low-risk environment (Fig. 3b). Holographic and augmented reality systems, such as head-mounted displays (Fig. 3c), now permit whole teams to rehearse rare or high stakes scenarios like mass casualty responses. In all these cases, the benefit is the same. Learners are exposed to accurate anatomy and realistic tasks in a format that is repeatable, observable by faculty, and adaptable to different skill levels.

To maximize educational value, 3D modeling activities should be linked to explicit learning objectives and to assessment. For example, an anatomy lab session that uses 3D-printed hearts should specify whether the objective is identification of surface landmarks, understanding of chamber relationships, or rehearsal of a surgical approach. Performance can then be assessed through labeled images, timed identification tasks, or checklists of procedural steps. When 3D models are incorporated in this structured way, they become part of competency-based training rather than optional visual aids.

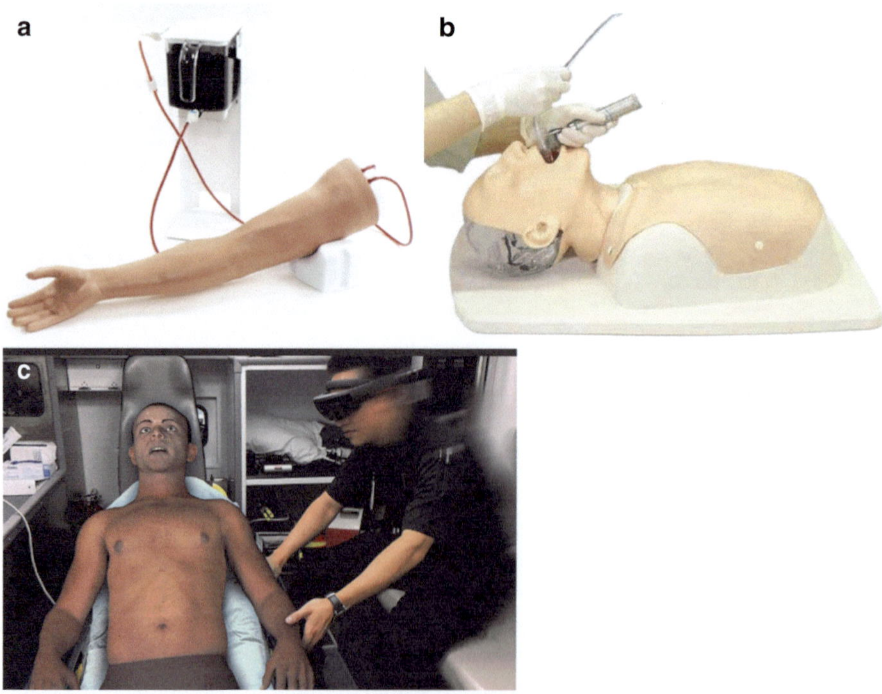

Fig. 3 (**a**) Model arm connected to pump to simulate veins for blood draw [5]. (**b**) Airway model for intubation practice [6]. (**c**) HoloLens augmented reality in an ambulance [7]

Virtual Reality

Virtual and augmented realities have added a new layer to technology-assisted medical education. Instead of only looking at a 3D model on a screen, learners can be placed inside a simulated clinical or procedural environment and asked to act as if they were in the operating room or in the emergency department. This immersion allows them to integrate what they see, hear, and do, which supports experiential learning. Virtual reality (VR) places the learner in a fully computer-generated environment viewed through a headset (Fig. 4a). Augmented reality (AR) keeps the real world visible and adds digital objects on top of it (Fig. 4b), for example a holographic heart or a bleeding trauma patient. Mixed reality (MR) sits in between. In medical training, VR is usually used for procedural practice and team-based simulations, while AR is useful for anatomic visualization during teaching rounds or in the operating room.

A major educational advantage of VR is that scenarios are repeatable. A student can practice the same laparoscopic cholecystectomy, coronary angiography, or difficult airway multiple times until performance improves. An instructor can watch the same scene on a monitor and provide immediate feedback on instrument handling, ergonomic, safety steps, or how to better expose the field of view in a 3D plane. This makes VR suitable for competency-based training. The simulation can automatically record completion time, number of errors, instrument collisions, and missed steps, and those metrics can be linked to learner milestones in surgery, anesthesia, or interventional cardiology.

VR is also valuable for nontechnical skills. A virtual patient encounter can be designed to require history taking, physical exam choice, interpretation of vital signs, and generation of a differential diagnosis. Because the learner is inside the scenario, cognitive load is closer to real practice than when reading a case on paper. For emergency medicine, VR can reproduce rare high stakes events such as cardiac arrest in a child or a mass casualty triage line. Learners can make decisions, see the consequences, and then repeat the scenario without putting patients at risk.

3D modeling enhances VR when the scenario is built from real patient data. A CT or MRI can be segmented, converted to a 3D model, and then imported into a

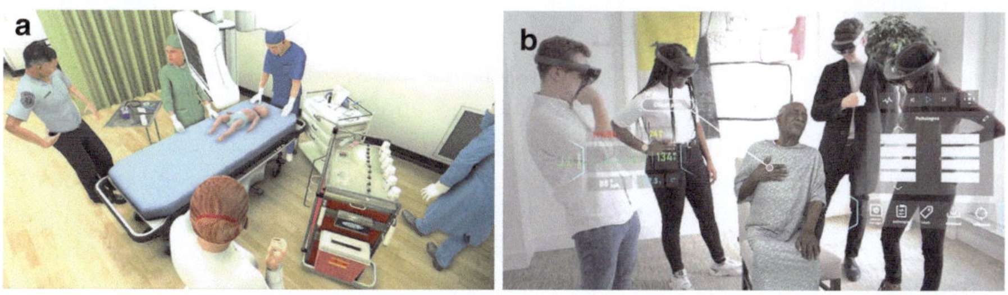

Fig. 4 (**a**) VR: A medical team practice saving a baby's life in a virtual word [8]. (**b**) AR: 3D video capture of a standardized holographic patient sitting in a chair being assessed by a group of medical students [9]

VR platform. The learner can then rehearse a procedure on an actual patient specific anatomy rather than on a generic model. This is particularly helpful in orthopedic, neurosurgical, and congenital cardiac cases where anatomic variation is large. It also supports preoperative team briefings, because anesthesiologists, surgeons, and nurses can view the same model in the same virtual space.

Despite these benefits, VR and AR need to be selected carefully. Not every task requires a headset. Low complexity tasks such as simple anatomic identification can be done on a desktop 3D viewer or on a printed model for less cost. VR is best reserved for procedures that require spatial judgment, coordination of more than one instrument, or practice in a time pressured setting. This is consistent with good curriculum design, where fidelity matches the task rather than the technology available. There are also limitations related to technological advancement and computing power. Some current systems have limited haptic feedback, so the learner can see tissue but cannot feel resistance. Motion sickness and discomfort from headsets can reduce session length for some learners. Building high-quality VR scenarios from real patient images requires trained personnel and time. In addition, when real patient data are used, programs must follow institutional policies for privacy and secure storage of imaging. When these factors are addressed, VR and AR can serve as effective companions to 3D modeling. Three-dimensional models teach accurate form. Virtual reality teaches accurate performance. Together they allow learners to move from recognizing anatomy, to manipulating it, to applying it in real clinical situations.

Resident Education

Resident training builds on the foundations developed in medical school but requires a higher level of anatomic precision, procedural confidence, and rehearsal of complex workflows. 3D modeling technology and simulation are well suited for this stage because residents are learning to translate knowledge into safe operative performance. Many surgical specialties now include simulation-based training on virtual or robotic platforms before residents operate on patients. In abdominal and pelvic surgery, for example, residents can practice on a Da Vinci 5 DV5 robotic simulator to remove a gallbladder or uterus in a virtual cavity using laparoscopy (Fig. 5). They can receive a force and haptic feedback which help them sense pull, and push forces exerted on patient tissue and apply precise energy. The system records time to completion, instrument collisions, dropped objects, and critical errors, and it generates an objective performance report that helps the trainees to improve their surgical skills and faculty can review. These metrics can be mapped to program milestones and used to determine whether a resident is ready to advance to live cases.

In surgical subspecialties, 3D modeling has transformed resident training by making technical skill acquisition more realistic. Orthopedic residents can practice placing vertebral pedicle screws or lag screws on sawbone models. These anatomic

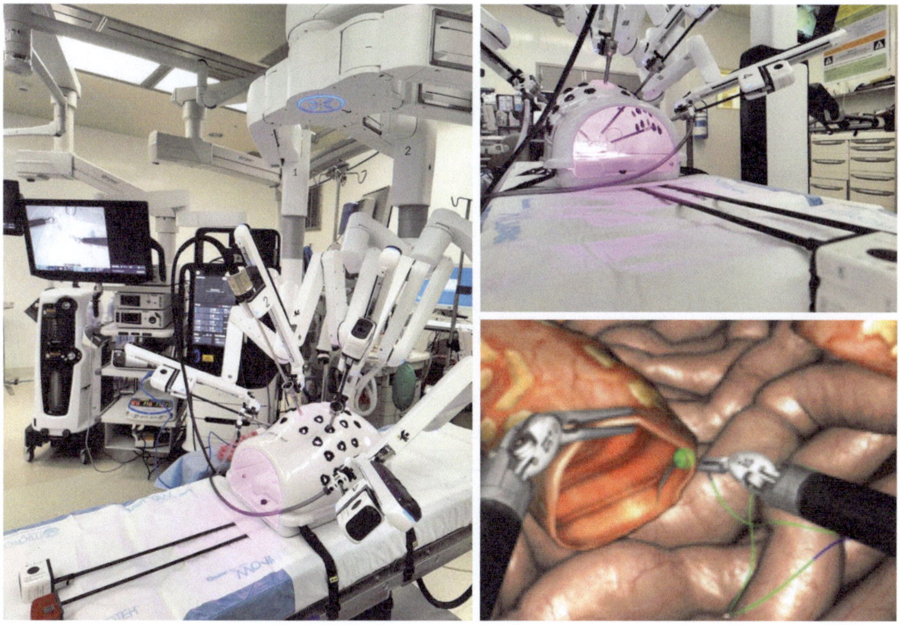

Fig. 5 DaVinci 5 robotic surgical and training system with intuitive simulation enables trainees to perform tube anastomosis and tube closure exercises [10, 11]

replicas reproduce the feel of drilling through cortical and cancellous bone from healthy or osteoporotic patients, which helps residents learn the appropriate pressure and angle before entering the operating room. Cardiothoracic and vascular surgery trainees use 3D-printed models of hearts and blood vessels to practice anastomoses, valve repairs, and canulation. Practicing on patient specific models helps residents understand individual anatomic variation rather than memorizing a single textbook version. This improves operative planning and reduces surprise in the operating room.

3D models are also useful for teaching minimally invasive techniques. Laparoscopic and arthroscopic procedures are difficult for beginners because of the 2D video view, the use of long instruments, and the need to operate through small portals. Training models that reproduce joint or abdominal cavities allow residents to improve hand eye coordination, triangulation, and tissue handling in a controlled setting. Faculty can observe from outside the field, pause the procedure, and demonstrate the correct movement using the same model.

After residency, physicians who enter interventional fellowships in radiology, cardiology, or endovascular surgery can continue to benefit from 3D-based simulation. Catheter-based procedures require planning of access routes, appreciation of vessel tortuosity, and anticipation of complications. When trainees rehearse on 3D reconstructions of real patients, their performance in the catheterization laboratory improves in terms of safety and efficiency, especially when simulation is added to traditional mentor-based training [12].

There are, however, considerations for implementation. High-fidelity printed models and robotic simulators have higher costs, so they should be reserved for procedures in which error carries high patient risk or where real cases are infrequent. Lower fidelity models can be used for basic psychomotor skills. Residents should be taught how to interpret 3D reconstructions and segmentation output so that they can recognize inaccuracies. When real patient imaging is used to generate models for training, residency programs must follow institutional policies for privacy and de-identification. When integrated thoughtfully, 3D modeling, VR and robotic simulation create a progression for residents. They begin with task trainers to learn basic movements, advance to patient specific 3D models to understand complex anatomy, and finally perform supervised procedures on real patients. This progression supports competency-based surgical education and produces graduates who are more confident and safer in the operating room.

Patient Education

Patients can easily feel overwhelmed when they are asked to understand a new diagnosis, especially when it involves anatomy they have never seen before. Physicians often rely on explanations and 2D images from X-ray, CT or MRI to describe the problem, which does not help in understanding their diagnosis. 3D models can help inform patients by making the problem visible and tangible. When a patient can hold or view a 3D model of their own anatomy, spatial relationships become easier to understand. A cardiothoracic surgeon can show the exact location of a septal defect or an outflow obstruction and then point to the path the surgeon plans to take (Fig. 6a). An orthopedic surgeon can display or print a 3D model of a complex fracture and indicate where plates and screws will be placed. The surgeon can show 3D models of disease progression to help manage expectations (Fig. 6b). This concrete demonstration helps patients see why a certain approach is needed and what the risks are. It can also reduce anxiety because the unknown becomes visible.

Patient-specific 3D models are especially useful in conditions that are complex, rare, or highly variable from person to person. Examples include congenital heart disease, craniofacial reconstruction, pelvic and acetabular fractures, and large bone or soft tissue tumors. In these situations, the usual 2D images are often difficult for patients and their families to understand. A 3D model allows the surgeon to explain the deformity or defect in simple language and to show the expected result after repair. This supports shared decision making because the patient is choosing between surgical options and outcomes that they can actually see.

Not every patient requires a 3D-printed model. There is a cost in time and materials to convert an image to a print, and not all patients will benefit to the same degree. A simple ankle fracture or a straightforward hernia repair can usually be explained with 2D images or diagrams. A good approach is to use patient specific 3D models

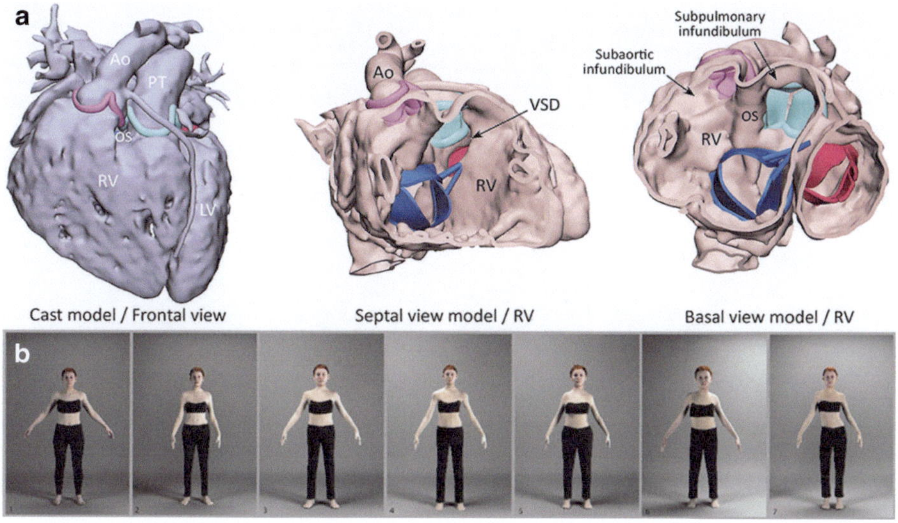

Fig. 6 (**a**) 3D modeling of cast and endocardial surface anatomy (middle and right-hand panels) for double outlet right ventricle with a subpulmonary ventricular septal defect (VSD) [13]. (**b**) VR avatars created using 3D scans of bodies of real female patients with thoracic scoliosis with different Cobb angles [14]

for cases in which the patient is undecided about surgery, in which the anatomy is unusual, or in which multiple specialists need to explain the same plan to the family. A physical model requires fewer technical words, and the clinician can point, trace, and compare normal and abnormal versions. Families can take photographs of the models to review later. This is important for pediatrics and for long or staged procedures where decisions are made over several visits. 3D models can transform a difficult counseling session into an understandable one. They help patients and families see the problem, understand the proposed solution, and participate in decisions about their care.

Innovation in Medical Care

3D modeling is no longer limited to classrooms and simulation labs. It has entered routine clinical workflows and is reshaping how prostheses are designed, how complex operations are planned, and how patient specific implants are manufactured. As healthcare moves toward precision medicine, 3D modeling provides the technical bridge between individual patient anatomy and individualized treatment. It does this by converting imaging data into accurate, modifiable digital objects that can be tested virtually and, when needed, produced physically (Fig. 7).

To understand its clinical value, it is helpful to think of the process in three steps (Fig. 8). First is acquisition, which is most often high-resolution CT or MRI

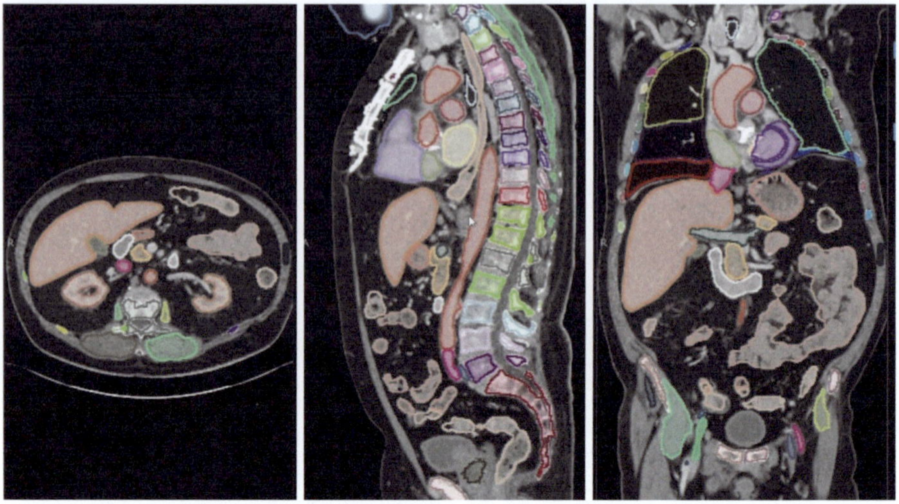

Fig. 7 Axial, sagittal, and coronal CT images with segmentation of structures via different colors [15]

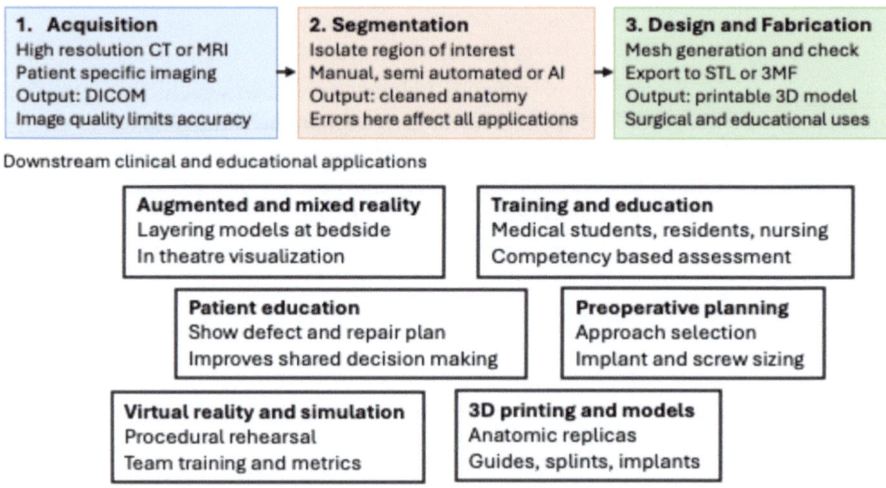

Fig. 8 Clinical 3D modeling pipeline and its downstream educational and surgical applications

images. Second is segmentation, in which the region of interest is isolated from surrounding tissues, sometimes manually, sometimes with semi-automated software, and increasingly with artificial intelligence (AI). Third is design and fabrication, in which the segmented volume is turned into a surface mesh, checked, and exported to a file format such as STL for visualization, education, virtual planning, or printing. Every later application in this section relies on the quality of these three steps.

If segmentation is inaccurate or imaging is incomplete, the model will also be inaccurate.

Surgical Planning and Patient Specific Instrumentation

Surgical planning is one of the areas where 3D modeling has shown the biggest benefit. Surgeons who perform complex reconstructions report that printed models help them understand spatial relationships, select the most appropriate surgical approach, and even reduce operating room time because instruments and implants can be chosen in advance. A survey of surgeons in complex cases found advantages in preoperative planning, economic savings, and better communication within the team when 3D models were used [16].

Virtual surgical planning (VSP) takes this further by allowing the entire procedure to be rehearsed on a computer. Imaging and 3D scans are imported, the defect or deformity is segmented, and the surgeon performs the planned cuts, reductions, or reconstructions virtually. In craniofacial and orthognathic surgery, VSP has been shown to decrease planning time and improve accuracy compared to traditional methods. Park and colleagues reported a 41 to 62% reduction in time when virtual planning was used for orthognathic surgery [17].

Prosthetics

Conventional prosthetic fabrication depended on manual casting, hand modification, and several rounds of patient fittings. This was effective but slow and it did not create a permanent digital record. 3D modeling and computer-aided design have changed this sequence. A prosthetist can now scan the residual limb with a handheld 3D scanner, generate a digital model of the stump, and design the socket around the actual patient geometry. Pressure points and load distribution can be evaluated in software and corrected before the fabrication of the prosthesis (Fig. 9). The final design is then printed in thermoplastic materials, sometimes with internal lattice structures that reduce weight without sacrificing strength. This workflow decreases material waste, makes it easier to reproduce a device later, and improves comfort because the socket is matched to the patient rather than to an estimated shape [19].

There are still limitations of this manufacturing process. Some high stress components such as those used in athletic or very active patients benefit from metals like titanium. Printers that can process titanium and other advanced materials are expensive and not widely available in low resource settings. In many developing countries, there are also challenges with scanner availability, maintenance of printers, and supply of printing materials.

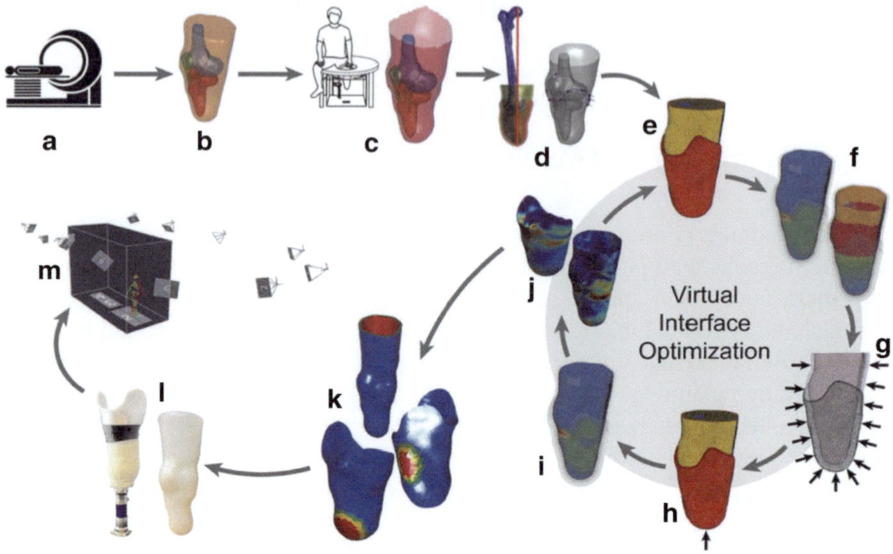

Fig. 9 Map of digital prosthetic interface design framework to evaluation, based on (**a**) 3D imaging via MRI or CT. (**b**) Biomechanical model reconstruction through segmentation. (**c**) Digital image. (**d**, **e**) Preliminary socket and liner design. (**f**) Pressure region definitions for the socket and the liner design. (**g**–**j**) Finite element simulation and optimization loop. (**k**) Further modification such as mesh manipulation and liner extension. (**l**) Fabrication by 3D printing. (**m**) Clinical evaluation [18]

Orthopedic Surgery

In orthopedic surgery, 3D modeling is used for presurgical planning as well as implant customization. Many fractures have complex 3D patterns that are difficult to appreciate on 2D X-ray images. Rendering CT data into a 3D model allows the surgeon to rotate, separate, and reduce individual fragments (Fig. 10a). 3D models can better evaluate the fracture's alignment, angulation, and rotation as well as the relationship between the bone and soft tissues. Plates and screws can be positioned virtually. Screw lengths and trajectories can be checked to make sure that joints and neurovascular structures are not violated. The same STL files can then be used to 3D print the bone, to prebend plates on a physical replica, or to manufacture patient specific cutting and drilling guides (Fig. 10b, c). This improves accuracy and can shorten operative time.

There are also many constraints in generating an accurate 3D model. Reconstruction depends on high-quality imaging and good segmentation. Errors early in the workflow are propagated to the printed model, to the guide, and to the implant. Custom devices require days to weeks to manufacture. That is acceptable for tumors or elective reconstructions but not for open fractures or septic joints where surgery must be done immediately. Institutions that wish to adopt 3D planning should therefore define which indications justify the extra time and cost.

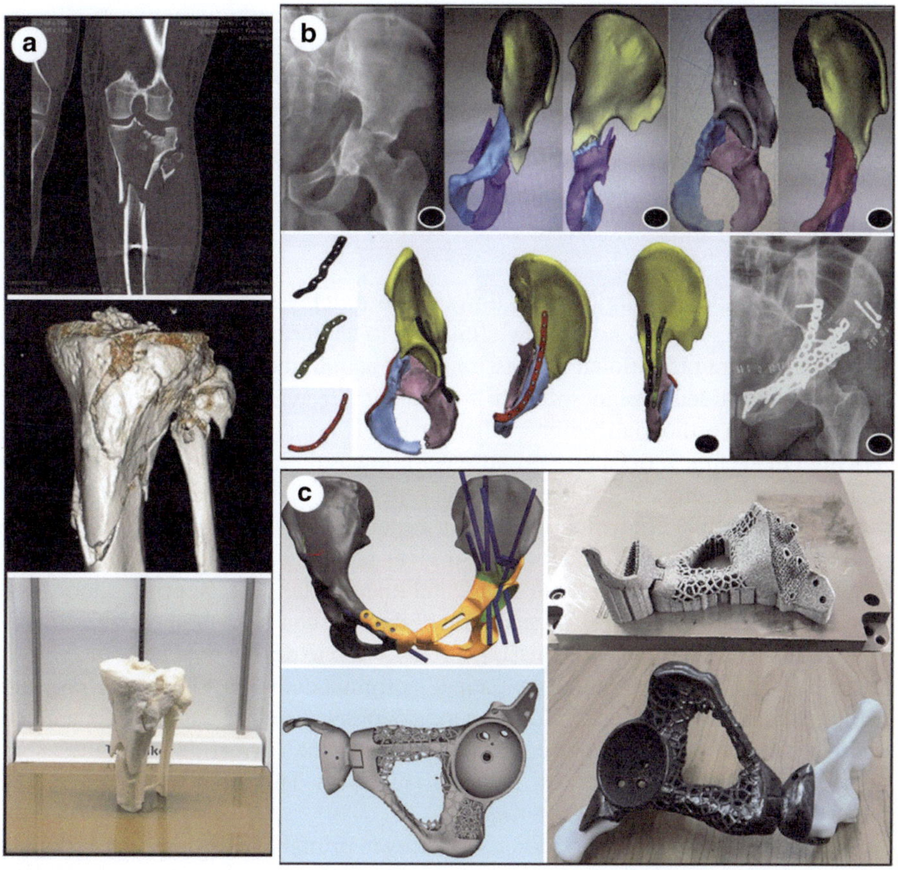

Fig. 10 (**a**) Coronal CT image, 3D reconstruction, and 3D-printed model of a left-sided tibial plateau fracture [20]. (**b**) X-ray of an acetabulum fracture with 3D model creation, and virtual hardware [21]. (**c**) A custom made pelvic implant for a chondrosarcoma resection [22]

Cardiovascular and Structural Heart Interventions

3D modeling is becoming an increasingly powerful tool in the world of cardiology, a field where understanding the anatomy and relationships of blood vessels, heart valves and chambers dictate the intervention and diagnosis. Echocardiography and CT scans can now be converted into 3D digital hearts that interventional teams will examine from any angle. In international surveys, most congenital heart surgeons agreed that these models improved their understanding of complex congenital lesions and believed that 3D models would become part of routine planning [23].

Patient specific models are particularly useful when standard access routes or device sizes are not possible. In one reported case, a stenotic bicuspid aortic valve and unusual subclavian anatomy made a standard transcatheter approach challenging. A 3D-printed model of the heart, and the nearby vasculature allowed the team to simulate the procedure and choose a surgical cut down to the axillary artery as the safest option (Fig. 11). This type of pre-operative planning and pre-training can prevent complications during the actual procedure [25].

Dentistry and Maxillofacial Restoration

Dentistry has adopted digital workflows more quickly than many other clinical fields. Intraoral scanners now allow clinicians to capture the dentition and gingiva in minutes without traditional impressions. The acquired data are imported directly into computer-aided design software to generate crowns, bridges, implant abutments, and even orthodontic aligners that can be 3D printed in the dentist clinic with very high fit accuracy. Because the entire workflow is digital, minor adjustments can be made and devices reprinted without repeating the impression step, which improves both clinic efficiency and patient experience.

3D modeling has also transformed surgical planning in oral and maxillofacial cases. When patients present with segmental mandibular defects, orbital floor loss, or post traumatic asymmetry, 3D scanning of the face can be combined with contralateral mirroring to recreate the missing anatomy and to design prosthetic or skeletal segments that closely reproduce the patient's original contours. Custom cutting and drilling guides can be produced for both the donor site, such as a fibula flap, and the recipient site, so that osteotomies are performed at the correct angle and the segments are seated in the planned position (Fig. 12). This reduces intraoperative guesswork and shortens operative time.

Beyond hard tissue reconstruction, advances in printable elastomers and silicone like materials now make it possible to fabricate external facial prostheses, including ears and noses, with more realistic texture and color [27]. When these are derived

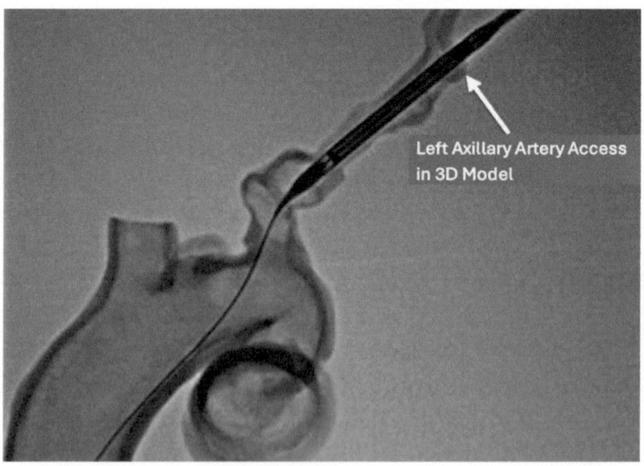

Fig. 11 X-ray showing catheter access to a 3D heart model from the left axillary artery [24]

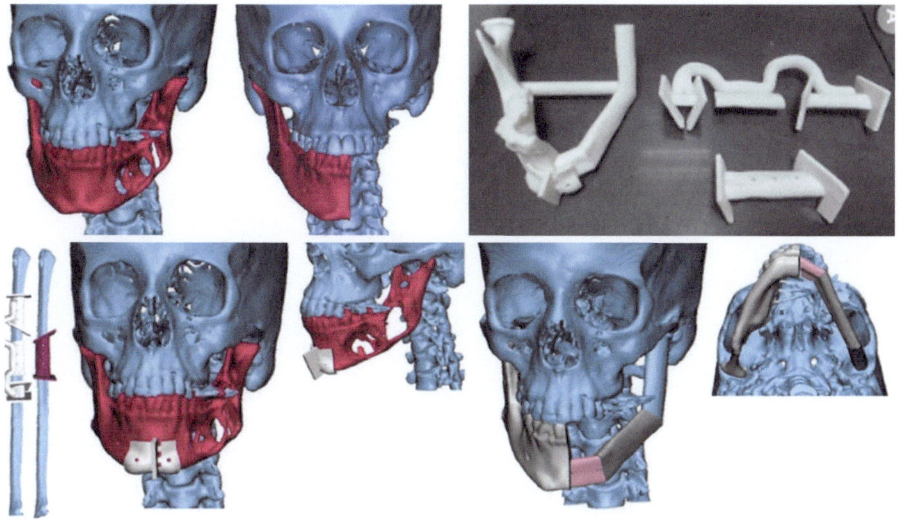

Fig. 12 3D virtual model of a craniofacial skeleton with planned mandibular resection, virtual model and 3D-printed patient-specific fibular and mandibular cutting guides [26]

from the patient's own facial scan, they integrate better cosmetically and functionally, supporting speech, mastication, and psychosocial recovery.

Therapeutic Virtual Reality

Pain management has traditionally relied on medications and physical therapy to treat both acute and chronic pain. Immersive virtual reality has been used as an adjunct for pain management, particularly in burn patients undergoing dressing changes, which are highly painful. By engaging patients in an interactive environment such as SnowWorld (Fig. 13), which allows patients to interact with snowmen, igloos and penguins via snowballs, attention is diverted, and pain scores decrease compared to standard care [29]. This is a good example of how 3D immersive environments can be therapeutic, not only educational.

Conclusion

The implementation of 3D modeling has become a powerful tool across medical care and education. For patients and their families, patient-specific 3D models make complex pathology visible, which improves understanding and decision making when a surgical intervention is considered. For medical students, residents, and other medical trainees, 3D models and related technologies such as VR, AR, and

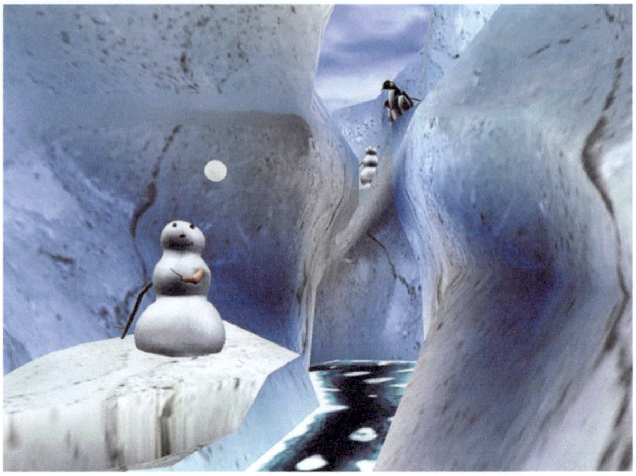

Fig. 13 SnowWorld virtual reality showing a snowman by an icy river with penguins on a cliff [28]

MR enhances comprehension of anatomy, strengthens procedural skills, and builds confidence before entering the operating room. Clinically, 3D modeling facilitates preoperative planning, improves prosthetic and implants design, and ultimately contributes to more efficient and precise medical care.

As 3D modeling technology continues to evolve, and its role in medicine will only expand, bridging education, innovation, and precision medicine into a more integrated form of healthcare.

References

1. Plastinated models. Available at https://doi.org/10.1186/s12909-022-03756-2. Accessed on 31 Oct 2025.
2. Boyajian MK, Lubner RJ, Roussel LO, Crozier JW, Ryder BA, Woo AS. A 3D printed suturing trainer for medical students. Clin Teach. 2020;17(6):650–4. https://doi.org/10.1111/tct.13176.
3. 3D anatomy models. Available at https://www.atomedge.com/. Accessed on 31 Oct 2025.
4. Lim KH, Loo ZY, Goldie SJ, Adams JW, McMenamin PG. Use of 3D printed models in medical education: a randomized control trial comparing 3D prints versus cadaveric materials for learning external cardiac anatomy. Anat Sci Educ. 2016;9(3):213–21. https://doi.org/10.1002/ase.1573.
5. Model arm. Available at https://limbsandthings.com/us/products/70304-basic-venipuncture-arm-light-skin-tone. Accessed on 31 Oct 2025.
6. Airway model. Available at https://www.gtsimulators.com/products/difficult-airway-management-simulator-kk-mw13?srsltid=AfmBOoqG0jJphM9ntSGyQnF6d8FW7Gn8yFPqCDJ1FzdQEAGWDgT3jMqh. Accessed on 31 Oct 2025.
7. Augmented reality. Available at https://www.verdict.co.uk/ar-training-medcognition/. Accessed on 31 Oct 2025.
8. Virtual reality with baby. Available at https://www.aamc.org/news/future-or-fad-virtual-reality-medical-education. Accessed on 31 Oct 2025.
9. Holographic patient. Available at https://doi.org/10.1080/10872981.2021.1953953. Accessed on 31 Oct 2025.

10. DaVinci robot. Available at https://www.chronicle1909.com/2024/08/22/robotics-rule-at-riverbend-new-surgical-robot-added-to-toolbox/. Accessed on 31 Oct 2025.
11. Bowel anastomosis simulation. Available at https://mimicsimulation.com/dv-trainer-software-upgrade-provides-surgeons-with-enhanced-performance-more-options-for-robotic-surgery-simulation-and-training/. Accessed on 31 Oct 2025.
12. Jensen UJ, Jensen J, Ahlberg G, Tornvall P. Virtual reality training in coronary angiography and its transfer effect to real-life catheterisation lab. EuroIntervention. 2016;11(13):1503–10. https://doi.org/10.4244/EIJY15M06_05.
13. 3D model of heart surface. Available at https://doi.org/10.3389/fped.2021.621672. Accessed on 31 Oct 2025.
14. Models of females with various scoliosis severities. Available at https://doi.org/10.3390/app13042374. Accessed on 31 Oct 2025.
15. CT images showing segmentation. Available at https://developer.nvidia.com/blog/computed-tomography-organ-and-disease-segmentation-using-the-nvidia-vista-3d-nim/. Accessed on 31 Oct 2025).
16. Thorn C, Ballard J, Lockhart C, Crone A, Aarvold A. The perioperative utility of 3D printed models in complex surgical care: feedback from 106 cases. Ann R Coll Surg Engl. 2023;105(8):747–53. https://doi.org/10.1308/rcsann.2022.0127. Epub 2023 Jan 9.
17. Park SY, Hwang DS, Song JM, Kim UK. Comparison of time and cost between conventional surgical planning and virtual surgical planning in orthognathic surgery in Korea. Maxillofac Plast Reconstr Surg. 2021;43(1):18. https://doi.org/10.1186/s40902-021-00305-7. Erratum in: Maxillofac Plast Reconstr Surg 2023;45(1):37. 10.1186/s40902-023-00404-7.
18. Lee DRC, Yang X, Riccio-Ackerman F, Alemón B, Ballesteros-Escamilla M, Solav D, Lipsitz SR, Moerman KM, Meyer CI, Jaeger AM, Huegel JC, Herr HM. A clinical comparison of a digital versus conventional design methodology for transtibial prosthetic interfaces. Sci Rep. 2024;14(1):25833. https://doi.org/10.1038/s41598-024-74504-3.
19. Hassan BB, Wong MS. Contemporary and future development of 3D printing technology in the field of assistive technology, orthotics and prosthetics. Can Prosthet Orthot J. 2023;6(2):42225. https://doi.org/10.33137/cpoj.v6i2.42225.
20. Tibial Plateau fracture imaging. Available at https://doi.org/10.1007/s00068-022-02055-1. Accessed on 31 Oct 2025.
21. Virtual pelvis fixation and final fixation. Available at https://doi.org/10.1016/j.cjtee.2019.07.006. Accessed on 31 Oct 2025.
22. Pelvic implant. Available at https://doi.org/10.1177/0300060520917275. Accessed on 31 Oct 2025.
23. Valverde I, Gomez-Ciriza G, et al. Three-dimensional printed models for surgical planning of complex congenital heart defects: an international multicentre study. Eur J Cardiothorac Surg. 2017;52(6):1139–48. https://doi.org/10.1093/ejcts/ezx208.
24. Catheter in 3D heart model. Available at https://doi.org/10.1016/j.jaccas.2020.01.021. Accessed on 31 Oct 2025.
25. Alasnag MA, Al-Nasser IM, Porqueddu MM, Ahmed WH, Al-Shaibi KF. 3D model guiding transcatheter aortic valve replacement in a patient with aortic coarctation. JACC Case Rep. 2020;2(3):352–7. https://doi.org/10.1016/j.jaccas.2020.01.021.
26. Mandible imaging for reconstruction. Available at https://doi.org/10.1186/s12885-022-10322-y. Accessed on 31 Oct 2025.
27. Nuseir A, Hatamleh MM, Alnazzawi A, Al-Rabab'ah M, Kamel B, Jaradat E. Direct 3D printing of flexible nasal prosthesis: optimized digital workflow from scan to fit. J Prosthodont. 2019;28(1):10–4. https://doi.org/10.1111/jopr.13001.
28. SnowWorld virtual reality. Available at https://doi.org/10.3389/fnhum.2019.00262. Accessed on 31 Oct 2025.

29. Hoffman HG, Rodriguez RA, Gonzalez M, Bernardy M, Peña R, Beck W, Patterson DR, Meyer WJ 3rd. Immersive virtual reality as an adjunctive non-opioid analgesic for pre-dominantly Latin American children with large severe burn wounds during burn wound cleaning in the intensive care unit: a pilot study. Front Hum Neurosci. 2019;13:262. https://doi.org/10.3389/fnhum.2019.00262.

Innovation in General Practice

Katie Joo, Michelle Vu, and Jocelyn Deleon

Introduction

Primary care is the cornerstone of effective health systems; however, it faces mounting challenges that strain its capacity to deliver comprehensive and equitable care. Central among these is the rising burden of chronic diseases, including diabetes, hypertension, cardiovascular disease, and COPD. These conditions account for most morbidity and mortality worldwide and demand sustained, coordinated management, which traditional episodic, physician-centric models are ill-suited to address.

Compounding this are persistent structural inequities rooted in socioeconomic disadvantage, racial and ethnic disparities, language barriers, and systemic racism. Populations with the greatest disease burden often face the highest barriers to timely, high-quality care, with social determinants, such as housing instability, food insecurity, and inequitable digital access, widening these gaps.

Access and patient engagement are major challenges. Brief in-person visits and fragmented follow-ups fail to meet the needs of patients managing complex conditions or navigating multiple social barriers. Workforce shortages, administrative complexity, and evolving expectations for more flexible and personalized care have intensified these challenges.

Addressing these interrelated challenges necessitates a comprehensive overhaul of primary care—one that is proactive, team-oriented, digitally integrated, and equity-centered. Innovations such as telehealth, remote patient monitoring, optimized EHRs, interprofessional collaboration, integrated behavioral health,

K. Joo · M. Vu · J. Deleon (✉)
Western Michigan University Homer Stryker M.D. School of Medicine, Kalamazoo, MI, USA
e-mail: Jocelyn.Deleon@wmed.edu

S. S. Chahin et al. (eds.), *Innovation in Medical Education and Clinical Practice*, https://doi.org/10.1007/978-3-032-19116-8_18

same-day access models, patient-centered medical homes, and group visits signal a shift toward more holistic, patient-centered, and sustainable models of care.

This chapter reviews how primary care physicians' roles have evolved in practice, setting the stage for the digital, team-based, and access innovations that follow.

The Evolving Role of Primary Care Physicians

Primary care physicians (PCPs) are the cornerstones of healthcare systems, providing comprehensive, longitudinal, and patient-centered care. Over recent decades, their role has undergone significant transformation in response to the rising prevalence of chronic diseases and widening health inequities. Thus, PCPs have integrated innovative approaches to better align with modern care delivery models, increase access, and improve quality of care. The evolution of general practice highlights the resilience of primary care and the critical role of innovation in ensuring its continued efficiency and efficacy.

Chronic diseases, such as diabetes, hypertension, cardiovascular disease, and chronic obstructive pulmonary disease, account for the majority of morbidity and mortality in the United States and globally. The Centers for Disease Control and Prevention estimates that six in ten adults in the United States live with at least one chronic condition, with four in ten experiencing two or more chronic conditions [1]. To manage complex, lifelong illnesses more efficiently, PCPs have transitioned toward a more proactive health management approach. Evidence-based care pathways, disease registries, and risk stratification tools are now commonly employed in general practice, and the adoption of team-based care models further allows sustained and efficient chronic disease management.

Beyond clinical care, PCPs play a central role in mitigating health inequities in Canada. Disparities in access and outcomes are often driven by social determinants of health (SDOH), such as socioeconomic status, education, housing, and systemic racism. Today, many PCPs routinely screen for social needs, such as food insecurity, transportation barriers, and housing instability, during visits. This practice has been supported by the integration of SDOH tools into electronic health records, allowing more standardized data collection and referrals to community resources. However, research shows that screening without robust referral pathways may exacerbate patient frustration, underscoring the need for closed-loop systems that ensure follow-through [2]. By addressing the broader determinants of health, PCPs extend their role beyond clinical treatment to encompass advocacy and holistic support.

In the ever-evolving digital age, PCPs continuously adapt to different care delivery models. The COVID-19 pandemic accelerated the adoption of telemedicine, patient portals, and secure messaging systems, fundamentally altering patient–provider interactions. PCPs have adjusted to offering flexible scheduling, virtual visits, and expanded channels of communication, enabling patients to engage more directly with their care. Digital health technologies, such as remote patient monitoring and integrated behavioral health platforms, allow PCPs to manage increasingly complex populations. Practice redesign models, such as the patient-centered medical home (PCMH) and accountable care organizations (ACOs), redistribute tasks among multidisciplinary teams, which enables physicians to focus on decision-making. These innovations address the pressing need for efficiency in managing chronic conditions, equity in access and outcomes, and alignment with patient expectations for convenience and quality. Without them, primary care risks fragmentation, patient dissatisfaction, and worsening inequities in health care.

Furthermore, shared decision-making and culturally responsive communication are hallmarks of effective general practice. Patients are more informed and engage in active participation in medical decisions, which requires PCPs to act as educators and partners in health rather than solely as authoritative figures in the medical field. These changes reflect a broader societal shift toward patient-centered care, reinforcing the relevance of general practice in the era of patient-driven healthcare [3].

The role of PCPs has evolved significantly in response to chronic diseases, health inequities, and patient expectations. General practice has shifted from episodic care to longitudinal, team-based, and socially responsive models of care. Technological and structural innovations have been central to this evolution, ensuring that primary care is effective and equitable. By embracing innovation and expanding their scope beyond traditional clinical care, PCPs can strengthen their role as the backbone of the health system and advocates for population health.

These role shifts are enabled by technology. These digital tools make proactive, coordinated, and equitable primary care possible in the future.

Digital Tools

Primary care has always been at the forefront of healthcare delivery. Over the past two decades, it has undergone a rapid digital transformation driven by the chronic disease burden, growing patient expectations, and long-standing barriers to healthcare access. Key tools in this transformation include electronic health records (EHRs), clinical decision support systems (CDSS), telehealth, and remote patient monitoring (RPM). These are increasingly vital to how healthcare teams deliver proactive, continuous, and patient-centered care. Patient portals and mobile applications further enable education, reminders, and two-way communication. Together, these innovations are reshaping workflows and outcomes in primary care, especially when implemented with mindful attention to usability, integration, and equity [4–7, 12].

Electronic health records (EHRs) help clinicians organize and access patient information efficiently. When correctly implemented, optimized electronic health records (EHRs) can empower primary care providers. However, if not mindfully constructed, EHRs can be more of a burden than a tool for the healthcare professionals. When streamlined, EHRs facilitate task delegation, internal messaging, and the use of structured templates so that nurses and medical assistants can collect symptom-specific data and initiate protocolized care, offloading physicians and supporting continuous management [8]. However, poorly designed systems can create problems, such as limited data tracking, weak care planning tools, and difficulties in sharing information between systems [8]. Recent evidence shows that greater time spent in the EHR among primary care physicians is associated with better performance on certain ambulatory quality measures, such as diabetes, blood pressure control, and screening. This demonstrates that portions of the EHR may reflect patient communication and thorough follow-up, which directly translates into quality improvements [9]. The goal is not to increase the time spent in the system but to make it more efficient by using features such as smarter inbox management, team-based charting, and automation to improve quality without increasing the burden [8, 9].

Clinical decision support systems (CDSS) are built on EHRs by converting patient data into actionable information. These systems deliver reminders, order sets, and population registries to the users. An overview study details the consistent benefits of CDSS for preventive care, chronic disease monitoring, and medication safety when systems are well-designed and integrated with the workflow. However, it also highlights the risks of "alert fatigue" and the importance of usability and governance [10]. For medication safety, linking primary and secondary care EHRs enables surveillance of prescribing and monitoring hazards at the population scale, revealing higher risks among older adults, those with polypharmacy, and practices serving more deprived communities. However, these concerns can be addressed through targeted outreach and monitoring prompts [11].

Telehealth, delivered through video, phone, and secure messaging, significantly expanded access to care during the COVID-19 pandemic. Video, telephone, and secure messaging visits expanded rapidly in 2020, converting a minority of encounters into the majority at the pandemic peak. In a national analysis, office-based primary care visits declined by 50.2% in Q2 2020 compared with Q2 2018–2019, while telemedicine rose from 1.1% of visits pre-pandemic to 35.3% in Q2 2020, illustrating telehealth's ability to preserve access to care when in-person care is disrupted [12]. Likewise, provider surveys document dramatic virtual care uptake, with respondents reporting an average of two-thirds of visits conducted virtually during the first wave, high satisfaction, and intentions to sustain meaningful levels of telehealth after the pandemic [5]. Beyond patient volume, patient outcomes and follow-up plans are crucial when considering the efficacy of telehealth. A large integrated system cohort study of patient-initiated primary care telemedicine for acute conditions found that treatment patterns and short-term safety events were comparable between digital and in-person modalities, with some differences between video and telephone, suggesting that virtual visits can safely substitute for many acute issues when embedded in existing primary care teams [4]. Taken together, these data support hybrid models that match modality to clinical need and patient preferences [4, 5, 12].

Remote patient monitoring (RPM) takes this a step further by bringing care into the patients' homes. Digital tools, such as telehealth and remote patient monitoring, are not isolated innovations; they are complementary components of a broader strategy to enhance access, improve quality, and drive better patient outcomes in primary care. RPM connects home devices, such as automated blood pressure cuffs and glucometers, to primary care teams, so physiologic data are seamlessly incorporated into the clinical workflow. Research shows that when large primary care networks utilize integrated hypertension telemonitoring programs that feed data directly into routine practice processes, there is a reduction in average patient blood pressure and a decreased need for office visits [6]. In Scotland's ScaleUp BP program across 75 practices ($n \approx 3200$), mean systolic and diastolic pressures fell by approximately 6.6/4.2 mmHg, with a 19% reduction in face-to-face appointments among participants compared with 11% among nonparticipants. The seamless integration of BP readings with routine results has been cited as crucial to its success [6]. Qualitative research with U.S. primary care physicians confirms that RPM can improve the quality of care for chronic conditions, particularly hypertension and diabetes; however, integration is restricted by data volume, workflow design, staff role clarity, digital/health literacy, and questions about financial sustainability [7]. Clinicians have described practical facilitators, such as unclear protocols, low staff support, and difficulties in integrating RPM into EMR, as operational barriers [7]. These findings underscore the insufficiency of RPM devices alone in improving care. Efficiency is achieved when RPM is coupled with redesigned workflows that define who reviews the data, when medications are adjusted, and how patients are coached depending on their data [6, 7].

Patient portals and mobile applications further support continuous care by providing patients with easy access to laboratory results, secure messaging, and reminders for testing, medication refills, or appointments. Portals also help sustain patient engagement after virtual or in-person visits are completed. In primary care systems that scaled telehealth quickly, secure asynchronous messaging was a major mode of virtual care and a key factor in continuity [5]. Studies of telemedicine visit content also suggest that virtual modalities can safely manage many acute complaints while enabling efficient follow-up through the EHR, portal, or phone to support timely reinforcement of education and adherence [4, 12]. For RPM programs, patient-facing apps that display trends and prompts, combined with provider outreach, are central to sustained engagement [6, 7].

The greatest impact occurs when these digital tools work together. The CDSS identifies gaps in care. Telehealth creates flexible access points for patients. RPM provides real-time health information. Portals support patient education and follow up. This integrated approach makes primary care more proactive and personalized. However, clinician interviews have warned that digital adaptations have the potential to exacerbate disparities if not intentionally designed. Connectivity, device access, and digital literacy remain barriers cited by both patients and clinicians. Practices serving disadvantaged communities experience more missed monitoring, thus emphasizing the need to pair digital tools with equity-focused workflows and community partnerships [5, 7, 11].

Digital tools are redefining primary care as a continuous, relationship-centered, and data-informed enterprise. RPM enables early intervention. Telehealth preserves access and continuity of care. EHR optimization and CDSS make data actionable, and patient portals support education and follow-up. Evidence shows that these beneficial results are attainable when systems are integrated into team workflows and backed by policies with equity considerations. Primary care organizations that invest in these pillars will be positioned to deliver safer, more equitable, and effective care in the coming years [4–12].

However, digital transformation also introduces new challenges. Managing data streams, coordinating care, and ensuring smooth workflows require more than individual clinician efforts. Primary care must embrace interprofessional collaboration to translate digital capacity into better outcomes. Teams that include physicians, nurses, pharmacists, social workers, behavioral health specialists, and community partners can share responsibilities, ensure seamless care transitions, and address medical and social needs. Thus, interprofessional teamwork is not just complementary to digital innovation; it is essential to realizing its full potential.

Interprofessional Collaboration: Team-Based Care and Behavioral Health Integration

An integral part of primary care innovation is its evolution toward models that broaden the care team and integrate behavioral health to meet patients' biopsychosocial needs, while advancing health equity. Team-based care and integrated behavioral health (IBH) are two complementary approaches fundamentally based on collaboration among nurses, social workers, pharmacists, mental health clinicians, and physicians. They are equipped with structured processes for identifying and addressing social determinants of health (SDoH) and linking patients to community resources to address SDoH. Evidence from case studies, trials, reviews, and implementation research demonstrates that interprofessional teamwork can improve care coordination and patient experience, while IBH improves pediatric behavioral outcomes. [13–21].

Team-based care aligns complementary expertise, such as nurses' care coordination, social workers' resource navigation, and pharmacists' medication management, around shared goals for patients. Nurses frequently orchestrate population management and care transitions, closing gaps in preventive and chronic care while coordinating with IBH clinicians for same-day concerns. Social workers contribute to psychosocial assessment, brief interventions, resource navigation, and often lead community linkage efforts or liaison roles [19–21]. Pharmacists embedded in teams improve medication reconciliation, adherence support, and deprescribing. In rural and underserved settings, the presence of pharmacists is specifically associated with fewer perceived drug-related problems [14]. Cross-training, standing orders, and shared registries enable these professions to operate at the top of their licenses and to hand off seamlessly within integrated workflows [13, 16].

In an underserved, predominantly rural U.S. setting, a multisite survey of clinicians found that interprofessional teams were perceived to improve patient outcomes, clinic efficiency, and care coordination. Importantly, teams that included a clinical pharmacist were perceived to prevent medication associated problems ($p < 0.0001$) [14]. A recent review of co-located, team-based primary care models concluded that, despite variability in design and reporting, these models generally showed benefits for both patients and providers. The successful implementation of team-based care relies on capable care managers, stable staffing, a shared vision, leadership, and shared data systems. Financing and workforce constraints are common barriers to implementing these strategies [16].

Embedding mental health providers in primary care settings improves access to common concerns, especially in the pediatric population. A meta-analysis of integrated medical-behavioral care for children found that, compared with usual primary care, integrated care produced superior behavioral and quality-of-life outcomes [17]. Qualitative research has demonstrated how IBH teams utilize brief problem-focused interventions, same-day consultations, and warm handoffs to integrate behavioral and medical care into a single encounter [13]. Studies further indicate that team-based models that co-locate IBH can improve patient and provider experiences. However, there is limited consistent evidence on costs, and implementation success largely depends on local contexts [16].

Notably, the everyday mechanics of team functioning play a vital role in its efficiency and efficacy. Research into integrated practices describes three recurrent interprofessional strategies of consulting, coordinating, and collaborating (the 3Cs) that clinicians use to share mental models, align plans, and match provider roles to patient needs [13]. These strategies are supported by tangible design choices, such as co-located workspaces, huddles, warm handoffs, and flexible staffing. However, research with primary care clinicians in large integrated systems highlights that integration can introduce distinctive stressors, such as administrative burden, referral 'dumping,' and perceived limits on autonomy. This highlights the need to design team-based care with attention to clinician well-being [15].

Team-based and integrated models are most impactful when they explicitly address the SDoH and link patients to community resources. A multisite qualitative study of health systems that created programs to help with patients' housing, transportation, and economic needs found that most programs-built case-management-style approaches anchored in referrals to community-based organizations (CBOs), with some programs providing higher-intensity assistance, such as form completion and home visits. This study found four major operational challenges in engaging CBOs: obtaining clinical buy-in, centering patients' perspectives, and sustaining programs [19]. Among older adults, a primary care liaison (PCL) model trained staff across patient-centered medical homes to assess unmet needs and broker services. Over the course of 1 year, the PCL counseled 327 recently discharged older patients and arranged support such as transportation, in-home care, and food, demonstrating the feasibility of cross-sector partnerships embedded in primary care [20]. From the patient perspective, interviews with 102 adults who participated in a clinic-based screening and resource referral program highlighted that warm handoffs, navigation assistance, and follow-up made resources realistically attainable and conveyed that the health system actually cared. Patients have described this relationship as therapeutic in its own right [21].

Implementing practical tools and workflows to address SDoH is essential. A recent review cataloged commonly used clinical screening instruments and referral platforms and emphasized the pairing of screening with closed-loop referral tracking and EHR integration [18]. Importantly, the same review underscores that screening must be coupled with trustworthy community linkages and attention to stigma, privacy, and patient preferences to emphasize and attain equity [18].

Several implementation themes recur across studies. First, the design for proximity and real-time communication, such as colocation, huddles, brief consultations, and warm handoffs, is crucial to the 3Cs of teamwork [13]. Second, care managers or liaisons should be designated to drive the social care workflow and maintain CBO relationships [16, 20]. Third, adopting SDoH screening tools and building closed-loop referrals into the EHR, with role clarity on who screens, who navigates, and who follows up [18–21]. Fourth, measuring what matters to patients and their teams. [18, 21]. Finally, anticipating clinician workload and autonomy concerns in integrated systems and address them with appropriate staffing, documentation support, and clear referral pathways [15].

Prior to the implementation of new models, deliberate thought must be put into the design to ensure patient equity. Team-based and IBH models can mitigate disparities by improving access to behavioral care, delivering culturally responsive brief interventions, and reducing barriers to community resources. However, inequities can widen if screening is universal while assistance is scarce, if referrals lack follow-through, or if workflows ignore language access, immigration-related fears, or disability accommodations. Evidence across reviews and qualitative studies points to strategies that promote equity, such as codesigning screening questions with communities to minimize stigma, hiring community health workers and culturally competent staff, prioritizing warm handoffs over paper referrals, and tracking completion of resource connections rather than screening alone [18–21].

Team-based primary care and integrated behavioral health are complementary strategies for delivering whole-person care. The literature shows that interprofessional collaboration improves coordination and addresses the safety of medications. Research demonstrates that IBH improves pediatric behavioral outcomes and that structured SDoH workflows with community partnerships can translate screening into tangible assistance. Clinics that design for the daily mechanics of the healthcare team, embed navigation and liaison roles, and build closed-loop referral infrastructure are best positioned to deliver equitable, person-centered care that reflects the realities of patients' lives [13–21].

Same Day Access and Team-Based Continuity

There have been two long-standing challenges in primary care: timely access and continuity of care. Same-day or walk-in appointment availability, particularly when integrated within a team-based model of care, might be a solution to these challenges. Same-day access may decrease the number of patients who delay seeking care, decrease the use of emergency services, and increase patient satisfaction in addressing acute needs in a timely manner. It has been a concern that this rapid access could decrease continuity of care, which is crucial to the patient-provider relationship as well as improved outcomes. However, recent literature has found that when there is a team-based framework, continuity and access can reinforce rather than compete with each other.

Forman et al. studied how academic primary care clinics provide continuity of care even while offering same-day appointments and examined what factors may contribute or be a detriment to their success. The study found that team-based continuity models allow patients to be seen quickly without losing the sense of an ongoing therapeutic relationship with the doctor. Most sites used NPs, RNs, and PAs as part of their team-based approaches. For example, when a resident's patient needed a same-day visit, but the resident was not in the clinic that day, another professional, whether another resident, attending physician, RN, NP, or PA, would be able to step in to fill that spot. Effective continuity of care also requires consistent communication across the team. Clinics used strategies such as electronic medical records, huddles, and structured communication processes to preserve communication efforts across different professionals. [22].

In addition to Forman et al.'s studies of team-based continuity, Burch et al. examined how appointment volume, type, and modality influenced the patient experience in 5000 general practices in England. From the data in the General Practice Patient Survey and NHS appointment records, they found that face-to-face visits with general practitioners were strongly associated with higher patient satisfaction, better continuity, and improved perceptions of support for long-term conditions. However, it was also revealed that more same-day appointments were associated with lower patient satisfaction, further emphasizing the fact that rapid access alone does not guarantee a positive patient experience. [23].

The findings from these two studies demonstrate an important tension. Forman et al. revealed that same-day access can be beneficial when paired with team-based coverage models to preserve continuity in patient care. In contrast, Burch et al. suggested that same-day access is not as important to patient experience but rather the opportunities for in-person relationship-centered care. Additionally, Burch et al. discovered a negative association between telephone appointments and patient experience, which further emphasizes the importance of face-to-face interactions over rapid access for patient satisfaction.

Together, these studies indicate that expanding same-day or walk-in access is not inherently positive or negative. The implementation of these innovations has proven to be important. It is crucial to consider team-based structures without the expense of face-to-face encounters or relational care when implementing same-day access to general practices. Innovations in access should be carefully balanced with relational and informational continuity to ensure that improvements in efficiency do not come at the expense of patient trust, satisfaction, or long-term outcomes. Team-based structures, such as those found in Patient-Centered Medical Homes (PCMHs), provide the organizational foundation needed to balance timely access with sustained, coordinated care.

Patient-Centered Medical Homes (PCMHs)

As general practice faces multitudes of challenges, from providing care for diverse populations to meeting the needs of rising rates of chronic illness, Patient-Centered Medical Homes (PCMH) have emerged as a possible way to redesign general practice. PCMHs allow for long-term relationships between patients and providers, as well as coordinated, comprehensive, and team-based care. This shifts general practice toward proactive, preventive, and population-oriented care. With the implementation of PCMH, general practice can work toward reducing avoidable hospitalizations, combat the barriers that populations must face to obtain healthcare, and improve overall outcomes for patients.

Chronic disease management is one of the main targets of PCMHs, as the process requires continuity, coordination, and patient engagement. John et al. (2020) compared PCMH-based care with standard primary care by conducting a systematic review and meta-analysis of randomized and non-randomized trials. The study's findings demonstrated significant improvements in biomedical outcomes, such as blood pressure, glycated hemoglobin, and low-density lipoprotein cholesterol. Additionally, this study found that the benefits of PCMH care extended beyond patients' physical health. Patients who received PCMH care had an increased quality of life, decreased depressive episodes, increased odds of remission rates, and overall improvement in self-management. Reductions in hospital admissions were also associated with patients receiving PCMH care. However, the PCMH model incurs higher costs of care than standard primary care visits. Overall, the evidence suggests that PCMHs are beneficial in delivering effective chronic disease care by integrating prevention, mental health support, and sustained follow-up within a team-based structure [24].

Kern et al. further demonstrates that the benefits of PCMH might not always be visible, but the long-term evidence suggests gains in efficiency. This study analyzed 5 years of data from practices in New York that had implemented PCMH models and compared them with standard practices that used EHRs and paper records. Initially, from 2008 to 2011, it seemed as if the quality of care appeared to be similar between these two groups. However, by 2012, there was a noticeable difference between PCMH and non-PCMH practices in hospitalizations in the PCMH group. This emphasizes that although PCMH transformation may be gradual, in the long term, the model can reduce reliance on costly acute care services, reflecting better continuity, care coordination, and proactive management of health conditions [25].

Finally, the PCMH has proven to address inequities in care, especially for populations with limited resources that have difficulty accessing preventive care and rely heavily on emergency departments. The study by Van den Berk-Clark et al. was a systematic review and meta-analysis of 33 studies examining PCMHs in low-income settings. They found that PCMH interventions consistently improved clinical outcomes and treatment adherence and reduced emergency department utilization. The study's results suggest that PCMH interventions are particularly valuable for economically disadvantaged patients who have less access to coordinated care and are more affected by chronic diseases. The study did note that there were limitations that did not address confounding variables. However, with the consistency of the positive effects of PCMHs in diverse contexts, there is good evidence for the benefits they provide in patient care [26].

These studies together illustrate the multi-dimensional benefits of the PCMH framework. There is evidence that PCMHs improve biomedical, mental health, and quality of life outcomes [24]. There is also evidence that the long-term implementation of PCMHs improves outcomes by reducing hospitalizations and system-wide efficiencies [25]. Lastly, PCMHs can even reduce healthcare access and outcome disparities for low-income populations, only adding to the benefit that PCMHs can provide for general care [26].

It is critical to recognize that relationships, continuity, and proactive management are as important as access alone. PCMHs are a longitudinal intervention that encompasses the goals of primary care, such as patient-centered care, preventive care, chronic disease management, and equity for underserved populations. However, their success depends on sustained commitment, including building infrastructure, aligning payment incentives, and investing in the workforce needed to deliver comprehensive, relationship-centered care. The PCMH is a critical model for revitalizing the foundation of the healthcare system. While PCMHs set the structure, many patients still need more time, education and peer support. These needs can be addressed through group visits and self-management programs.

Group Visits and Chronic Disease Self-Management

Diabetes, hypertension, and heart failure are just some examples of chronic diseases that account for a significant part of healthcare costs, morbidity, and mortality worldwide. Long-term conditions have been hard for patients to manage due to primary care lacking the support that patients need to manage these conditions, such as education or longitudinal care rather than brief one-on-one appointments. Group medical visits (GMVs) and other self-management programs are recent innovations in primary care. These visits group patients with similar conditions together and encourage them to take a more active role in their care. This innovation emphasizes health literacy, peer-to-peer support, and improved clinical outcomes.

Group visits typically involve 8–20 patients who meet with one or more physicians for sessions that include not only individualized medical assessments but also patient health education and teaching. During these sessions, physicians provide information to patients about disease processes, treatment options, lifestyle modification, and self-monitoring skills. The session provides a group dynamic that encourages patients to share their challenges, ask questions, build a community, and establish accountability.

Cunningham et al. systematically reviewed randomized controlled trials that compared group medical care to individual care. This study mainly focused on pregnancy, diabetes, and other chronic health conditions. Group visits improve patient experiences, outcomes, and costs for many different health conditions. There was a consistent improvement in patient knowledge and satisfaction with care, while also reducing emergency department hospitalizations in some populations. The results of the different studies reviewed varied, but all found that group visits did not result in worse clinical outcomes than usual care, suggesting that they could be used as a beneficial addition to traditional general care models [27].

One of the strongest arguments for the implementation of group visits appears when discussing underserved populations, where the need for continuity of care and health literacy is most pronounced. Korenhof et al. conducted a prospective cohort study targeting adults with chronic conditions and their caregivers with low socioeconomic status. These participants were enrolled in a 6-week community-based Chronic Disease Self-Management Program (CDSMP) and reported their outcomes in a self-administered questionnaire at a 6-month follow-up. The reported improvements included improvements in confidence, self-management skills, and perceived social support. This is particularly significant in emphasizing that CDSMPs can increase engagement and empowerment, even among patients who usually face challenges in getting the care they need [28].

Group visits improve patient outcomes through three main mechanisms. First, they provide extended time for education and building of the patient–physician relationship, which is often difficult in normal, quick primary care visits. With this, patients gain a better understanding of their condition and become more directly involved in their care. Second, there is a development of community and support when patients see others facing similar struggles and can share their strategies for management. The stigma surrounding chronic diseases is also reduced through group visits. Finally, group visits support a holistic care experience for patients, with interdisciplinary care that includes nurses and dietitians.

There are also challenges that come with implementation of group visits. Many patients may be uncomfortable sharing their personal health information in a group setting, and people may not be able to participate in these visits fully. Other barriers may include insufficient physicians trained in group facilitation sessions, staffing shortages, and scheduling complications that come with trying to coordinate large groups. Additionally, the research demonstrates that there is difficulty in assessing outcomes based on the conditions being addressed. Group visits improve patient empowerment and healthcare experience, but their ability to improve hard clinical outcomes is not well measured. Studies currently only suggest some improvement or no difference compared to individual visits.

Group visits and chronic disease self-management programs combine medical management with education and peer support to allow patients to take a more active role in managing their health care. There was a clear improvement in patient knowledge and satisfaction with this implementation, as well as a reduction in emergency and hospital visits. These visits particularly benefit underserved populations, as they provide patients with increased access to medical care in a more supportive environment. However, the implementation of group visits and chronic disease self-management programs in primary care will require adequate training for facilitators and reinforcement of patient comfort. With the recent shift in healthcare that focuses on the patient experience, group visits are a good addition that offers a patient-centered method for managing chronic diseases and addressing overall patient health concerns. To move from promising pilots to routine practice, innovations require sustainment strategies, such as measurement, leadership, payment alignment, workforce development, and infrastructure.

Sustaining Innovation and Improving Access

With innovation in general practice, there is a need for not only successful implementation but also the sustainment of these innovations in the long term. Although there are many promising innovations, such as PCMHs and group visits, their long-term success depends on continuous investment in quality improvement, supportive leadership, and alignment with broader health policies. This can be achieved by ensuring that innovations are adaptable, scalable, and relevant to all diverse populations.

Several continuous quality improvement (CQI) frameworks can ensure that innovations continue to serve their purpose of benefiting patient care in general practice. There are different methods to CQI, including frameworks such as Plan-Do-Study-Act (PDSA) cycles that help with keeping innovations in check by monitoring outcomes, refining processes, and testing the innervations appropriately. The Agency for Healthcare Research and Quality (AHRQ) emphasizes that CQI is most effective when integrated into an interdisciplinary team, organized system, and appropriate leadership [29]. As discussed previously, Kern et al. demonstrated in their study that the reductions in hospitalizations resulting from PCMHs only emerged in long-term assessments [25]. With CQI, innovations can persist through the potential risks that come with implementing long-term changes.

Strong leadership support is as important as CQI for innovations in general practice. Leaders who can advocate for and prioritize changes can acquire more resources and compliance from other staff. When leaders view innovation as part of their mission, the organization is more likely to embrace new models of care. Additionally, leaders promote structured communication and fair division of work and accountability, which is clearly demonstrated as an important factor of effectiveness in the study of same-day access clinics by Forman et al. [22]. Leadership is important for innovation, as it is viewed as an opportunity rather than burdens.

Finances are also an essential factor to consider when sustaining innovation. Value-based care models that reward prevention and equity are essential for practices to adopt innovations that improve outcomes rather than increase visit volume and ensure long-term sustainment. Etz et al. stated that innovations must be embedded in systems of accountability and enabling policies to be sustained. It emphasizes the alignment of small clinic changes with broader system policies, such as quality metrics [30]. Furthermore, Van den Berk-Clark et al. highlighted that adequate resources and reimbursement were critical for reaching low-income patients with PCMHs [26]. Sustained innovation depends on finances that align with broader system incentives and recognize the long-term cost savings of these new ways of care.

Workforce development plays a role in innovation by ensuring its replicability and scalability. Physicians and staff involved in these innovations need to adopt new skills in areas such as cultural competence, effective interdisciplinary communication, and patient engagement, which are required for the expansion of innovations beyond traditional general practice. Yano et al. highlighted the significance of training and mentorship for the VA staff to adapt to the PCMH's patient-centered approach [31]. Similarly, Etz et al. argued that capacity-building strategies that prepare physicians and staff to learn and improve their skills to respond to these new innovations are factors on which sustainment will depend [30]. Workforce development is a key player in sustaining innovations and ensuring that the staff in practice feel prepared and supported.

Innovations that go beyond traditional visits can only be scaled and adapted through infrastructure. Infrastructure includes EHRs, data systems, and telehealth platforms, but also extends to the redistribution of tasks among staff or figuring out locations for visits, such as group visits. Frikha et al. highlighted that co-located team-based care models depended on more than just physical proximity but needed infrastructure that enabled real-time communication and coordination and efficient workflows. The study also demonstrated the importance of role clarity, structured team meetings, and organizational support in the effectiveness of clinics, which further characterizes infrastructure as both a technological and cultural resource. Etz et al. also highlights the role of infrastructures by arguing that innovation is rarely sustained when left to individual practices. Instead, infrastructures of support, such as standardized performance metrics, peer learning networks, and policy frameworks, help embed innovations into existing care. Especially for long-term care, infrastructure is key in fostering accountability, shared learning, and adaptation over time [30]. Infrastructure plays a major role in allowing innovations to persist and thrive across diverse contexts.

Finally, innovations should address barriers faced by underserved communities, some of which may include lack of transportation, insurance, and technology access. Innovations should support these populations rather than exacerbate their problems. A good example of this is Korenhof et al.'s study of community-based group interventions that improved the management of medical problems among underserved patients. This demonstrates that innovations can be equity-focused and benefit overall healthcare equity in general practice [28]. The benefits of innovations should aim to reach all populations, including those that are marginalized, and equity should be the central idea for design and implementation.

Sustaining innovation in general practice requires many different elements to ensure that the benefits of these changes are consistent for all patients. With all these components, innovations can change primary care into a patient-centered system that is capable of delivering higher-quality care. These system levers succeed when clinical leaders support them. Therefore, we conclude with the broader role of general practitioners in driving system-wide changes and accountability.

Role of General Practitioners in System-Wide Change

The role of general practitioners continues to change and adapt over time, but they continue to sit at the heart of modern health systems. General practitioners have a unique position that allows them to be physicians, educators, innovators, leaders, and advocates. Their role in being responsible for a wide scope of practice, continuity of care, and connecting to the community makes general practitioners essential to system-wide changes in health systems.

Schäfer et al. argue that general practitioners bridge the physical, mental and social aspects of health because they are able to provide long-term patient-centered care unlike specialists who focus on certain organ systems. The broad scope of general practitioners allows them to recognize more areas for improvement in the healthcare system and create solutions to these gaps [32]. General practices are not only the patient's first point of contact but also the first point of contact for new explorations and innovations in health care. Stange et al. expanded on this by highlighting general practice as a critical factor in population health. They discuss the "primary care paradox" in which health systems have better population outcomes, improved equity, and lower costs if they provide more primary care. These benefits, which are seen as a part of the "primary care paradox", are due to the distinctive role of general practitioners as broad-scope, life-long providers [33]. General practitioners heavily influence population health improvements through their positions in the integration of health, innovation, and community.

However, once again, equity is emphasized with the discussion of innovations in general practice. Eissa et al. reviewed the National Academies of Sciences, Engineering, and Medicine (NASEM) 2021 report and argued that the impact on underserved communities needs to be considered when implementing innovations in general practice, such as workforce training and redesigned payment systems [34]. General practitioners are in the ideal role to integrate and advocate for innovations that benefit marginalized groups and prioritize equity. As witnesses to the consequences of inequity, they have the responsibility and insight to ensure that innovations address equity along with efficiency.

The role of general practitioners in system-wide change goes further to address effective and efficient data collection during these changes. Jones et al. stressed that implementing high-quality care requires collection of data on factors such as patient experience, equity outcomes, access and continuity of care. Therefore, in general practice, there should be methods for engaging in data evaluation and transparency in data reporting. This provides evidence that innovation is beneficial and helps policymakers and physicians identify which strategies work and under what circumstances [35].

From all these perspectives, there is a consistent theme that general practitioners are a valuable part of advocacy and care. They can use their close connection to the community and their patients to influence policies that will promote valuable funding, workforce distribution, and health equity. General practice is a setting that allows the piloting and adaptation of new models that can later be scaled across other health systems. In all its different roles, general practice bridges the connection between healthcare workers, patients, advancements in medicine, and the community.

Conclusion

Primary care advances most effectively when innovations function as integrated systems rather than isolated initiatives. Digital tools, including electronic health records, telehealth platforms, remote monitoring technologies, and patient portals, extend care beyond traditional office visits and enable timely data-informed clinical action. Interprofessional teams translate these capabilities into coordinated, person-centered care that addresses physical, behavioral, and social needs in a unified way. Access strategies, such as same-day scheduling paired with team continuity, enhance responsiveness while preserving trusted and therapeutic relationships. Organizational models, such as patient-centered care structures, provide the foundation for population health management and planned care, whereas group visits and self-management programs enhance patient engagement, health literacy, and peer support. Sustained impact depends on continuous quality improvement, payment models aligned with team-based care, workforce development and interoperable information systems that support seamless communication.

This integrated approach represents a deliberate shift from episodic, clinician-centered encounters to continuous, patient-centered, efficient, and equity-focused primary care. Access expands through multiple coordinated channels; quality improves as teams close preventive and chronic care gaps; outcomes improve through proactive monitoring and early intervention; and equity deepens through language access, culturally responsive communication, and reliable connections to community resources.

References

1. Centers for Disease Control and Prevention. About chronic diseases. CDC. Updated July 3, 2023. Accessed 19 Aug 2025. https://www.cdc.gov/chronic-disease/about/index.htm.
2. Garg A, Boynton-Jarrett R, Dworkin PH. Avoiding the unintended consequences of screening for social determinants of health. JAMA. 2016;316(8):813–4. https://doi.org/10.1001/jama.2016.9282.
3. Shanafelt TD, Noseworthy JH. Executive leadership and physician well-being: nine organizational strategies to promote engagement and reduce burnout. Mayo Clin Proc. 2017;92(1):129–46. https://doi.org/10.1016/j.mayocp.2016.10.004.
4. Reed M, Huang J, Graetz I, et al. Treatment and follow-up care associated with patient-initiated telemedicine visits for acute primary care illnesses. JAMA Netw Open. 2021;4(12):e2138719. Available at: https://jamanetwork.com/journals/jamanetworkopen/fullarticle/2786184.
5. Mohammed HT, Hyseni L, Bui V, et al. Exploring the use and challenges of implementing virtual visits during COVID-19 in primary care and lessons for sustained use. PLoS

One. 2021;16(6):e0253665. https://pmc.ncbi.nlm.nih.gov/articles/PMC8224904/. PMCID: PMC8224904.

6. Hammersley V, Parker R, Paterson M, et al. Telemonitoring at scale for hypertension in primary care: an implementation study. PLoS Med. 2020;17(7):e1003137. https://pmc.ncbi.nlm.nih.gov/articles/PMC7299318/. PMCID: PMC7299318.
7. Hailu R, Sousa J, Tang M, Mehrotra A, Uscher-Pines L. Challenges and facilitators in implementing remote patient monitoring programs in primary care. J Gen Intern Med. 2024;39(13):2471–7. https://pmc.ncbi.nlm.nih.gov/articles/PMC11436674/. PMCID: PMC11436674.
8. O'Malley AS, Draper K, Gourevitch R, Cross DA, Scholle SH. Electronic health records and support for primary care teamwork. J Am Med Inform Assoc. 2015;22(2):426–34. https://pmc.ncbi.nlm.nih.gov/articles/PMC4394968/. PMCID: PMC4394968.
9. Rotenstein LS, Adrashi A, Balageorge GB, et al. Association between electronic health record time and quality of care metrics in primary care. JAMA Netw Open. 2022;5(10):e2237086. Available at: https://jamanetwork.com/journals/jamanetworkopen/fullarticle/2797453.
10. Sutton RT, Pincock D, Baumgart DC, et al. An overview of clinical decision support systems: benefits, risks, and strategies for success. J Eval Clin Pract. 2020;26(1):40–9. https://onlinelibrary.wiley.com/doi/10.1111/jep.12535
11. Khunti K, Zaccardi F, van Marwijk H, et al. Primary care medication safety surveillance with integrated primary and secondary care electronic health records: a cross-sectional study. Drug Saf. 2015;38(7):689–703. https://pmc.ncbi.nlm.nih.gov/articles/PMC4486763/. PMCID: PMC4486763.
12. Alexander GC, Tajanlangit M, Heyward J, Mansour O, Qato DM, Stafford RS. Use and content of primary care office-based vs telemedicine care visits during the COVID-19 pandemic in the US. JAMA Netw Open. 2020;3(10):e2021476. https://pmc.ncbi.nlm.nih.gov/articles/PMC7532385/. PMCID: PMC7532385.
13. Cohen DJ, et al. Integrating behavioral health and primary care: consulting, coordinating and collaborating among professionals. J Am Board Fam Med. 2015;28(Suppl 1):S21–31. PMCID: PMC7304937.
14. Wan S, Teichman PG, Latif D, et al. Healthcare provider perceptions of the role of interprofessional care in access to and outcomes of primary care in an underserved area. J Interprof Care. 2018;32(2):220–3. PMCID: PMC6368170.
15. Anderson E, Solch AK, Fincke BG, et al. Concerns of primary care clinicians practicing in an integrated health system: a qualitative study. J Gen Intern Med. 2020;35(11):3218–26. PMCID: PMC7661604.
16. Fortin Y, Foisy A, Cauchy C, et al. Transformation of primary care settings implementing a co-located teambased care model: a scoping review. BMC Health Serv Res. 2024;24(1):890. PMCID: PMC11299417.
17. Asarnow JR, Rozenman M, Wiblin J, Zeltzer L. Integrated medical-behavioral care compared with usual primary care for child and adolescent behavioral health: a meta-analysis. JAMA Pediatr. 2015;169(10):929–37. (Article ID 2422331).
18. AbuGhada R, et al. Integrating social care into healthcare: a review on applying the social determinants of health in clinical settings. Healthcare (Basel). 2023;11(20):2771. PMCID: PMC10573056.
19. Fraze TK, Beidler LB, Fichtenberg C, Brewster AL, Gottlieb LM. Resource brokering: efforts to assist patients with housing, transportation, and economic needs in primary care settings. Ann Fam Med. 2021;19(6):507–14. PMCID: PMC8575510
20. Kim J, Pacino V, Wang H, et al. System redesign: the value of a primary care liaison model to address unmet social needs among older primary care patients. Int J Environ Res Public Health. 2021;18(21):11135. PMCID: PMC8582881.
21. Hsu C, Cruz S, Placzek H, et al. Patient perspectives on addressing social needs in primary care using a screening and resource referral intervention. J Gen Intern Med. 2020;35(2):481–9. PMCID: PMC7018904.

22. Forman JH, Robinson CH, Krein SL. Striving toward team-based continuity: provision of same-day access and continuity in academic primary care clinics. BMC Health Serv Res. 2019;19(1):145.
23. Burch P, Whittaker W, Lau Y-S. Relationship between the volume and type of appointments in general practice and patient experience: an observational study in England. Br J Gen Pract. 2025;75(754):e375–81. https://doi.org/10.3399/BJGP.2024.0276.
24. John JR, Jani H, Peters K, Agho K, Tannous WK. The effectiveness of patient-centred medical home-based models of care versus standard primary care in chronic disease management: a systematic review and meta-analysis of randomised and non-randomised controlled trials. Int J Environ Res Public Health. 2020;17(18):6886.
25. Kern LM, Edwards A, Kaushal R. The patient-centered medical home and associations with health care quality and utilization: a 5-year cohort study. Ann Intern Med. 2016;164(6):395–405.
26. van den Berk-Clark C, Doucette E, Rottnek F, Hughes R, Manard W, Lawrence T, et al. Do patient-centered medical homes improve health behaviors, outcomes and experiences of low income patients? A systematic review and meta-analysis. Health Serv Res. 2018;53(3):1777–98.
27. Cunningham SD, Sutherland RA, Yee CW, Bohnenkamp JH, Thomas JD, Lewis JB, et al. Group medical care: a systematic review of health service performance. Int J Environ Res Public Health. 2021;18(23):12726.
28. Korenhof SA, Rouwet EV, Elstgeest LEM, van Halteren AR, Robben SHM, Schers HJ, et al. The effect of a community-based group intervention on chronic disease self-management in a vulnerable population. Front Public Health. 2023;11:1221675.
29. Agency for Healthcare Research and Quality (AHRQ). Continuous quality improvement (CQI) strategies to optimize your practice. In: Primary care practice facilitation curriculum [Internet]. Rockville: Agency for Healthcare Research and Quality (US); 2013. [cited 2025 Feb 6]. Available from: https://www.ncbi.nlm.nih.gov/books/NBK599556/.
30. Etz RS, Zyzanski SJ, Sweeney SA, Stange KC. Sustaining innovation in health care delivery: a framework for implementation and scale-up. Ann Fam Med. 2025;23(1):16–23.
31. Yano EM, Maciejewski ML, Klein S, Barker A, Chapman B, Hastings SN, et al. Primary care transformation: a qualitative study of implementation of the patient-centered medical home in the Veterans Health Administration. J Gen Intern Med. 2022;37(8):1958–68.
32. Schäfer WLA, van den Berg MJ, Groenewegen PP. The role of general practice in complex health care systems. BMC Prim Care. 2023;24(1):16.
33. Stange KC, Miller WL, Etz RS. The role of primary Care in Improving Population Health. Milbank Q. 2023;101(S1):795–840.
34. Eissa A, Rowe R, Pinto AD, Okoli GN, Campbell KM, Washington JC, et al. Implementing high-quality primary care through a health equity lens. Ann Fam Med. 2022;20(2):164–9.
35. Jones C, Westfall JM, Stange KC, Parchman ML, Liaw W, Etz RS. Measuring implementation of high-quality primary care: a roadmap for improvement. Ann Fam Med. 2023;21(6):520–6.

Introduction to Telehealth in Psychological Services

Lowell Bouchard, Anna Nungester, Farzana Zafreen, and Summer S. Chahin

The Emergence of Telehealth

Telehealth, is a broad term used to capture the use of telecommunication technologies to deliver health-related services across distances [1]. Over time telehealth has transformed from a peripheral innovation into a central component of modern healthcare delivery [2]. Within psychology, this modality is commonly referred to as telepsychology and encompasses remote assessment, intervention, consultation, and supervision, which is delivered through digital technologies such as telephone and videoconferencing [3, 4]. These services encompass a wide range of activities, including but not limited to clinical care (e.g., psychological and neuropsychological assessments, interventions, and treatments), professional collaboration (e.g., consultations, supervision, and communication), as well as education, training, and research [2, 4]. However, terms describing these services are not well agreed upon. A systematic review identified at least 14 different terms used to describe behavioral health service adaptations during COVID-19 (i.e., telehealth, telemedicine, telemental health, telepsychiatry, teletherapy, telebehavioral health, telepsychology, virtual delivery, videoconferencing psychotherapy, telephone-based psychotherapy, teleconsultation, video telehealth, digital health, unguided mental health program) underscoring the need for clearer definitions and standardized language [5]. Throughout this chapter, we will use the terms telehealth and telepsychology interchangeably to refer to psychological services offered through virtual means due to

L. Bouchard · A. Nungester · F. Zafreen
Western Michigan University, Kalamazoo, MI, USA
e-mail: lowell.bouchard@wmed.edu

S. S. Chahin (✉)
Western Michigan University Homer Stryker M.D. School of Medicine, Kalamazoo, MI, USA
e-mail: Summer.chahin@wmed.edu

S. S. Chahin et al. (eds.), *Innovation in Medical Education and Clinical Practice*, https://doi.org/10.1007/978-3-032-19116-8_19

considerable research using both interchangeably, inconsistency with term usage, and to offer clarity as well as ease of reading.

The historical trajectory of telehealth demonstrates recurrent cycles of experimentation, decline, and resurgence. Its integration into psychological care has unfolded in several distinct waves. From 1950s to the 1970s, early initiatives such as the University of Nebraska's use of closed-circuit television to deliver psychiatric consultations across hospitals illustrated the potential utility of remote care, but high costs and infrastructure limitations curtailed widespread adoption [2, 6]. During the 1980s, interest was renewed in military and correctional institutions, where telehealth reduced transportation costs and improved access to specialized services [2]. By the 1990s, national telecommunications initiatives such as federally funded demonstration projects and statewide telemedicine networks expanded the feasibility of remote care by reducing infrastructure barriers and legitimizing telehealth within healthcare policy [2]. At the same time, the rise of the internet and advances in video conferencing standards provided the technological backbone for scalable and affordable service delivery [7]. In the 2000s–2010s, advances in digital and internet-based videoconferencing standards and platforms facilitated broader integration of remote services [7]. The 2020s marked a decisive turning point, as the COVID-19 pandemic transformed telepsychology into a primary mode of service delivery. In this way, the COVID-19 pandemic acted as a decisive catalyst for telepsychology use and application. As telehealth evolved the questions shifted from feasibility to fairness and fit. The focus now turns to who can equitably access high-quality telepsychology, under what conditions it works best, and where barriers and risks remain.

Equity considerations are particularly important, as broadband access, digital literacy, and socioeconomic status strongly shape who can equitably benefit from telehealth. Research shows that telemedicine improves access and outcomes more broadly across patient populations [8]. The current literature highlights key advantages of telepsychology including expanded access for underserved and stigmatized populations, enhanced convenience, and continuity of care during crises, while accumulating evidence further supports its efficacy across diverse groups, including veterans, individuals facing geographic barriers, and other underserved populations [3, 9–12]. At the same time, challenges remain. These include challenges establishing rapport and inequities tied to technological literacy, device and internet access, and dependence on others to facilitate telehealth visits [13]. It is important to also highlight the differences among mental health professions (e.g., psychiatry, psychology, nursing, and social work) in how they engage with telehealth which can further complicate implementation, revealing systemic hierarchies and power dynamics that influence adoption [12]. Additionally, significant gaps remain in addressing long-term outcomes beyond cross-professional differences in implementation such as the adequacy of regulatory protections [12, 14]. Looking ahead, the evolving field of digital mental health, including smartphone apps, virtual reality, and artificial intelligence, offers new opportunities for integration into hybrid models of care, though concerns about evidence, engagement, and equity remain central [15].

Efficacy of Telepsychology Versus In-Person Psychotherapy

A substantial body of research supports the clinical efficacy of telepsychology compared to in-person psychotherapy across diverse conditions, populations, and treatment settings. In a comprehensive meta-analysis, Batastini and colleagues [16] examined 57 empirical studies of videoconferencing technologies (VCTs) and found that mental and behavioral health interventions delivered remotely produced treatment effects largely equivalent to those delivered face-to-face across 281 individual outcomes and 4336 clients. This suggests that videoconferencing represents a viable and effective treatment for mental health services. This efficacy appears to carry over to specific symptom reduction. Berryhill and colleagues [17] conducted a systematic review of 33 studies on videoconferencing psychotherapy (VCP) for depression, finding significant symptom reductions with effect sizes ranging from medium to large. Similarly, Giovanetti and colleagues [18] found no significant differences in depressive symptom reduction between teletherapy and in-person psychotherapy across randomized controlled trials. Beyond symptom reduction and treatment equivalence, researchers have also examined the therapeutic alliance (i.e., the collaborative and affective bond between client and therapist), which is widely recognized as a key determinant of treatment success) [19]. Davis and colleagues [20] used a non-inferiority design with matched clinical samples and demonstrated that both therapeutic alliance and symptom outcomes in teletherapy were statistically non-inferior to those observed in in-person psychotherapy.

For youth and young-adult populations, Lehtimäki et al. [21] synthesized 18 systematic reviews and meta-analyses and concluded that computerized cognitive-behavioral therapy (cCBT) shows the strongest and most consistent evidence for reducing anxiety and depression among individuals aged 10–24 years, with small-to-moderate pooled effects relative to nonactive controls. Similarly, Şahin and colleagues [22] demonstrated that telemedicine interventions yield significant improvements in mental health outcomes among older adults. These findings offer support for telepsychology's utility across age groups. Overall, evidence indicates that telepsychology achieves comparable clinical outcomes to in-person psychotherapy, with effectiveness influenced by contextual factors such as modality, population, and infrastructure, supporting its viability as an effective modality for delivering mental health care across diverse populations and treatment contexts [16, 19–26].

The Role of COVID-19

The COVID-19 pandemic has served as a critical turning point in the widespread adoption of telehealth, particularly in mental and behavioral health care. With the need for social distancing and lockdowns, telehealth became the primary means of delivering mental health services, and this shift resulted in several key findings.

Rapid Pivot to Telehealth During the Pandemic

The COVID-19 pandemic showcased a rapid pivot to telehealth across healthcare domains, including mental health. Researchers emphasize that the pandemic "redefined the delivery of healthcare" by accelerating adoption of telehealth in aging care, demonstrating both feasibility and patient acceptance but also underscoring persistent challenges related to digital literacy and equity [27]. Arafat and colleagues [28] reported that telemedicine interventions during the pandemic significantly improved mental health outcomes. Others provide empirical evidence of this shift in the context of a university counseling center, where a sudden transition from in-person to videoconference therapy created a natural experiment [20]. Their findings demonstrated that teletherapy was noninferior to in-person psychotherapy with respect to therapeutic alliance and outcomes, suggesting that the rapid pivot did not compromise quality of care [20].

Temporary Regulatory Changes and Licensure Flexibility

During the pandemic, many U.S. state licensing boards relaxed licensure requirements for telehealth, allowing providers to practice across state lines [21, 23]. This temporary regulatory flexibility made it possible to maintain access to mental health care despite geographical restrictions [21, 23]. Researchers highlight system- and policy-level barriers such as affordability, accessibility, and security that influence telehealth adoption, calling for structural reforms to support equitable access in aging care [27]. Similarly, others review pre-pandemic policy activity, including proposed Centers for Medicare and Medicaid Services rules and state-level initiatives, noting that policy changes were key to enabling broader telehealth implementation [25]. Others situate their counseling center's shift to teletherapy within broader operational challenges but do not focus on licensure or regulatory specifics [20]. Policy support is recognized as critical and directly facilitated the rapid scaling of telehealth during COVID-19.

Surge in Demand for Mental Health Services

As the pandemic took its toll on mental health, there was a large increase in demand for mental health services, with telehealth being the primary modality [25]. This surge highlighted the need for scalable mental health interventions, which telehealth is uniquely positioned to offer. Some situate their noninferiority study within the broader mental health crisis facing college students during the pandemic, noting that the sharp rise in service demand made the adoption of teletherapy both necessary for infection control and critical for meeting increased need [20].

Growth of Telehealth and Digital Mental Health Tools Post-Pandemic

Across the literature, there is consensus that telehealth has grown substantially and will remain a durable feature of healthcare delivery. Some researchers document steady pre-pandemic growth in evidence for telemental health and telerehabilitation, noting that outcomes were often equivalent to in-person care [25]. Others further emphasize that the pandemic normalized the use of videoconference therapy and broadened acceptance of digital mental health tools among both providers and clients [20]. They note that clinician attitudes toward teletherapy became more favorable after widespread exposure during COVID-19, while clients valued its flexibility and convenience.

Advantages and Limitations of Telepsychology

The literature on telepsychology underscores both significant advantages and limitations that shape its role within contemporary mental health care. On one hand, research highlights the potential of virtual modalities to expand access, enhance convenience, reduce stigma, and ensure continuity of services across diverse populations and settings. On the other, persistent challenges remain, including technological barriers, inequities in access, concerns about privacy and data security, and questions regarding clinical suitability. Therefore, telepsychology should not be viewed as a wholesale substitute for traditional therapy, but rather as a complementary model whose effectiveness depends on thoughtful integration within broader systems of care. Its success ultimately rests on attention to contextual, ethical, and cultural factors.

Advantages

Increased Accessibility and Flexibility

Telepsychology reduces traditional barriers to care, making services available to rural, disabled, and marginalized populations. Systematic reviews emphasize how telehealth can improve access to care and potentially mitigate geographic inequities, particularly in non-urban and underserved settings [23, 29, 30]. Additionally, telepsychology expands the reach of providers, enabling them to serve clients across broader regions. This capacity is particularly valuable in areas with shortages of mental health professionals or specialized expertise. Reviews emphasize that cross-regional service delivery is one of telehealth's defining advantages, broadening the impact of psychological services and extending care to previously underserved populations [29, 30]. Another advantage of telehealth is the flexibility it offers to both clients and providers. Flexible telepsychological models allow clinicians to deliver timely, coordinated interventions while reducing barriers such as travel burdens [23]. These features contribute to greater acceptance for telepsychology for clients who perceive it as useful, accessible, and convenient [31]. In a comprehensive meta-analysis, Abuyadek and colleagues [32] reported pooled acceptability rates of 71% among tele-mental health users and 66% among providers, with usability significantly higher among patients. This highlights that telehealth is broadly well-received and feasible, with higher acceptance rates from clients compared to providers. This may be partly attributed to the alleviation of burdens that telehealth provides. In a scoping review of 29 systematic reviews, Zhang et al. [27] examined the benefits of telehealth in aging care and found that telehealth can remove geographic and time barriers and extends care from hospitals to home and community settings, thereby improving access for socially isolated or physically homebound older adults. Moreover, telehealth maintained comparable clinical outcomes, symptom reduction, and self-reported quality-of-life improvements to in person care during the COVID-19 pandemic [20, 26].

Reduced Stigma

Beyond accessibility and convenience, one of telepsychology's most meaningful advantages lies in its potential to reduce the stigma often associated with seeking mental health care in person [15, 33–35]. Stigma has been found to reduce the therapeutic alliance, which is an important element in the therapeutic process [36]. Research suggests that a strong therapeutic alliance can be successfully established in text-based digital psychotherapy and that this alliance positively influences treatment outcomes [37]. Moreover, telepsychology may reduce key stigma-related barriers to help-seeking, particularly those tied to disclosure fears, shame, and social identity threats, by providing a form of care that allows individuals to seek support without the public visibility or labeling often attached to in-person services [38]. By allowing clients to engage in therapy from the privacy of their own homes, teletherapy offers a sense of safety and discretion that can make help-seeking more approachable for many individuals. These privacy and accessibility benefits may be especially important in smaller or tightly knit communities, where cultural responsiveness and adaptation are essential to address stigma and ensure equitable engagement [39, 40].

Cost-Effectiveness

Telehealth helps reduce costs associated with traditional therapy, such as travel and lost wages [24]. This can make mental health services more accessible to individuals who might otherwise be unable to afford in-person care. Research suggests that telehealth services can expand access to care and alleviate financial strain for patients. However, the evidence base for cost-effectiveness in telepsychology is still emerging. Findings from broader telehealth research suggest that while remote interventions can reduce individual costs, such as travel and time away from work, the evidence remains limited in scope and rigor [27]. Research suggests that telepsychology and other digital mental health approaches are clinically effective and potentially cost-efficient and generally cost-effective, especially when used in integrated or stepped-care systems that rely on lower-cost tools like phone, email, or text-based services, but economic research is lagging behind [23, 41].

Limitations

Technology as a Barrier

Despite its many advantages, telepsychology continues to face significant technological barriers that limit equitable access and effectiveness. Access to appropriate devices, reliable internet connections, and basic digital literacy are among the most consistent obstacles to the widespread adoption of remote care. These challenges disproportionately affect individuals from lower socioeconomic backgrounds, rural areas, and marginalized communities, which may contribute to rather than reduce existing health disparities [29, 42]. Digital literacy and technological proficiency are particularly critical for effective telehealth participation. Wind and colleagues [11] note that both patients and mental health professionals often face steep learning curves when adopting digital platforms for therapy, which can slow engagement and hinder the broader implementation of these services. Similarly, limited digital literacy, and basic technology barriers (for example, bandwidth and device usability) often make it difficult for older adults to use telehealth, leading to resistance or dropout [27]. These barriers highlight that telepsychology's success depends not only on availability but also on the usability and accessibility of technology across populations.

Beyond access, the quality and stability of internet connections can directly affect clinical reliability and assessment outcomes. Shaver (2022) observed that poor connectivity and inconsistent audiovisual quality may compromise the accuracy of neurocognitive testing and the flow of therapy sessions. Such technical disruptions may erode trust in the therapeutic process, particularly when combined with concerns about data privacy and confidentiality. Clients frequently express worries about being overheard in shared living spaces, while clinicians face the added responsibility of maintaining secure communication channels and data management practices [30, 31]. Research also suggests that the impact of these technological barriers varies across settings and is of particular concern to providers. For example, while university students reported few access-related difficulties and valued the convenience of virtual sessions, providers remained concerned about technological reliability and confidentiality [20].

Privacy Concerns

Despite the security of most telehealth platforms, some patients may still worry about the confidentiality of their sessions. Concerns may arise regarding the security of video calls, the potential for technical disruptions, or the risk of their personal information being exposed, which is particularly relevant for individuals living in shared spaces or using public internet access [25]. Confidentiality and security remain recurring concerns in telehealth implementation after the COVID-19 pandemic surge. Concerns about data security and privacy are consistently identified as key barriers to telehealth implementation and continued use. Patients have generally reported positive experiences with telemedicine, though some have expressed concerns about data security and privacy [25]. Reviews of telehealth in aging care identify privacy and data security as policy- and system-level concerns that influence whether older adults are willing to adopt and continue using telehealth [27]. Broader analyses likewise highlight that technical issues, distrust in telehealth systems, and concerns about data security and privacy remain among the most commonly reported barriers to telehealth use [42, 43]. Overall, ensuring confidentiality and robust data security appears to be a key challenge for the long-term sustainability of telehealth.

Specific Mental Health Concerns and Modalities

Across studies of depression, anxiety, and trauma-related disorders, telehealth-delivered cognitive-behavioral and exposure-based treatments produced significant symptom reductions with no consistent differences from face-to-face care [10, 17, 44]. However, research on suicidality and high-risk mental health conditions remains limited and mixed. Tenso et al. (2025) found that a higher proportion of virtual mental health visits was associated with a lower likelihood of suicide-related events. In contrast, Accorsi and colleagues [45] reported that evidence is insufficient to support full remote management for patients at high suicide risk and recommended immediate in-person evaluation, with continued remote monitoring and family involvement until care transfer is completed. Similarly, evidence for more complex interventions remains limited. Van Leeuwen et al. [46] reported that most tele-DBT (Dialectical Behavior Therapy) research focuses on feasibility and clinician/patient acceptability, not on controlled tests of clinical efficacy. They found little quantitative evidence that online or blended DBT can match standard, in-person DBT, especially for high-risk presentations (e.g., suicidality, borderline personality disorder), and concluded that switching videoconferencing or online training is not advised if face-to-face is an option [46]. Similarly, a review by Lehtimäki et al. [21] found that digital mental health interventions, particularly computerized CBT, can modestly reduce anxiety and depression in youth, but evidence for other formats remains weak. Most studies were small, methodologically limited, and conducted in high-income countries, leaving cost-effectiveness and generalizability unclear [21]. Overall, while telepsychology shows promise across common mental health conditions, current evidence remains uneven, with limited data for severe or complex presentations.

Cultural, Linguistic, and Equity Considerations

Linguistic and cultural considerations are fundamental to ensuring that telepsychology promotes equity rather than perpetuating existing disparities. Without intentional adaptation to clients' cultural contexts, digital mental health interventions risk reproducing inequities in both access and effectiveness. Structural barriers, such as limited broadband access, lack of culturally tailored content, and low digital literacy, disproportionately affect marginalized populations, including racial and ethnic minorities, immigrant and refugee communities, LGBTQ+ individuals, and those in rural or low-income areas [29, 32, 42, 47]. Tele-mental health is viewed as acceptable across diverse groups, including refugees and racial/ethnic minorities, and it can extend services across geographic and language boundaries; however, issues like privacy, safety, and usability still need to be addressed before broad implementation, especially for vulnerable populations [32]. Wang et al. [29] noted that cultural and linguistic barriers, including differences in traditional beliefs and mistrust of technology, limit telehealth's inclusiveness and highlight the need for culturally sensitive design and community-specific adaptation. Ethical responsiveness in virtual care thus must extend to include culturally congruent metaphors, relational dynamics, and collective values. Greenup and Best [48] emphasize that culturally attuned telepsychology integrates family and community participation and aligns therapeutic approaches with clients' cultural worldviews to promote trust and engagement.

Telepsychology may also amplify disparities when intersecting forms of marginalization (e.g., race, gender, sexual orientation, and socioeconomic status) are overlooked [39, 49]. For example, clients living in shared or unsupportive home environments may lack privacy during sessions, while culturally and linguistically diverse clients may experience telehealth platforms as impersonal or culturally detached [42]. Rural residents face additional barriers, including limited facilities, transportation challenges, and a shortage of culturally competent professionals [47, 50, 51]. Broadband access remains a pressing issue: 18% of individuals living on tribal lands lack broadband compared to 4% on non-tribal lands [52]. Even where the internet is available, cost and device limitations, especially among LatinX and Black communities who rely more on smartphones than home broadband, constrain access [53, 54]. Digital literacy further compounds disparities. Older adults and individuals with limited English proficiency may find online portals inaccessible, while varying insurance coverage and state licensure laws restrict service availability. For example, the Psychology Interjurisdictional Compact (PSYPACT) now allows licensed psychologists to provide telehealth across 43 states, reducing some regulatory barriers [55, 56].

Ethically, psychologists are bound by the APA principles of justice and respect for people's rights and dignity [57]. Inequitable care undermines these standards, especially when teletherapy platforms fail to ensure privacy, professionalism, or cost transparency [58]. Addressing these inequities requires a multi-level approach. At the system level, policies should support broadband expansion, linguistic access, and reimbursement for culturally adapted care [49, 52]. At the provider level, clinicians must receive training in culturally responsive telepractice, communication awareness, and ethical interpreter use [39, 59]. Internet-based training has been shown to improve therapists' transcultural competence [60]. Community-driven and participatory design models, engaging patients, advocacy groups, and local leaders, can help create linguistically and culturally tailored telehealth tools [29]. Efforts should also include patient-centered adaptations: for instance, integrating spirituality and community references in care for Native American patients [51], or using familiar media (e.g., WhatsApp, YouTube) to reach LatinX clients [54].

Unconscious bias also remains a significant concern in digital contexts. Studies reveal racial disparities in pain assessment and treatment decisions [51, 61, 62], underscoring the importance of culturally adapted assessment tools and continued provider education [59]. Expanding research, infrastructure, and funding, particularly for underrepresented groups, will be vital to achieving equity in telepsychology and preventing digital technologies from deepening existing divides [47, 50, 52, 54]. Telehealth has immense potential to bridge the gap in accessing healthcare services and improve health outcomes [40]. During the COVID-19 pandemic, the increased use of telehealth platforms provided an opportunity to view them as a tool to minimize the barriers to accessing care. Nevertheless, due to several obstacles, the feasibility of this reality is constricted [40]. Healthcare inequalities and disparities are well-established and thoroughly documented via numerous studies [47]. It is often accounted for based on geographical locations, such as between rural and urban areas, particularly in regions with underprivileged communities, including racial, ethnic, sexual, gender, and romantic minorities, the elderly population, and groups in lower socioeconomic levels [47].

Ethical and Legal Considerations

There are multiple ethical and legal issues to consider in teletherapy. The American Psychological Association (APA) has published ethical principles and a code of conduct for psychologists [57] and guidelines for the practice of telepsychology [4]. In terms of the practice of telepsychology, APA has provided 11 guidelines to ensure the dissemination of ethical, legal, and safe telepsychology practices that are evidence-based [4, 63]. These are the revised version of the eight guidelines published in 2013, and involve topics, such as competency of the psychologist (both content and technical competencies); informed consent; data security, management, and transmission; data disposal; documentation (both clinical and administrative documentation); interjurisdictional practice; clinical best practices; testing and assessment (for diverse populations and special practices); emergencies; supervision/training; and emerging technologies [4, 63]. Those who are credentialed with PSYPACT also have a requirement to complete CEs in ethics in telehealth/telepsychology practices. It is expected that telehealth practitioners will maintain the same ethical standards as those observed during in-person meetings, as asserted by the APA [64, 65].

Based on the guidelines, during telepsychology services, psychologists are required to operate within the scope of their professional education, training, and skills. They should provide a transparent and comprehensive explanation of the policies and processes of the technological service delivery. The informed consent should also include the unique risks or benefits, the cost of the service, and any limitations of the platform and services. Psychologists should be extremely cautious about data security, storage, management, and disposal. There can be multiple issues, such as computer malware, loss of hard drives, involvement of third-party services without proper data security, saving files in unsecured locations, etc., that can jeopardize the privacy and security of the service holder. Professionals should properly document services and always be aware of the laws and regulations of the state in which they and their patients are located. Moreover, mental health service providers should offer treatment and assessment services grounded in evidence-based standards. The guidelines also specify that psychologists should have safety plans in place for emergencies and undergo continuous training and supervision.

In 2025, APA published its proposed draft of the revised ethical principles and code of conduct of psychologists. It includes a new segment on technology. The proposed contents include ethical guidelines for psychologists regarding technological competencies, the use of technologies, confidentiality, privacy, security, transmission, and disposal of electronic data, as well as various social media and online platforms [66]. Once finalized and published, this will also serve as a guide for professionals to ensure ethical practices. Teletherapy or telepsychology is subject to HIPAA compliance. The Health Insurance Portability and Accountability ACT of 1996 (HIPAA) preserves individuals' electronic "protected health information (PHI)" and "personally identifiable information (PII)". Any violation of this act will lead to monetary penalties or criminal penalties, depending on the severity of the contravention [4, 67]. Furthermore, states may have their own laws and regulations to protect individuals' rights and privacy, which professionals should be aware of [67].

Privacy and confidentiality can be a significant concern in teletherapy, especially for LGBTQIA+ patients [50, 63, 68]. LGBTQIA+ patients may not have disclosed their identity to others. So, if confidentiality of the teletherapy session is not established, they may not feel safe to discuss sensitive information [68]. It is pivotal to obtain the patient's consent in the documentation process to avoid discrimination and stigma. Patients should be asked whether they approve or disapprove of medical documentation and disclosure of information related to their identities [69]. Some other ethical obligations are associated with insufficient evidence regarding the efficacy of teletherapy compared to face-to-face therapy in a varied range of symptoms [70]. Scholars have criticized its limitations in monitoring non-verbal behaviors, especially during assessments [71, 72]. The shortcomings of missing non-verbal cues, such as undetected subtle signs and bodily cues (e.g., fidgeting, poor hygiene, signs of intoxication), result in an incomplete assessment of psychological distress, leading to misdiagnosis or overlooking crucial information necessary for effective treatment [72, 73]. Multiple studies showed that telehealth psychological services are as effective as in-person sessions for various behavioral health conditions, such as depression and anxiety [26, 70, 74]. However, there is a lack of support for its effectiveness in reducing complex mental health issues, such as bipolar disorder and schizophrenia [70].

Implementation and Best Practices

Professionals providing telepsychology should abide by ethical guidelines, interstate laws, and HIPAA regulations to avoid legal and/or professional consequences. They should use user-friendly teletherapy apps that promote professionalism, transparency, fair costs, and continuous care for patients [58]. The unique set of skills needed for effective telehealth delivery involves both clinical competencies and technological proficiency. A consistent limitation in telehealth research is the inadequate preparation of mental health providers to deliver effective virtual care. Although telepsychology has become widespread since the COVID-19 pandemic, many clinicians report limited training in telehealth technology, remote communication, and online therapeutic methods. Fernández-Batanero et al. [75] found that teletherapy quality varies greatly with providers' technological competence and ability to engage clients virtually, while Mercadal Rotger and Cabré [76] observed lower therapeutic-alliance ratings online than in person. Marriott et al. [77] similarly noted that therapist confidence in trauma-focused telehealth relies on structured supervision and telehealth-specific training. More broadly, Gajarawala and Pelkowski [78] reported that telehealth adoption has outpaced clinician training, leading to gaps in confidence related to troubleshooting, privacy, and safety. Collectively, these findings underscore the need for standardized competencies and continuing education to strengthen both the technical and interpersonal skills required for effective digital care.

Graduate and postdoctoral programs should include a curriculum focused on telehealth-specific skill development, such as ethical guidelines for telehealth platforms, privacy limitations, managing technological constraints, and effective communication patterns. This curriculum should also encompass effective psychological assessments and treatments using teletherapy applications. Psychology programs should also involve proper supervision in telehealth contexts. Supervisors who will be providing supervision for teletherapy should collaboratively decide if they will engage in traditional in-person (face-to-face) supervision or tele-supervision. In addition to the general competencies required for supervising a trainee, the supervisor must be competent in telecommunication modality, privacy, laws, and specific guidelines related to ethical and best practices in telepsychology. Supervisors should discuss the particular challenges and requirements (e.g., longer screen time and self-care) necessary for effective telepsychology practice.

Government programs should be implemented that focus on training both clients and professionals in digital privacy, safety, and security. There needs to be federal and state-level policies placed targeting cybersecurity and privacy concerns regarding digital platforms [50]. Mental healthcare professionals should keep in mind that best practices may not fit everyone the same. For instance, privacy concerns may pose a significant issue for individuals from lower SES backgrounds who are living in overcrowded homes. To them, the telephone will be a more suitable option for telepsychology than utilizing video-conference platforms. This will create more flexibility, allowing them to move to a comparatively quiet and private space. Hence, the best practice will require considering unique factors involving the individual. Moreover, changing regulations may create significant billing issues and make the complex reimbursement process more challenging for providers. For instance, reimbursement may vary by state and health insurance plan. Providers will be required to check individual insurers to determine the eligibility of services and reimbursements [79].

Additionally, to increase engagement of LGBTQIA+ patients, a telehealth version of the drop-in care model can be considered [68]. Telehealth providers should operate HIPAA-compliant platforms to ensure the privacy and protection of their data. Additionally, to secure protected health information (PHI) and personally identifiable information (PII), psychologists must take preventive measures, such as using a secure network, sitting in a private location, using headphones, implementing an automated risk detection system, utilizing personal and network firewalls, employing strong passwords and encryption, avoiding fraud and malpractice, etc. Professionals should be careful when using third-party services to dispose of data [63]. In the post-pandemic era, many flexible conditions have either been terminated or modified. Teletherapy professionals should consciously get acquainted with the new requirements and regulations and carefully document their notes to avoid any compliance and liability-related issues. Lastly, to establish an effective, standardized service, psychologists should undergo continuous training and frequently evaluate their clinical effectiveness using outcome measures. The outcome measures may involve standardized instruments regarding clinical outcome, therapeutic alliance, and patient satisfaction [80].

Therapeutic Alliance and Training

Therapeutic alliance, which refers to the working relationship between therapist and client, is a key predictor of treatment outcomes [19, 23]. Teletherapy can successfully foster strong therapeutic relationships despite the remote nature of the medium [19, 20]. Moreover, telehealth services have been shown to enhance access, continuity, and patient engagement in treatment [25]. In addition to technological innovations, therapeutic alliance remains a critical factor in the success of telepsychology.

While previous research has demonstrated that teletherapy can maintain or even enhance the therapeutic alliance, this is dependent on several factors, including clinician training, platform quality, and patient readiness [19, 20]. In a large-scale quantitative analysis, Eichenberg and colleagues [81] found that therapeutic alliance scores were statistically comparable across online and face-to-face psychotherapy. However, Norwood and colleagues [34] found that working alliance scores were slightly lower in videoconferencing psychotherapy compared to face-to-face therapy, but symptom reduction outcomes were non-inferior across modalities. Similarly, meta-analyses and non-inferiority trials have consistently shown equivalent alliance strength and clinical efficacy [16, 17, 19, 20]. As telepsychology expands, ensuring that therapists are trained in remote communication skills and rapport-building techniques will be crucial to fostering a strong therapeutic alliance.

Telehealth Case Examples and Clinical Applications

The following fictional vignettes illustrate how telepsychology can be applied across populations and interventions, showing both its potential benefits and its challenges in practice.

Case 1: María

María, a 27-year-old Latina graduate student, who sought help for social anxiety that had intensified during the pandemic. In her telehealth-based CBT program, she and her therapist built an exposure hierarchy to address feared social situations. For her first assignment, María went to a café and attempted to order a coffee from the barista while keeping her therapist connected by video. Having the therapist "on the line" made the task feel less daunting, but it also served as a safety behavior, providing reassurance that blunted the learning opportunity. In later sessions, the therapist helped María understand that avoidance and safety behaviors maintain anxiety in the long term. Together, they decided that future exposures would be completed independently, with María reporting back in session. At first, her anxiety spiked and she considered leaving, but she managed to complete the conversation. She recognized that handling the situation without immediate support was a turning point. Although her therapist could not directly observe, María's growing independence highlighted the value of balancing support with the need to reduce reliance on safety behaviors.

Case 2: Daniel

Daniel, a 42-year-old White single father of four, began telepsychology to address frequent depressive symptoms. His therapist introduced a behavioral activation approach, emphasizing the importance of scheduling activities that increased both pleasure and access to natural reinforcers. Together, they created weekly plans that included short walks during his lunch break, cooking dinner with his children, and gradually re-engaging with a long-neglected hobby. Telehealth provided the flexibility to schedule sessions after his children's bedtime, an accommodation that would have been nearly impossible with in-person care. Between sessions, Daniel used a mood-tracking app and shared his activity logs through the virtual platform, which helped him monitor progress and link mood improvements to increased activity. Attendance was more consistent than in his prior in-person therapy, though at first, he found it harder to feel emotionally connected over video. He also raised concerns about the security of his personal data. Over time, however, Daniel described telehealth as "the only way therapy could fit into my life right now," noting that the structure of behavioral activation gave him practical tools to combat inactivity and isolation.

Across these cases, telepsychology demonstrated clear advantages in enhancing accessibility, reducing logistical barriers, and supporting continuity of care. María's case illustrated how telehealth can bring structured CBT exposures into real-world environments, while Daniel's case highlighted how flexible scheduling and digital tools can improve adherence and reinforce behavioral activation strategies. At the same time, these examples reveal common challenges, including the risk of unique vitrail safety behaviors during exposures and ongoing concerns about data security. Together, the cases present how telepsychology despite some obstacles can be a valuable and adaptable means of delivering evidence-based care; one that requires thoughtful tailoring to client needs, resources, and contexts to maximize its effectiveness.

Future Directions in Telepsychology

The future of telepsychology holds immense potential, with emerging technologies and integrative models that may transform mental health care delivery. Key areas of advancement include integrative and interdisciplinary care, virtual reality, artificial intelligence, and hybrid care models.

Integrative and Interdisciplinary Care

Telepsychology is increasingly converging with other therapeutic modalities, creating opportunities for integrative and team-based care. Embedding digital interventions within established evidence-based treatments such as CBT, family-based interventions, and multisystemic approaches has shown promise [82]. For example, telehealth platforms have extended parent management training and trauma-focused therapies into underserved communities, with preliminary evidence of sustained engagement [82]. Heinsch and colleagues [12] emphasized that integration requires understanding profession-specific differences in telehealth engagement; psychiatrists, psychologists, nurses, and social workers vary in how they perceive and implement remote care due to distinct training models and systemic hierarchies. Within pediatric and family-based contexts, remote behavioral interventions allow coordinated treatment among therapists, parents, and schools, while reducing logistical barriers to care delivery [82]. Similarly, integration into occupational therapy has supported clients with developmental or sensory processing challenges through joint online sessions that combine behavioral coaching with adaptive environmental modifications [83].

Virtual Reality and Artificial Intelligence

Virtual reality (VR) and artificial intelligence (AI) represent rapidly expanding frontiers in telepsychology, offering innovative ways to enhance engagement, accessibility, and personalization of care. VR involves the use of computer-generated, three-dimensional settings that can range from simple visual displays to fully immersive, multisensory experiences, which enable users to interact with or move through them, often by controlling virtual objects or characters [84]. VR-based therapies, particularly for exposure-based treatments, have shown strong efficacy in reducing anxiety, phobic avoidance, and PTSD symptoms [85–87]. Meta-analytic findings confirm robust effects across randomized controlled trials, and younger clients often show high engagement with gamified, interactive formats [86, 87]. Beyond exposure therapy, VR applications now extend to mood, anxiety, and neurodevelopmental disorders, improving emotional regulation and treatment adherence [88, 89]. Mobile, 5G-enabled VR platforms have demonstrated feasibility and preliminary effectiveness for adolescents in rural areas [89]. Despite promising results, sustaining long-term engagement and tailoring content to individual users remain ongoing challenges [90, 91].

AI, computer systems that learn from data to recognize patterns and make predictions [91–93], is increasingly shaping mental health innovation. Machine-learning models can detect and predict psychological symptoms by analyzing speech, language, facial expressions, and wearable data [94, 95]. These tools have demonstrated diagnostic accuracy rates exceeding 80% for major depressive disorder using biological and cognitive markers [96]. Natural language processing (NLP) further allows real-time analysis of client speech or text to identify depressive thinking patterns, monitor emotion, or summarize therapy notes [94, 95, 97]. Similarly, conversational AI systems powered by large language models can simulate therapeutic dialogue using cognitive-behavioral and motivational interviewing principles, supporting users' self-monitoring and coping skills [91, 95]. Researchers emphasize that AI should augment, not replace, clinical judgment [91, 93, 98, 99]. While AI can streamline assessment, documentation, and monitoring, human oversight remains critical for ethical and empathic care. Barriers to adoption include limited clinician training, data bias, and privacy concerns, underscoring the need for transparency, safety, and equity standards [93, 99].

Hybrid Care

The next phase of telepsychology likely involves hybrid systems that integrate AI-driven tools with traditional therapy [100, 101]. Mobile apps, wearable sensors, and predictive algorithms can track behavioral and physiological data, such as sleep, heart rate, and speech, to detect early signs of distress and enable timely clinician intervention [102, 103]. Evidence suggests these models enhance engagement, reduce dropout, and make care more continuous and individualized [43, 101]. However, achieving equitable implementation will require intentional design, clinician training, and robust ethical frameworks to ensure these technologies serve all populations fairly [49, 83, 104].

Discussion

The rapid evolution of telepsychology has reshaped both the conceptual and practical boundaries of psychological care. Across modalities, populations, and contexts, evidence increasingly supports the clinical efficacy of telepsychology comparable to in-person psychotherapy in-person psychotherapy for common mental health concerns such as depression and anxiety [16–18]. Meta-analyses and large-scale reviews demonstrate that core therapeutic processes, including alliance, engagement, and outcome, can be preserved when interventions are delivered via secure video, phone, or digital platforms [19, 20, 34, 76]. These findings, while encouraging, must be interpreted in light of significant contextual and systemic factors that shape who benefits from telepsychology and how it is implemented.

From a systems perspective, telepsychology has succeeded in reducing geographic, financial, and logistical barriers to mental health services [2, 29, 105]. During and after the COVID-19 pandemic, this expansion improved access for rural clients and accelerated policy reforms enabling interstate practice and reimbursement parity [11, 52, 55–57, 64]. At the same time, the literature highlights persistent inequities: low digital literacy, limited broadband access, and language mismatches which continue to exclude marginalized populations from equitable participation [8, 40, 47, 49, 50, 52–54]. Culturally and linguistically diverse communities, particularly refugees, immigrants, and Indigenous groups, remain disproportionately underserved, underscoring the need for culturally adapted telepsychological frameworks [39, 49, 60, 106]. Addressing these disparities requires more than technical accessibility, it demands integration of informed cultural and ethical practice.

Therapeutic alliance remains a central determinant of telepsychology outcomes. Studies consistently find that alliance strength in videoconferencing psychotherapy is statistically non-inferior to in-person formats when supported by appropriate technological infrastructure and clinician training [19, 20, 34, 76, 81]. Training in telepresence may be necessary to sustain alliance quality. Moreover, therapists report variable confidence in adapting evidence-based protocols to remote delivery particularly for exposure-based and trauma-focused interventions [77, 82]. Competence models and supervision structures must therefore evolve to address the cognitive, emotional, and ethical complexities unique to digital care [60, 63, 83].

Ethical considerations have become increasingly salient as telepsychology expands across jurisdictions. Issues of confidentiality, informed consent, emergency response, and cross-state practice are complicated by evolving legal frameworks such as PSYPACT and HIPAA's digital provisions [57, 63–67]. Ethical decision-making now extends to encompass data privacy, algorithmic transparency, and the responsible use of artificial intelligence. AI-enabled systems show promise in enhancing diagnostic precision, monitoring client progress, and delivering personalized interventions [92–98], yet they raise profound concerns about bias, accountability, and human oversight [93, 99]. The integration of AI into telepsychology will require rigorous ethical guidelines, interdisciplinary collaboration, and ongoing empirical validation to ensure these tools augment rather than replace clinical judgment.

Beyond technology, telepsychology's future depends on its ability to sustain human connection across distance. Emerging models such as hybrid care, blended interventions, and virtual reality-based therapies illustrate how digital and in-person modalities can complement one another rather than compete [43, 85–89]. Hybrid systems may offer the flexibility of remote access while preserving the relational depth of face-to-face encounters. Similarly, virtual reality and interactive digital environments are expanding possibilities for exposure therapy, relaxation training, and immersive psychoeducation, especially for youth and anxiety-related disorders [85–89, 107–109]. These innovations mark a paradigm shift from telepsychology as a crisis adaptation to telepsychology as a permanent, evidence-based component of integrated behavioral health care.

However, significant research gaps persist. Most telepsychology studies have focused on high-income contexts, brief treatments, and common disorders; less is known about long-term outcomes, comorbid conditions, and culturally diverse populations. Methodological heterogeneity (i.e., varying platforms, outcome measures, and clinician expertise) limits comparability across studies. Future research should prioritize longitudinal designs, process-based analyses, and equity-focused implementation. Clinically, the challenge lies in training practitioners not merely to use digital tools, but to conceptualize telepsychology as an evolving relational space requiring technological literacy, cultural humility, and ethical reflexivity. In sum, the accumulated evidence positions telepsychology as a mature and indispensable extension of contemporary psychological practice. Its efficacy is now well-established, its ethical and legal foundations are consolidating, and its technological horizon continues to expand through. The next decade will determine whether telepsychology fulfills its transformative potential; to democratize access, enhance cultural inclusion, and reimagine psychological care for a digitally connected world.

References

1. Centers for Disease Control and Prevention. Research anthology: telehealth and telemedicine [Internet]. Atlanta: CDC; 2024 [cited 2025 Sep 21]. Available from: https://www.cdc.gov/phlp/php/publications/research-anthology-telehealth-and-telemedicine.html.
2. Nickelson DW. Telehealth and the evolving health care system: strategic opportunities for professional psychology. Prof Psychol Res Pract. 1998;29(6):527–35.
3. Cooper SE, Campbell LF, Smucker BS. Telepsychology: a primer for counseling psychologists. Couns Psychol. 2019;47(8):1074–114. https://doi.org/10.1177/0011000019895276.
4. American Psychological Association. Guidelines for the practice of telepsychology [Internet]. Washington, DC: American Psychological Association; 2024 [cited 2025 Oct 18]. Available from: https://www.apa.org/about/policy/telepsychology-revisions.
5. Elliott KS, Nabulsi EH, Sims-Rhodes N, Dubre V, Barena E, Yuen N, et al. Modality and terminology changes for behavioral health service delivery during the COVID-19 pandemic: a systematic review. Front Psychiatry. 2024;14:1265087. https://doi.org/10.3389/fpsyt.2023.1265087.
6. Benschoter RA, Wittson CL, Ingham JG. Two-way television in group therapy. Dis Nerv Syst. 1965;26:66–70.
7. Joskowicz J. Video conferencing technologies: past, present and future. TechRxiv. 2023. https://doi.org/10.36227/techrxiv.24669051.v1.
8. Ezeamii MI, Kumar R, Ojemeni MT, Al-Balas M, Osei-Tutu E, Okpala PU, et al. Telehealth and health equity: understanding the barriers to equitable healthcare delivery. 2022;31(1):60–66.
9. Abrams Z. How well is telepsychology working? Monit Psychol. 2020;51(5):46–55.
10. Sablone S, Bellino M, Lagona V, Franco TP, Groicher M, Risola R, et al. Telepsychology revolution in the mental health care delivery: a global overview of emerging clinical and legal issues. Forensic Sci Res. 2024;9(3):owae008. https://doi.org/10.1093/fsr/owae008.
11. Wind TR, Rijkeboer M, Andersson G, Riper H. The COVID-19 pandemic: the 'black swan' for mental health care and a turning point for e-health. Internet Interv. 2020;20:100317. https://doi.org/10.1016/j.invent.2020.100317.
12. Heinsch M, Tickner C, Betts D, Brosnan C, Vincent K, Canty J. Differences in the use and perception of telehealth across four mental health professions: insights from a secondary analysis of qualitative data. Qual Health Res. 2025;35(6):601–10. https://doi.org/10.1177/10497323241271960.
13. Franzosa E, Gorbenko K, Brody AA, Leff B, Ritchie C, Kinosian B, et al. Telehealth use among older adults in home-based primary care during COVID-19: a qualitative study. J Am Geriatr Soc. 2021;69(9):2598–606.
14. McBain RK, Schuler MS, Qureshi N, Matthews S, Kofner A, Breslau J, et al. Expansion of telehealth availability for mental health care after state-level policy changes from 2019

to 2022. Focus (Am Psychiatr Publ). 2025;23(3):353–61. https://doi.org/10.1176/appi.focus.25023019.
15. Torous J, Linardon J, Goldberg SB, Sun S, Bell I, Nicholas J, et al. The evolving field of digital mental health: current evidence and implementation issues for smartphone apps, generative artificial intelligence, and virtual reality. World Psychiatry. 2025;24(2):156–74.
16. Batastini AB, Paprzycki P, Jones ACT, MacLean N. Are videoconferenced mental and behavioral health services just as good as in-person? A meta-analysis of a fast-growing practice. Clin Psychol Rev. 2021;83:101944. https://doi.org/10.1016/j.cpr.2020.101944.
17. Berryhill MB, Culmer N, Williams N, et al. Videoconferencing psychotherapy and depression: a systematic review. Telemed J E Health. 2018;25(6):435–46. https://doi.org/10.1089/tmj.2018.0058.
18. Giovanetti AK, Punt SEW, Nelson EL, Ilardi SS. Teletherapy versus in-person psychotherapy for depression: a meta-analysis of randomized controlled trials. Telemed J E Health. 2022;28(8):1077–89. https://doi.org/10.1089/tmj.2021.0294.
19. Aafjes-van Doorn K, Spina DS, Horne SJ, Békés V. The association between quality of therapeutic alliance and treatment outcomes in teletherapy: a systematic review and meta-analysis. Clin Psychol Rev. 2024;110:102430. https://doi.org/10.1016/j.cpr.2024.102430.
20. Davis KA, Zhao F, Janis RA, Castonguay LG, Hayes JA, Scofield BE. Therapeutic alliance and clinical outcomes in teletherapy and in-person psychotherapy: a noninferiority study during the COVID-19 pandemic. Psychother Res. 2024;34(5):589–600. https://doi.org/10.1080/10503307.2023.2229505.
21. Lehtimäki S, Martic J, Wahl B, Foster KT, Schwalbe N. Evidence on digital mental health interventions for adolescents and young people: systematic overview. JMIR Ment Health. 2021;8(4):e25847. https://doi.org/10.2196/25847.
22. Şahin E, Yavuz Veizi BG, Naharci MI. Telemedicine interventions for older adults: a systematic review. J Telemed Telecare. 2024;30(2):305–19. https://doi.org/10.1177/1357633X211058340.
23. Hilty DM, Sunderji N, Suo S, Chan S, McCarron RM. Telepsychiatry and other technologies for integrated care: evidence base, best practice models and competencies. Int Rev Psychiatry. 2018;30(6):292–309. https://doi.org/10.1080/09540261.2019.1571483.
24. Shigekawa E, Fix M, Corbett G, Roby DH, Coffman J. The current state of telehealth evidence: a rapid review. Health Aff (Millwood). 2018;37(12):1975–82. https://doi.org/10.1377/hlthaff.2018.05132.
25. Shaver J. The state of telehealth before and after the COVID-19 pandemic. Prim Care. 2022;49(4):517–30. https://doi.org/10.1016/j.pop.2022.04.002.
26. Bulkes NZ, Davis K, Kay B, Riemann BC. Comparing efficacy of telehealth to in-person mental health care in intensive-treatment-seeking adults. J Psychiatr Res. 2022;145:347–52. https://doi.org/10.1016/j.jpsychires.2021.11.003.
27. Zhang Y, Leuk JS, Teo WP. Domains, feasibility, effectiveness, cost, and acceptability of telehealth in aging care: scoping review of systematic reviews. JMIR Aging. 2023;6:e40460. https://doi.org/10.2196/40460.
28. Arafat MY, Zaman S, Hawlader MDH. Telemedicine improves mental health in COVID-19 pandemic. J Glob Health. 2021;11:03004. https://doi.org/10.7189/jogh.11.03004.
29. Wang S, von Huben A, Sivaprakash PP, Saurman E, Norris S, Wilson A. Addressing health service equity through telehealth: a systematic review of reviews. Digit Health. 2025;11:1–13. https://doi.org/10.1177/20552076251326233.
30. Langarizadeh M, Tabatabaei MS, Tavakol K, Naghipour M, Rostami A, Moghbeli F. Telemental health care, advantages, disadvantages, and ethical issues: a narrative review. Acta Inform Med. 2017;25(3):205–12. https://doi.org/10.5455/aim.2017.25.205-212.
31. Sora B, Nieto R, Montesano A, Armayones M. Acceptance and use of telepsychology from the clients' perspective: questionnaire study to document perceived advantages and barriers. JMIR Ment Health. 2021;8(10):e22199. https://doi.org/10.2196/22199.

32. Abuyadek RM, Hammouda EA, Elrewany E, Elmalawany DH, Ashmawy R, Zeina S, et al. Acceptability of tele-mental health services among users: a systematic review and meta-analysis. BMC Public Health. 2024;24:1143. https://doi.org/10.1186/s12889-024-18436-7.
33. Tenso K, Strombotne K, Garrido MM, et al. Virtual mental health care and suicide-related events. JAMA Netw Open. 2024;7(11):e2443054. https://doi.org/10.1001/jamanetworkopen.2024.43054.
34. Norwood C, Moghaddam NG, Malins S, Sabin-Farrell R. Working alliance and outcome effectiveness in videoconferencing psychotherapy: a systematic review and noninferiority meta-analysis. Clin Psychol Psychother. 2018;25(6):797–808. https://doi.org/10.1002/cpp.2315.
35. Fletcher TL, Hogan JB, Keegan F, Davis ML, Wassef M, Day S, et al. Recent advances in delivering mental health treatment via video to home. Curr Psychiatry Rep. 2018;20(8):56. https://doi.org/10.1007/s11920-018-0922-y.
36. Seidman AJ, Vogel DL, Lannin DG. Examining between- and within-person effects of the self-stigma of seeking psychological help on the therapeutic working alliance: the moderating role of psychological distress. Psychotherapy. 2023;60(2):206–11. https://doi.org/10.1037/pst0000482.
37. van Lotringen C, van der Vaart R, Wiersma JE, van Gemert-Pijnen JE, Riper H. Text-based alliance in digital psychotherapy: a scoping review. Front Digit Health. 2021;3:767728. https://doi.org/10.3389/fdgth.2021.767728.
38. Clement S, Schauman O, Graham T, Maggioni F, Evans-Lacko S, Bezborodovs N, et al. What is the impact of mental health-related stigma on help-seeking? A systematic review of quantitative and qualitative studies. Psychol Med. 2015;45(1):11–27.
39. Willis HA, Gonzalez JC, Call CC, Quezada D, Scholars for Elevating Equity and Diversity (SEED), Galán CA. Culturally responsive telepsychology & mHealth interventions for racial-ethnic minoritized youth: research gaps and future directions. J Clin Child Adolesc Psychol. 2022;51(6):1053–69. https://doi.org/10.1080/15374416.2022.2124516.
40. Cortelyou-Ward K, Atkins DN, Noblin A, Rotarius T, White P, Carey C. Navigating the digital divide: barriers to telehealth in rural areas. J Health Care Poor Underserved. 2020;31(4):1546–56. https://doi.org/10.1353/hpu.2020.0116.
41. Hilty DM, Serhal E, Crawford A. A telehealth and telepsychiatry economic cost analysis framework: scoping review. Telemed J E Health. 2023;29(1):23–37. https://doi.org/10.1089/tmj.2022.0016.
42. Kemp E, et al. Barriers and disparities in telehealth uptake and use: scoping review. JAMIA Open. 2025;8(2):ooaf019. https://doi.org/10.1093/jamiaopen/ooaf019.
43. Greenway T, Patel R, Singh A, Gega L. Blended and hybrid models of telepsychology: emerging evidence and practice considerations. Curr Opin Psychol. 2024;56:101597. https://doi.org/10.1016/j.copsyc.2024.101597.
44. Swint J, Fischer M, Zhang W, Zhang X. Therapy without borders: a systematic review on telehealth's role in expanding mental health access. medRxiv [Preprint]. 2024. https://doi.org/10.1101/2024.07.30.24311208.
45. Accorsi TAD, Lima KA, Köhler KF, Cordioli E, Pedrotti CHS. Assessment of suicidal ideation via telemedicine: a case report and management suggestions. Int J Emerg Med. 2023;16:84. https://doi.org/10.1186/s12245-023-00557-2.
46. van Leeuwen H, Sinnaeve R, Witteveen U, Van Daele T, Ossewaarde L, Egger JIM, et al. Reviewing the availability, efficacy and clinical utility of telepsychology in dialectical behavior therapy (Tele-DBT). Borderline Personal Disord Emot Dysregul. 2021;8(1):26. https://doi.org/10.1186/s40479-021-00165-7.
47. Edmiston K, AlZuBi J. Trends in telehealth and its implications for health disparities. NAIC Center for Insurance Policy and Research (CIPR); 2022 [cited 2025 Oct 5]. https://doi.org/10.52227/25241.2022.

48. Greenup EP, Best D. Systematic review and meta-analysis of no show or non-attendance rates among telehealth and in-person models of care. BMC Health Serv Res. 2025;25:663. https://doi.org/10.1186/s12913-025-12826-2.
49. Gallegos-Rejas VM, De Guzman KR, Kelly JT, Smith AC, Thomas EE. Strategies to improve telehealth access for culturally and linguistically diverse communities: a systematic review. J Public Health (Oxf). 2025;47(3):e374–90. https://doi.org/10.1093/pubmed/fdaf030.
50. Afni N. Disparities in healthcare access: addressing systemic barriers in urban and rural communities. J Health Lit Qual Res. 2023;3(2):112–22. https://doi.org/10.61194/jhlqr.v3i2.543.
51. Kruse CS, Bouffard S, Dougherty M, Parro JS. Telemedicine use in rural Native American communities in the era of the ACA: a systematic literature review. J Med Syst. 2016;40(6):145. https://doi.org/10.1007/s10916-016-0503-8.
52. U.S. Government Accountability Office. Closing the digital divide for the millions of Americans without broadband [Internet]. 2023 [cited 2025 Oct 5]. Available from: https://www.gao.gov/blog/closing-digital-divide-millions-americans-without-broadband.
53. Iasiello JA, Rajan A, Zervos E, Parikh AA, Snyder RA. Racial differences in patient-reported access to telehealth: an important and unmeasured social determinant of health. JCO Oncol Pract. 2023;19(12):1215–23. https://doi.org/10.1200/OP.23.00006.
54. Anaya YB, Hernandez GD, Hernandez SA, Hayes-Bautista DE. Meeting them where they are on the web: addressing structural barriers for Latinos in telehealth care. J Am Med Inform Assoc. 2021;28(10):2301–5. https://doi.org/10.1093/jamia/ocab155.
55. US Health News. PSYPACT gets an A (for access, among other things) [Internet]. 2025 [cited 2025 Oct 5]. Available from: https://www.mercer.com/en-us/insights/us-health-news/psypact-gets-an-a-for-access-among-other-things/.
56. PSYPACTMap. PSYPACT [Internet]. [cited 2025 Oct 5]. Available from: https://psypact.gov/page/psypactmap.
57. American Psychological Association. Ethical principles of psychologists and code of conduct (2002; amended 2010 Jun 1 and 2017 Jan 1) [Internet]. 2017 [cited 2025 Oct 5]. Available from: https://www.apa.org/ethics/code/.
58. Jo E, Kouaho WJ, Schueller SM, Epstein DA. Exploring user perspectives of and ethical experiences with teletherapy apps: qualitative analysis of user reviews. JMIR Ment Health. 2023;10:e49684. https://doi.org/10.2196/49684.
59. Young AN. Guide to providing culturally competent behavioral health services via telehealth. Pract Innov. 2022;7(3):170–7. https://doi.org/10.1037/pri0000173.
60. Atzor M-C, Andersson G, von Lersner U, Weise C. Effectiveness of Internet-based training on psychotherapists' transcultural competence: a randomized controlled trial. J Cross-Cult Psychol. 2024;55(3):260–77. https://doi.org/10.1177/00220221231221095.
61. Hoffman KM, Trawalter S, Axt JR, Oliver MN. Racial bias in pain assessment and treatment recommendations, and false beliefs about biological differences between blacks and whites. Proc Natl Acad Sci USA. 2016;113(16):4296–301. https://doi.org/10.1073/pnas.1516047113.
62. Rambachan A, Noorulhuda H, Fang MC, Bazinski M, Manuel S, Hubbard C, Prasad P. Pain assessment disparities by race, ethnicity, and language in adult hospitalized patients. Pain Manag Nurs. 2023;24(4):393–9. https://doi.org/10.1016/j.pmn.2023.03.012.
63. Perle JG, Smucker-Barnwell S, Morland LA, Villalobos BT, Moore HD, Frye WS, et al. A compendium for the 2024 APA guidelines for the practice of telepsychology: guideline applications and resources. Am Psychol. 2025. https://doi.org/10.1037/amp0001579.
64. Telehealth Certification Institute. PSYPACT allows for telepsychology across state lines [Internet]. [cited 2025 Oct 5]. Available from: https://www.telementalhealthtraining.com/psychology/psypact-allows-for-telepsychology-across-state-lines.
65. Cowan M. Ethical considerations for interjurisdictional practice [Internet]. 2024 [cited 2025 Oct 5]. Available from: https://cdn.ymaws.com/www.papsy.org/resource/collection/1D2A9876-938B-4567-9D3A-7500D0D24015/W26_-_Ethical_Telepsychology_and_Interjurisdic.pdf.

66. American Psychological Association. Ethical principles of psychologists and code of conduct (proposed draft) [Internet]. 2025 [cited 2025 Oct 5]. Available from: https://apps.apa.org/APACommentingPortal/CommentSite?SiteNum=125&PersonID=0.
67. U.S. Department of Health and Human Services. Summary of the HIPAA privacy rule [Internet]. 2025 [cited 2025 Oct 5]. Available from: https://www.hhs.gov/hipaa/for-professionals/privacy/laws-regulations/index.html.
68. National LGBTQIA+ Health Education Center. Patient-centered telehealth for LGBTQIA+ communities [Internet]. 2024 [cited 2025 Oct 5]. Available from: https://www.lgbtqiahealtheducation.org/publication/patient-centered-telehealth-for-lgbtqia-communities/.
69. Alpert AB, Mehringer JE, Orta SJ, Redwood E, Hernandez T, Rivers L, et al. Experiences of transgender people reviewing their electronic health records: a qualitative study. J Gen Intern Med. 2023;38(4):970–7. https://doi.org/10.1007/s11606-022-07671-6.
70. Greenwood H, Krzyzaniak N, Peiris R, Clark J, Scott AM, Cardona M, et al. Telehealth versus face-to-face psychotherapy for less common mental health conditions: systematic review and meta-analysis of randomized controlled trials. JMIR Ment Health. 2022;9(3):e31780. https://doi.org/10.2196/31780.
71. Martin AC. Legal, clinical, and ethical issues in teletherapy. In: Scharff JS, editor. Psychoanalysis online: mental health, teletherapy and training. 1st ed. London: Routledge; 2013. p. 75–84.
72. Lin T, Anderson T. Reduced therapeutic skill in teletherapy versus in-person therapy: the role of non-verbal communication. Couns Psychother Res. 2024;24(1):317–27. https://doi.org/10.1002/capr.12666.
73. Foley GN, Gentile JP. Nonverbal communication in psychotherapy. Psychiatry (Edgmont). 2010;7(6):38–44.
74. Bellanti DM, Kelber MS, Workman DE, Beech EH, Belsher BE. Rapid review on the effectiveness of telehealth interventions for the treatment of behavioral health disorders. Mil Med. 2022;187(5–6):e577–88. https://doi.org/10.1093/milmed/usab318.
75. Fernández-Batanero JM, Fernández-Cerero J, Montenegro-Rueda M, Fernández-Cerero D. Effectiveness of digital mental health interventions for children and adolescents. Children (Basel). 2025;12(3):353. https://doi.org/10.3390/children12030353.
76. Mercadal Rotger J, Cabré V. Therapeutic alliance in online and face-to-face psychological treatment: comparative study. JMIR Ment Health. 2022;9(5):e36775. https://doi.org/10.2196/36775.
77. Marriott BR, Peer S, Wade S, Hanson RF. Therapists' perceived competence in delivering trauma-focused cognitive behavioral therapy during statewide learning collaboratives. J Behav Health Serv Res. 2023;50(4):500–13. https://doi.org/10.1007/s11414-023-09847-2.
78. Gajarawala SN, Pelkowski JN. Telehealth benefits and barriers. J Nurse Pract. 2021;17(2):218–21. https://doi.org/10.1016/j.nurpra.2020.09.013.
79. Telehealth.HHS.gov. Telehealth policy updates [Internet]. [cited 2025 Oct 5]. Available from: https://telehealth.hhs.gov/providers/telehealth-policy/telehealth-policy-updates.
80. Chuo J, Macy ML, Lorch SA. Strategies for evaluating telehealth. Pediatrics. 2020;146(5):e20201781. https://doi.org/10.1542/peds.2020-1781.
81. Eichenberg C, Aranyi G, Rach P, Winter L. Therapeutic alliance in psychotherapy across online and face-to-face settings: a quantitative analysis. Internet Interv. 2022;29:100556. https://doi.org/10.1016/j.invent.2022.100556.
82. Dopp AR, Lippe M, Parisi KE, Hui S, Beasley LO, Silovsky JF. A game-based telehealth intervention for young children with disruptive behavior problems. J Clin Child Adolesc Psychol. 2021;50(6):840–54. https://doi.org/10.1080/15374416.2020.1867993.
83. McCord C, Bernhard P, Walsh M, Rosner C, Console K. A consolidated model for telepsychology practice. J Clin Psychol. 2020;76(6):1060–82. https://doi.org/10.1002/jclp.22954.
84. Essoe JKY, Reggente N, Ohno AA, Baek YH, Dell'Italia J, Rissman J. Enhancing learning and retention with distinctive virtual reality environments and mental context reinstatement. NPJ Sci Learn. 2022;7:31. https://doi.org/10.1038/s41539-022-00147-6.

85. Freeman D, Lambe S, Kabir T, et al. Automated virtual reality therapy to treat agoraphobic avoidance and distress in patients with psychosis (gameChange): a multicentre, parallel-group, single-blind, randomised, controlled trial in England with mediation and moderation analyses. Lancet Psychiatry. 2022;9(5):375–88. https://doi.org/10.1016/S2215-0366(22)00060-8.
86. Carl E, Stein AT, Levihn-Coon A, Pogue JR, Rothbaum B, Emmelkamp P, et al. Virtual reality exposure therapy for anxiety and related disorders: a meta-analysis of randomized controlled trials. J Anxiety Disord. 2019;61:27–36.
87. Seinfeld S, Montesano A. Virtual reality in psychotherapy: a commentary on strategies, interventions, and perspectives from five clinical reports. J Clin Psychol. 2025;81(9):888–94. https://doi.org/10.1002/jclp.23813.
88. Pedram S, Piatkowski T. Exploring the potential of virtual reality (VR) in mental healthcare: a systematic literature review. Virtual Real. 2025;29:135. https://doi.org/10.1007/s10055-025-01181-6.
89. Sarrió-Colas L, Reverté-Villarroya S, Castellà-Culvi AB, Barberà-Roig D, Gas-Prades C, Coello-Segura A, Adell-Lleixà M. Immersive virtual reality in psychotherapeutic interventions for youth with eating disorders: a pilot study in a rural context. Appl Sci. 2025;15(16):9013. https://doi.org/10.3390/app15169013.
90. Wiederhold BK. Addressing stress-related disorders and resilience building with digital tools and virtual reality. Cyberpsychol Behav Soc Netw. 2023;26(1):1–3. https://doi.org/10.1089/cyber.2023.29230.editorial.
91. Nie J, Shao HV, Fan Y, Shao Q, You H, Preindl M, et al. LLM-based conversational AI therapist for daily functioning screening and psychotherapeutic intervention via everyday smart devices. ACM Trans Interact Intell Syst. 2024:1–30. https://doi.org/10.1145/3712299.
92. Olawade O, Adepoju A, Adisa O, Akinola A. Digital mental health interventions for low-resource settings: a scoping review. BMC Psychiatry. 2024;24:412. https://doi.org/10.1186/s12888-024-05623-9.
93. Mansoor M, Ansari A. Ethical concerns in artificial intelligence-driven mental healthcare: bias, transparency, and accountability. Ethics Med Public Health. 2025;23:100927. https://doi.org/10.1016/j.jemep.2025.100927.
94. Cruz-Gonzalez P, He AW-J, Lam EP, Ng IMC, Li MW, Hou R, et al. Artificial intelligence in mental health care: a systematic review of diagnosis, monitoring, and intervention applications. Psychol Med. 2025;55:e18. 1–52. https://doi.org/10.1017/S0033291724003295.
95. Chen Y, Zhang C, Li H, Wang J, Liu F. Machine learning for major depressive disorder diagnosis using multimodal data: a clinical validation study. J Affect Disord. 2024;352:1–10. https://doi.org/10.1016/j.jad.2024.03.015.
96. Zhang X, Jiang J, Li H, Zhao C, Wang Q, Zhang Y, et al. Exploring the role of artificial intelligence in mental health interventions: a systematic review of clinical applications and ethical considerations. Front Psychiatry. 2025;16:1523843. https://doi.org/10.3389/fpsyt.2025.1523843.
97. Ni J, Jia H. Artificial intelligence and digital health equity: opportunities and challenges in global mental healthcare. Int J Environ Res Public Health. 2025;22(2):334. https://doi.org/10.3390/ijerph22020334.
98. Graham S, Depp C, Lee EE, et al. Artificial intelligence for mental health and mental illnesses: an overview. Curr Psychiatry Rep. 2019;21(11):116. https://doi.org/10.1007/s11920-019-1094-0.
99. Cecil J, Kleine A-K, Lermer E, Gaube S. Mental health practitioners' perceptions and adoption intentions of AI-enabled technologies: an international mixed-methods study. BMC Health Serv Res. 2025;25:556. https://doi.org/10.1186/s12913-025-12715-8.
100. Zhou Y, Li J, Gao Y, Luo X. Telehealth in cognitive behavioral therapy: applications, challenges, and future directions. Front Psychol. 2022;13:884213. https://doi.org/10.3389/fpsyg.2022.884213.
101. Cascella M, Schiavo D, Grizzuti M, Romano MC, Coluccia S, Bimonte S, Cuomo A. Implementation of a hybrid care model for telemedicine-based cancer pain management

at the Cancer Center of Naples, Italy: a cohort study. In Vivo. 2023;37(1):385–92. https://doi.org/10.21873/invivo.13090.
102. Borghare P, Kadam A, Raut S. Wearable health devices and artificial intelligence in mental health monitoring: current trends and future opportunities. Health Technol (Berl). 2024;14(3):345–60. https://doi.org/10.1007/s12553-024-00789-1.
103. Tang S, Sun J, Zhang L, Wang H. Internet of Things-based wearable devices for monitoring psychological and physiological health: a review. JMIR Mhealth Uhealth. 2022;10(7):e36221. https://doi.org/10.2196/36221.
104. Nelson D, Inghels M, Kenny A, Skinner S, McCranor T, Wyatt S, et al. Mental health professionals and telehealth in a rural setting: a cross sectional survey. BMC Health Serv Res. 2023;23:200. https://doi.org/10.1186/s12913-023-09083-6.
105. World Health Organization. WHO guideline: recommendations on digital interventions for health system strengthening. Geneva: World Health Organization; 2020.
106. Spanhel K, Balci S, Feldhahn F, Bengel J, Baumeister H, Sander LB. Cultural adaptation of internet- and mobile-based interventions for mental disorders: a systematic review. NPJ Digit Med. 2021;4:128. https://doi.org/10.1038/s41746-021-00498-1.
107. Emmelkamp PMG, Meyerbröker K. Virtual reality therapy in mental health. Annu Rev Clin Psychol. 2021;17:495–519. https://doi.org/10.1146/annurev-clinpsy-081219-115923.
108. Cieślik B. Mechanisms of virtual reality-based relaxation in older adults: a scoping review. J Clin Med. 2025;14(17):6126. https://doi.org/10.3390/jcm14176126.
109. Kuleli D, Tyson P, Davies NH, Zeng B. Examining the comparative effectiveness of virtual reality and in-vivo exposure therapy on social anxiety and specific phobia: a systematic review and meta-analysis. J Behav Cogn Ther. 2025;35:100524. https://doi.org/10.1016/j.jbct.2025.100524.

Uses of Technology in Psychological Assessment Practices

Eva R. Lieberman and Summer Chahin

History of Assessment

Until recently, psychological assessment has historically been a process that has remained unchanged since its inception. Written and printed materials were administered to participants in person and hand scored by the examiner. While the nature of printing, mass production of assessment measures, and normative scoring may have evolved, technology has really only been utilized in testing in the twenty-first century. Efforts to test human ability, like intelligence testing, date back to at least 2000 BC, when the Chinese emperor began implementing learning examinations [1].

Formal written testing is first observed in the Han Dynasty, around 200 BC—200 AD [1]. These initial efforts to prioritize a merit-based system were used to select civil servants and appoint government officials [2]. In the 1100s, European education systems and universities also began implementing testing to ensure learning based on desired societal standards and also promote meritocracy [3]. In the 1800s, testing became a more efficient process as access to education broadened [3]. The world wars provided a new context for testing, where large amounts of people were researching and applying testing for varying reasons.

Personality tests originated in the 1910s to help screen for soldiers more likely to experience "nervous breakdowns" or "shell shock" during and after military service [4]. The Army Alpha and Beta tests originated around the same era to test intellectual competency of recruits and classify their ability [1]. Since World War 1, the military has widely adopted assessment and testing as recruitment tools, screening tools for enlistment, and aptitude testing as a prerequisite to certain roles and

E. R. Lieberman · S. Chahin (✉)
Western Michigan University Homer Stryker M.D. School of Medicine,
Kalamazoo, MI, USA
e-mail: Eva.lieberman@wmed.edu; Summer.chahin@wmed.edu

S. S. Chahin et al. (eds.), *Innovation in Medical Education and Clinical Practice*, https://doi.org/10.1007/978-3-032-19116-8_20

positions [5]. The technology boom of the twenty-first century spans only about the last 30 years, which is a small portion of the many years psychological assessment has been utilized. This brief summary of the history of testing and assessment demonstrates the widely varying functions of testing, the contexts in which testing has been used, and the development of tools to attempt to best understand human psychology. The evolution of psychological testing now leads to new developments and contemporary goals for which the assessment and testing process need to be adapted, specifically through the integration of technology throughout the assessment process. Psychological assessment is the process by which we integrate testing results, clinical interviews, behavioral observations, and several other types of data into a comprehensive report which is used to diagnose a patient, describe or explain behavior, and provide recommendations [6–10].

Psychological assessment is categorically different from psychological testing, in that testing is the administration and scoring of a particular measure [9, 10]. Psychological assessment encompasses testing but adds to the testing process by integrating results from multiple tests [6, 8, 10, 11]. There is great variety in the tools that are available for psychological assessment and variety in the functionality of assessments used within an array of contexts. There are many purposes for psychological assessment and some of the most common assessment purposes include personality assessment, neuropsychological assessment, forensic assessment, intelligence and achievement assessment, and many others [7].

The assessment process for these varying purposes includes a battery of tests, but sometimes psychological assessment uses brief screeners to acquire information and inform treatment, intervention, or provides evidence for further testing. Screeners are often used in therapy intake appointments, within primary care settings, and in the initial steps of a larger psychological assessment. Some commonly used screeners in varying contexts include a depression screener (PHQ-9), anxiety (GAD-7), suicide risk screener (CSSRS), screening for autism spectrum disorders (M-CHAT), and screeners for cognitive decline (MOCA). Many of these screening tools are used to initially assess the need for further discussion or investigation. When individuals complete the screener and score above a certain threshold, that indicates further information is needed to appropriately diagnose, treat, or refer.

One of the primary benefits of using mental health screeners in primary care is their ability to identify mental health conditions early, even before they reach a level of severity that requires crisis intervention. Depression, anxiety, and alcohol use disorders often go undiagnosed in primary care because patients may be reluctant to discuss mental health concerns. Screeners help normalize these conversations by encouraging patients to reflect on their symptoms and behaviors, often leading to earlier diagnoses and more timely treatment [12]. Implementing consistent screening has gotten easier to work into the clinic flow as these are often digitized and can be given to patients in the waiting room on an iPad and can even be sent to their electronic health record to be completed before the visit to allow for provider efficiency.

Mental health screeners in primary care settings help bridge the gap between physical and mental health care. By identifying patients who are experiencing mental health challenges, primary care providers can offer or refer for appropriate treatments, such as medication, counseling, or referrals to mental health specialists. This is particularly beneficial for individuals who may not have access to specialized mental health services but receive care regularly in primary care settings. Integrating mental health care into primary care promotes a holistic approach to patient well-being, reducing the stigma often associated with seeking mental health treatment in more specialized settings [13].

The high prevalence of untreated mental health issues is a major concern in healthcare. Left undiagnosed, conditions like depression and anxiety can interfere with a patient's ability to manage chronic physical conditions, engage in work or social activities, and maintain quality of life. Furthermore, untreated mental health conditions can lead to increased healthcare utilization, including more frequent visits to emergency departments. By screening for mental health issues, primary care providers can intervene early to reduce the burden of untreated illness and improve overall patient outcomes [14].

Using structured mental health screeners in routine care helps establish a framework for discussing mental health in a way that is comfortable and nonjudgmental. It allows patients to see that mental health is an integral part of their overall health, helping to normalize discussions about emotional well-being. When patients are routinely asked about their mental health, they may be more likely to share concerns they would otherwise hesitate to bring up. This enhances the provider-patient relationship and can lead to better treatment adherence and outcomes [15].

Primary care practices that routinely implement mental health screenings can contribute to improving population health by identifying trends in mental health conditions within specific communities. This enables better resource allocation, early intervention, and targeted public health initiatives. For instance, if a practice identifies a higher-than-average rate of depression or anxiety among its patients, it may implement specific interventions, such as offering counseling or increasing access to mental health specialists, in response to the identified need.

Mental health screeners in primary care settings are an essential tool for early identification, diagnosis, and treatment of mental health conditions. They allow primary care providers to address a wide range of psychological issues efficiently, reduce the stigma associated with mental health care, and ensure that patients receive the appropriate care. By incorporating mental health screenings into routine care, primary care providers play a critical role in addressing the mental health needs of their patients, improving overall health outcomes, decrease healthcare costs with early intervention, and promoting a more integrated approach to healthcare.

Even within the most commonly used testing tools, there is constant research and progress toward improving the tools, leading to updates, changes, and adaptations to measures, subtests, and administration.

The Wechsler series of tests for intelligence and achievement have developed and improved as the need for assessment has increased and the populations being served have expanded. The Wechsler–Bellevue test, developed around WWII to assess soldiers, used subtests developed and included for the Army Alpha and Beta tests [16, 17]. Many of these subtests used in these early Wechsler tests still have general consistencies with modern subtests, including subtests like arithmetic, information, and comprehension [16]. Though these tests were taken from items and measures used primarily in military populations, they were adapted into tests used with the general population. A second form of this measure was created, and form II of the Wechsler–Bellevue test was standardized among a population of 18- to 40-year-old males [16]. Interestingly, form II was then revised and used as a children's version of the measure, leading to the creation of the WISC, which is now a commonly used intelligence test for children, currently on its fifth edition (WISC-V) [16]. Modern revisions of the Wechsler series (WAIS and WISC) include updated subtests, added subtests, and standardized norms for a broader population than the US military [16]. The Wechsler tests are just one example of measures that have been progressively updated, but this process is similar for many of the assessment tools used today.

Importantly, left out of this process is an adaptation and standardization process for minority populations. This chapter will also later discuss how assessment has historically been used as a tool to further marginalize individuals from the non-dominant culture. In terms of history and development of psychological assessment tools, the field has generally done a poor job in recognizing bias in administration and scoring for minoritized groups. People of color historically scored significantly below white individuals on measures of cognitive functioning, and intelligence, scoring between 7–8 points lower than white peers on measures of intelligence [18, 19]. Psychological assessment is one of the slowest developing fields of psychology. Major changes have occurred across many areas of psychology and technological development has progressed at a rapid pace; assessment development has failed to maintain similar progress [16, 17]. We continue to use tests and measures created for a specific population, but as access to testing has increased and more individuals are seeking psychological testing, the historical roots of assessment are ever present and overcoming these historical barriers should be a priority.

Barriers and Challenges of Assessment

Traditionally, assessment practices were paper and pencil measures, scored by hand, and administered exclusively in person. Testing materials for these paper versions include administration manuals, scoring manuals, record forms, scoring keys, and documents that fill filing cabinets. These materials are expensive to buy and cumbersome to store and keep in good condition. Additionally, a significant amount of space is required to store assessment protocols after the patient has completed their assessment, given that the requirement to store materials can be upwards of 10 years and varies by state or federal law and regulating body [20]. The time to administer these measures is extensive. Scoring these paper measures requires math done by hand, which needs to be checked and rechecked. This presents many opportunities for human error in scoring, then impacting results and interpretation. Report writing is another laborious process that, prior to the integration of technology, was extremely effortful and required tedious precision [7, 21].

In addition to the time-consuming process, assessments are typically provided in person during normal working business hours. This limits the ability of employed individuals to attend testing sessions for several hours a day instead of work. This barrier to access impedes opportunities that are gained from assessment results, including important diagnoses and supports that could benefit work performance. Not only would individuals miss out on payment for the day they miss, but this barrier is compounded for parents of children who need testing. Children would need to miss school for a day, and parents would need to miss work in order to bring their children, which many families cannot afford to do. Assessment only occurring during normal business hours then hinders children from getting the support they need if their parents are unable to miss work. Psychological assessment is also fairly restrictive in terms of available providers. There are often long waitlists that can range between several weeks to a year to get in for their initial appointment, and 2–3 years for those seeking Autism testing. This further extends the period of time that people are unable to receive important information provided by assessment, referrals for treatment, or accommodations for work or school. For example, it is recommended that Autism testing, and diagnosis occurs as early as possible, but if children and their families are waiting 2–3 years to be evaluated then they are missing out on important preventative care, treatment, and ABA services for years during an important time of development. Additionally, assessment is expensive. Health insurance may sometimes cover these expenses, but without coverage, the assessment process is limited to those who can afford hundreds or thousands of dollars [22].

A restrictive process in terms of time, money, and energy; psychological assessment is also historically restrictive toward minoritized populations [23–25]. Psychological assessment has a history rooted in discrimination, upholding white supremacy, and maintaining segregation [23]. While Benet's intelligence test was originally developed to help identify children needing academic assistance, this test was quickly co-opted and used as a tool to justify and promote eugenics [26, 27]. Psychological tests were also used to exclude immigrants to the United States and as evidence promoting segregation in schools [26]. Even still, psychological tests were created and validated with bias toward the dominant culture (white, English speaking, European Americans) and results of these tests lead to overdiagnosis, incorrect classroom placement, and a, reasonably so, mistrust in intelligence testing within minority communities and people of color [24, 26]. For example, children from minoritized communities were often misclassified as intellectually disabled or placed in lower educational tracks, which hindered their academic growth and future opportunities, reinforcing racial and class-based inequalities.

Additionally, intelligence testing was sometimes used to justify harsher sentences for people of color, reflecting the broader societal biases embedded in psychological assessment practices [28]. Further, psychological assessment also served as a barrier to care, where access to health care was limited and only allowed after assessment results demonstrated a need. Psychological testing was used to determine eligibility and access to social services, including welfare and disability benefits. Individuals from minoritized groups often faced systemic barriers and bias in these assessments, which were tailored to the dominant cultural norms, thus exacerbating disparities in access to basic needs.

As the values of psychologists have shifted, modernizing assessment has also meant working against the history of discriminatory practice [29]. Efforts to address these historical issues have led to the development of culturally sensitive assessments that are more inclusive and accurate. The American Psychological Association (APA) and other organizations have taken steps to implement fairness guidelines in psychological testing, aiming to reduce cultural biases in both test design and administration. Ongoing critiques note implicit bias and lack of diversity in research samples used to create and validate assessment tools.

Despite some modern advancements, the field continues to face challenges in fully eliminating bias. Critics argue that many current psychological assessments still lack sufficient representation of minoritized populations in their development, which means cultural bias remains an ongoing concern in clinical practice. However, as society increasingly values diversity and inclusion, psychological assessment has gradually adapted to better reflect cultural and societal shifts. These changes are evident in the growing emphasis on understanding not just cognitive ability, but also emotional and social intelligence, with tests designed to account for a wider range of experiences and identities.

Moves Toward Modernization

Modernizing psychological assessment has meant using the process of assessment for all populations and using assessment results to help improve functioning and psychological well-being, instead of upholding systems of oppression. Additionally, by dismantling this historical bias, modernizing assessment to include the use of technology broadens access to psychological assessment, bringing more people the benefits that the process affords. Psychological assessment has greatly changed since its formalized beginnings in the nineteenth century, not only through modernizing assessment practices, but resulting in evolution of function, form, and outcomes.

Modernization is not isolated to psychological assessment. General psychological practice has gone a long way in incorporating technology into practice. Virtual and telehealth therapy as standard practice has a body of literature that began to grow in the early 2000's, but use of this tool has exploded since the Covid-19 pandemic in 2020 [30–33]. Not only was this evolution necessary during the pandemic, but due to the many benefits associated with telehealth, this mode of service has become integral in many practices. Among those many benefits that have ingrained telehealth in the mainstream procurement methods of psychological services, telepsychology has broadened access on an incredible scale, allowing those who may have previously been irregular attenders, those without transportation, or those in areas with few providers locally to have access to therapy.

Additionally, the inclusion of technology is present in the treatment process. Inclusion of virtual reality has been introduced for treatment protocols like exposure therapy and pain management [34–36]. Virtual Reality (VR) has become an innovative tool in exposure therapy, helping treat conditions such as anxiety, PTSD, phobias, and other anxiety-related disorders. By creating controlled, immersive simulations of real-world scenarios, VR allows for safe, gradual exposure without the risks of in-person settings. Several studies demonstrate that VR exposure therapy can be as effective, if not more so, than traditional methods [37, 38]. The technology enables tailored experiences that can adjust in intensity, making it possible to personalize therapy based on each patient's progress and needs.

One of the key benefits of VR in exposure therapy is its ability to offer a highly controlled environment, allowing patients to confront fears at their own pace. For instance, someone with a fear of flying can start with a basic airplane simulation and gradually progress to more complex experiences, such as turbulence or the sounds of engines. This gradual approach ensures that therapy is manageable and reduces the risk of overwhelming patients. Furthermore, VR's immersive nature increases patient engagement and motivation, leading to higher satisfaction and better completion rates in treatment [39].

VR also enhances accessibility, making exposure therapy more available to individuals who might face barriers to traditional therapy, such as those living in rural areas or with mobility issues. Patients can engage in therapy from the comfort of their homes, using a variety of devices. This added convenience, combined with the anonymity VR provides, reduces stigma and encourages more individuals to seek treatment. Overall, VR's ability to provide tailored, engaging, and accessible therapy holds great potential for improving outcomes in mental health care, particularly for patients with anxiety, PTSD, and phobias.

Technology has also expansively been included in psychological research, ranging from brain scanning, survey research administered online, and development of new technology to improve psychological well-being [40–45]. Similar to the benefits of VR in the intervention realm, ecological momentary assessment (EMA) had been increasingly used as a research tool to provide richer data than self-report. Assessment data, like self-report screeners previously discussed, often relies on accurate reporting from the participant. Self-report is not a particularly accurate method of data collection. As technology, specifically mobile phones, became an integral part of everyday life, EMA presented an opportunity to collect behavioral data in the moment [46]. EMA consists of a variety of methods, but generally, EMA generally is repeated, real time data collection [46]. This may look like receiving text reminders on your phone with a link to complete a brief survey or report on current behaviors. EMA is a revolutionary tool in assessment, as reporting on mood and behavior for the week or month on a screener like the PHQ-9 or a screener for smoking, is retrospective and often inaccurate and biased based on recency. EMA not only provides opportunities for more accurate data, but because of the wide accessibility of cell phones, EMA offers increased accessibility, improved accuracy, and rich real-time information about functioning. As it pertains to psychological assessment, technology has progressed and been integrated in each step of the assessment process.

Integration of Technology into the Process

Even in initial steps like referrals and scheduling, technology is an integral part of how modern psychological assessment is conducted. Using email, virtual intake appointments, and scheduling applications in this introductory phase sets up the process to clearly integrate technology. Electronic medical records also help in these initial steps. Paper charts used to mean finding, filing, printing, and faxing documents. Now, all of the patient information is accessible by computer. Resources for patient contact can be found in the chart, referrals are easily sent to and from providers, and documentation of scheduling, initial sessions, and subsequent testing can all be located in the electronic medical record. Once a testing appointment is scheduled, a clinical interview is typically the next phase of the assessment process. The clinical interview provides important historical and contextual information about the testing patient. Technology is often integrated in this process through virtual appointments, where both the patient and interviewing provider are connected through (HIPPA compliant) software and video conferencing. We have had video conferencing capabilities for many years, and as previously discussed, since the Covid-19 pandemic, the use of this particular technological tool has drastically increased.

Additionally, awareness of video conferencing, ease of access, and ease of use have also made this tool highly popular within psychological assessment, the field of psychology, and generally popular within society. Secondary to the clinical interview, testing is the next phase of the assessment process. We previously mentioned that testing used to be a strictly paper and pencil process. Some testing included scoring tools within the assessment, including perforations and pages to transpose test answers onto in order to ease the hand-scoring process. While many of these types of tests are still in use, and some testing is still primarily done in this manner (i.e., IQ and achievement tests), the ease of computerized testing is quickly overtaking the paper and pencil forms.

Computerized testing now takes both test administration and scoring to a computer or tablet. Websites and organizations have made a variety of computerized administration available. This includes on screen assessments, where the participant takes a test on a computer or tablet in the presence of the examiner, remote on-screen assessment, where a link to a private test is emailed or electronically sent to the participant for them to take at home, and manual entry, where the test is administered by hand and the examiner transfers the test results to the computerized scoring program. Brief screeners and longer form tests administered on screen or remotely can easily be completed on tablets or phones and scored immediately. This is useful in many ways, including in medical and primary care settings where providers can initially assess psychological distress through a brief screener.

Further, long self-report measures that require proctoring (i.e., MMPI), can not only be administered virtually using an administration program like a previously mentioned remote on-screen administration, but can also be virtually proctored using video conferencing. Some measures have greatly benefited from the use of technology. For example, processing speed and inhibition tasks that require a respondent to very quickly respond or not respond. These tasks are extremely accurate due to computerized administration and function at speeds and with accuracy that human administration and scoring is incapable of. Other tests have incorporated tablet use and the use of touch screens to adequately adapt the test to be administered through technology.

Additional measures that are required to be completed by parents, guardians, teachers, or other important individuals are also much more easily distributed and collected by using technology. After all testing is completed, technology use in the scoring of the testing measures is an incredible tool. Administration programs also have scoring integrated into the software (i.e., QGlobal). Using technology in scoring provides a great number of advantages. Automated and computerized scoring happens behind the scenes, with only a few clicks from the examiner. This not only increased examiner productivity as they can use time that would have been spent scoring doing other things, but computerized scoring also increased accuracy of computations required for results, and reduce human error [11]. The final step in the assessment process is providing feedback. Similarly, to intakes and diagnostic interviews, these feedback appointments can be done through video conferencing applications, and reports sent through a number of virtual methods. As access to computers, tablets, and administration and scoring software has increased, the use of technology in administration and scoring of assessment has also risen, resulting in widespread use of these methods across the field.

Benefits of Integrating Technology

The increase in use of technology in the psychological assessment process has provided immense benefits in a variety of ways for both administrators and participants. In addition to some previously mentioned benefits, like time effectiveness for scoring tests, computerized testing greatly improves ease of use for a great number of individuals. For examiners who are comfortable with technology already, there is very little learning involved to be able to successfully administer and score a test. There may be some new workflow associated with what buttons to click and what options to select, but otherwise, technology literate folks likely have improved ease of use. The integration of technology in assessment may also be more cost effective. While the upfront cost of a licensing fee may be expensive, the cost may be offset when compared to how expensive acquisition of paper materials and manuals might cost, given that a single IQ test can cost up to $2000–3000 for the initial materials.

Other cost effectiveness associated with use of technology might be travel expenses saved by virtual appointments, printing expenses, and paid time for examiners and scorers. Many of these benefits also apply to the patient or testing parties, where travel time is reduced from virtual sessions, wait time to get a report is reduced due to computerized scoring, and access to electronic versions of the assessment report provides increased ease of distribution to relevant persons.

Costs and Concerns of Technology

The increased accessibility of virtual appointments has generally been overwhelmingly positive. While there are many benefits to integrating technology into this process, there are some negative aspects to the incorporation of technology in psychological assessment. However, once this option is made available, some assessment participants want virtual sessions, regardless of the purpose of the appointment. Some tests still need to be administered in person, so virtual appointments are not an option. This is an inconvenience for patients who want the convenience of a virtual appointment, but who need a comprehensive test battery, including in person tests.

The increased accessibility associated with technology is also a barrier for others. Technological literacy is a skill and often times, older adults or individuals unfamiliar with the rapid advances in technology are not equipped to take advantage of technology in assessment. Those who have difficulty with computers, web-based video applications, or other methods of testing that include technology may not only have decreased accessibility, but their difficulty with these tools may impact their testing ability, therefore impact their scores on testing measures. This presents a challenge for interpreting results, as their scores may not be an accurate reflection of their abilities, and instead a measure of their technological literacy. Additional disadvantages that come with the use of the internet are that it affords testing patients the ability to look up measures and potentially prepare or study for their assessment.

Tests in psychological assessment batteries are generally protected material to reduce any bias that may come with participants studying or preparing for the test. While increasing accessibility is often a benefit, in this situation, increased ease of access can cause damage to the validity of the testing measures. Other important concerns of technology in testing include the automated scoring process. While a time saving and effort saving process, automated scoring allows professionals to bypass learning how to hand score the testing measures. This may hinder their understanding of the calculations that go into scoring, the theory behind the scoring, and what goes into the scores presented to the testing participant.

Of course, with these advancements in the testing process, there will be challenges to overcome. As this integration of technology has rapidly accelerated in the last decade, the problems associated with rapidly changing methods and tools will continue to be present. It is critical that we continue to acknowledge, investigate, and work to improve some of these disadvantages in order to have the best assessment process possible. The speed at which technology continues to advance makes anticipating change a challenge for assessment, and for psychology as a whole. It is our responsibility to monitor this rapidly changing resource to ensure best practices are maintained and updated when new advances and tools become available.

References

1. Gregory RJ. Psychological testing: history, principles, and applications. Pearson Education India; 2004.
2. Min H, Xiuwen Y. Educational assessment in China: lessons from history and future prospects. Assess Educ Princ Policy Pract. 2001;8(1):5–10.
3. Brown GT. The past, present and future of educational assessment: a transdisciplinary perspective. Front Educ. 2022;7:1060633.
4. Gibby RE, Zickar MJ. A history of the early days of personality testing in American industry: an obsession with adjustment. Hist Psychol. 2008;11(3):164.
5. Nwafor CE, Atalor A. Psychological testing and assessment in the military. Practicum Psychologia. 2014;4(1)
6. Bornstein RF. Evidence-based psychological assessment. J Pers Assess. 2017;99(4):435–45.
7. Groth-Marnat G. Handbook of psychological assessment. Wiley; 2009.
8. Matarazzo JD. Psychological assessment versus psychological testing: validation from Binet to the school, clinic, and courtroom. Am Psychol. 1990;45(9):999.
9. Meyer GJ, Finn SE, Eyde LD, Kay GG, Moreland KL, Dies RR, Eisman EJ, Kubiszyn TW, Reed GM. Psychological testing and psychological assessment: a review of evidence and issues. Am Psychol. 2001;56(2):128.
10. Wright AJ, Chávez L, Edelstein BA, Grus CL, Krishnamurthy R, Lieb R, Mihura JL, Pincus AL, Wilson M. Education and training guidelines for psychological assessment in health service psychology. Am Psychol. 2021;76(5):794.
11. Naglieri JA, Drasgow F, Schmit M, Handler L, Prifitera A, Margolis A, Velasquez R. Psychological testing on the internet: new problems, old issues. Am Psychol. 2004;59(3):150.
12. Moussavi S, Chatterji S, Verdes E, Tandon A, Patel V, Ustun B. Depression, chronic diseases, and decrements in health: results from the world health surveys. Lancet. 2007;370(9590):851–8.
13. Walker EA, Katon W, Ciechanowski P. Integrating physical and mental health care: a model for the future. Prim Care Companion CNS Disord. 2015;17(4)
14. Katon W, Lin EH, Kroenke K. The association of depression and anxiety with medical symptom burden in patients with chronic medical illness. Gen Hosp Psychiatry. 2007;29(2):147–55.
15. Dobscha SK, Heagerty P, Brown G. Mental health screening in primary care: the case for integration. J Gen Intern Med. 2009;24(3):282–8.
16. Boake C. From the Binet–Simon to the Wechsler–Bellevue: tracing the history of intelligence testing. J Clin Exp Neuropsychol. 2002;24(3):383–405.
17. Pade H. The evolution of psychological testing: embarking on the age of digital assessment. In: Valle R, Klimo J, editors. *The changing faces of therapy: Innovative perspectives on clinical issues and assessment*; 2014. Retrieved from http://www.helloq.com/content/dam/ped/ani/us/helloq/media/The_Evolution_of_Psych_Testing_Embark_on_Digital_Assess_Pade_Final.pdf.
18. Gasquoine PG. Race-norming of neuropsychological tests. Neuropsychol Rev. 2009;19:250–62.
19. Nicolai KM, Kaplan RM. Student workbook for Kaplan and Saccuzzo's psychological testing: principles, applications and Issues. Thomson/Wadsworth; 2005.

20. Drogin EY, Connell M, Foote WE, Sturm CA. The American Psychological Association's revised "record keeping guidelines": implications for the practitioner. Prof Psychol Res Pract. 2010;41(3):236.
21. Barak A, English N. Prospects and limitations of psychological testing on the Internet. J Technol Hum Serv. 2002;19(2–3):65–89.
22. Eisman EJ, Dies RR, Finn SE, Eyde LD, Kay GG, Kubiszyn TW, Meyer GJ, Moreland KL. Problems and limitations in using psychological assessment in the contemporary health care delivery system. Prof Psychol Res Pract. 2000;31(2):131.
23. Brown RT, Reynolds CR, Whitaker JS. Bias in mental testing since bias in mental testing. Sch Psychol Q. 1999;14(3):208.
24. Reynolds CR, Suzuki LA. Bias in psychological assessment: an empirical review and recommendations. In: Handbook of psychology, Second Edition, vol. 10; 2012.
25. Poortinga YH. Cultural bias in assessment: historical and thematic issues. Eur J Psychol Assess. 1995;11(3):140–6.
26. Sayegh P, Vivian D, Heller MB, Kirk S, Kelly K. Racial, cultural, and social injustice in psychological assessment: a brief review, call to action, and resources to help reduce inequities and harm. Train Educ Prof Psychol. 2023;17(4):366.
27. Walters AS. The contribution of psychological assessment to systemic racism. Brown Univ Child Adolesc Behav Lett. 2021;37(9):8.
28. Auguste E, Bowdring M, Kasparek SW, McPhee J, Tabachnick AR, Tung I, Scholars for Elevating Equity and Diversity (SEED), Galán CA. Psychology's contributions to anti-blackness in the United States within psychological research, criminal justice, and mental health. Perspect Psychol Sci. 2023;18(6):1282–305.
29. Laher S, Cockcroft K. Moving from culturally biased to culturally responsive assessment practices in low-resource, multicultural settings. Prof Psychol Res Pract. 2017;48(2):115.
30. Maheu MM, Pulier ML, McMenamin JP, Posen L. Future of telepsychology, telehealth, and various technologies in psychological research and practice. Prof Psychol Res Pract. 2012;43(6):613.
31. Nelson EL, Bui TN, Velasquez SE. Telepsychology: research and practice overview. Child Adolesc Psychiatr Clin. 2011;20(1):67–79.
32. Carrillo de Albornoz S, Sia KL, Harris A. The effectiveness of teleconsultations in primary care: systematic review. Fam Pract. 2022;39(1):168–82.
33. Perrin PB, Rybarczyk BD, Pierce BS, Jones HA, Shaffer C, Islam L. Rapid telepsychology deployment during the COVID-19 pandemic: a special issue commentary and lessons from primary care psychology training. J Clin Psychol. 2020;76(6):1173–85.
34. Thomas D, Phillips AS. Virtual reality for psychological assessment in clinical practice. Pract Innov. 2016;1(3):197.
35. Li A, Montaño Z, Chen VJ, Gold JI. Virtual reality and pain management: current trends and future directions. Pain Manag. 2011;1(2):147–57.
36. Pourmand A, Davis S, Marchak A, Whiteside T, Sikka N. Virtual reality as a clinical tool for pain management. Curr Pain Headache Rep. 2018;22:1–6.
37. Rizzo A, Reger G, Gahm G, Difede J, Rothbaum BO. Virtual reality exposure therapy for combat-related PTSD. In: Post-traumatic stress disorder: basic science and clinical practice; 2009. p. 375–99.
38. Freeman D, Reeve S, Robinson A, Ehlers A, Clark D, Spanlang B, Slater M. Virtual reality in the assessment, understanding, and treatment of mental health disorders. Psychol Med. 2017;47(14):2393–400.
39. Maples-Keller JL, Bunnell BE, Kim SJ, Rothbaum BO. The use of virtual reality technology in the treatment of anxiety and other psychiatric disorders. Harv Rev Psychiatry. 2017;25(3):103–13.
40. Dev A, Roy N, Islam MK, Biswas C, Ahmed HU, Amin MA, Sarker F, Vaidyanathan R, Mamun KA. Exploration of EEG-based depression biomarkers identification techniques and their applications: a systematic review. IEEe Access. 2022;10:16756–81.

41. Picó-Pérez M, Fullana MA, Albajes-Eizagirre A, Vega D, Marco-Pallarés J, Vilar A, Chamorro J, Felmingham KL, Harrison BJ, Radua J, Soriano-Mas C. Neural predictors of cognitive-behavior therapy outcome in anxiety-related disorders: a meta-analysis of task-based fMRI studies. Psychol Med. 2023;53(8):3387–95.
42. Griffin M, Martino RJ, LoSchiavo C, Comer-Carruthers C, Krause KD, Stults CB, Halkitis PN. Ensuring survey research data integrity in the era of internet bots. Qual Quant. 2021;56:2841–52.
43. McBride DM. The process of research in psychology. Sage Publications; 2023.
44. Kjell ON, Kjell K, Schwartz HA. Beyond rating scales: with targeted evaluation, large language models are poised for psychological assessment. Psychiatry Res. 2024;333:115667.
45. Russell MA, Gajos JM. Annual research review: ecological momentary assessment studies in child psychology and psychiatry. J Child Psychol Psychiatry. 2020;61(3):376–94.
46. Shiffman S, Stone AA, Hufford MR. Ecological momentary assessment. Annu Rev Clin Psychol. 2008;4(1):1–32.

Surgical Innovations

Nicole Alvarez, Autumn Bennitt, and Lisa Miller

Introduction

Throughout history, surgeons have stood at the forefront of medical innovation. Long before the development of antibiotics, advanced imaging, or precise surgical instruments, surgeons were developing new tools, techniques, and approaches to treat injuries and diseases. From the earliest known surgical procedures in ancient civilization to today's minimally invasive robotic-assisted procedures and artificial intelligence-guided advancements, the field of surgery has been a never-ending source of innovation and evolution.

With the first documented leg amputation occurring over 31,000 years ago [1], this chapter traces the arc of surgical innovation across millennia, beginning with prehistoric societies, through the rapid breakthroughs of the nineteenth and twentieth centuries, and into the future. It examines the technological revolutions including laparoscopy, robotics, and transplantation techniques. The chapter finishes with a look at how changes in surgical education shape modern-day surgeons.

By exploring both the history and horizon of surgical practice, this chapter emphasizes that surgery is a constantly evolving field, driven by the surgeon's relentless pursuit of better care for their patients.

N. Alvarez · A. Bennitt · L. Miller (✉)
Western Michigan University Homer Stryker M.D. School of Medicine,
Kalamazoo, MI, USA
e-mail: nicole.alvarez@wmed.edu; Autumn.bennitt@wmed.edu; Lisa.miller@wmed.edu

S. S. Chahin et al. (eds.), *Innovation in Medical Education and Clinical Practice*, https://doi.org/10.1007/978-3-032-19116-8_21

Ancient Surgical History

Trepanation

Outside of a single documented leg amputation performed 31,000 years ago [1], the oldest known surgical procedure is known as trepanation, which involved drilling or scraping a hole into the skull. Evidence for this procedure traces back as far as 7000–10,000 years ago [2].

Trephined skulls have been found on every continent where prehistoric societies existed, suggesting that humans throughout the world independently saw a need for this procedure [3]. Whether used to relieve headaches, treat trauma, or address perceived spiritual or psychological ailments [3], we know that the earliest surgical innovators saw a need for this type of procedure.

Despite the lack of advanced tools or knowledge of germ theory, trepanned skulls with significant healing have been discovered [2, 3], suggesting that early surgeons had some understanding of hemostasis and wound care. They likely relied on herbal remedies and natural disinfectants to promote patient healing and survival, even without scientific understanding of their effects.

The techniques used for trepanation varied throughout cultures; however, it seems that there was an awareness of avoiding damage into the dura mater [2, 4]. While this procedure may seem brutal, it demonstrates the deep desire of surgeons to intervene in settings of disease or trauma.

Endoscopy

Endoscopy is defined as "a medical operation in which an endoscope is put into a person's body so that the parts inside can be seen." [5] As of 2017, approximately 75 million endoscopic procedures are performed annually [6]. Now using modern sedation techniques with high-definition images, this incredibly common procedure has very humble beginnings traced all the way back to 450 BC. The earliest documented use of this technique was by Hippocrates, when he used a rectal speculum to view a fistula [7]. At the time, the greatest challenges were lack of light and inability to see very far into the GI tract. Around 1000 AD, Albukisim, an Arabian surgeon and chemist, used a glass mirror to reflect light at the vulva to see into the vaginal canal [8]. These early discoveries in endoscopy laid the critical groundwork for the eventual development of laparoscopic surgery. The fundamental idea of gaining direct visual access to the interior of the body without making large incisions was born with tools like the rectal speculum and the use of reflected light. These techniques introduced the revolutionary concept that internal organs could be examined in vivo, opening an entirely new realm of diagnostic and therapeutic possibilities.

Over the centuries, innovations continued to build on this foundation. The invention of better lighting sources, particularly the electric light bulb in the late nineteenth century, dramatically expanded what could be visualized [9]. Coupled with the development of flexible and rigid scopes, physicians were able to examine deeper structures with greater clarity and less patient discomfort. These advancements made endoscopy increasingly practical and safe. The foundations of endoscopy led to the development of laparoscopy and the creation of the field of minimally invasive surgery.

Suturing

It is estimated that upward of 8% of emergency room visits each year are related to lacerations, with sutures being one of the most common methods of hemostasis and closure of these wounds [10]. While this technique is now ubiquitous in modern medicine, its origins can be traced back thousands of years. The earliest records of suturing techniques date back to ancient Egypt, around 3000 BC, where linen threads were used to close wounds [11]. Surgical papyri, documenting these developments, describe the act of stitching as well as the materials used. These documents reflect an early understanding that deliberately closing wounds could promote healing and prevent further harm.

Ancient Indian and Greek physicians, including Sushruta and Galen, two major figures in the history of surgical innovation, also described suture techniques [12, 13]. Sushruta, often referred to as the "father of surgery" wrote extensively about using natural materials such as plant fibers, animal sinews, and even human hair to tie bleeding vessels and close skin [12]. These early sutures, though rudimentary, represented a major step in transforming surgery from a last-resort intervention into a more viable and survivable treatment.

In Greece, Galen contributed to suturing technique by advancing anatomical knowledge and expanding the use of suture ligation. He described numerous different suture materials as well as knotting techniques [14]. These surgeons helped shift the perception of surgery from a brutal, desperate measure to a controlled art.

Despite these advancements, limitations remained. Early sutures came with significant risks: poor hygiene, non-absorbable materials, and imprecise techniques often led to infection and poor wound healing. Over time, techniques improved, including the rise of antiseptic techniques, which greatly reduced the risks involved with wound closure. Even today, new materials are frequently being developed, leading to improved outcomes and safer surgery.

Modern Surgical Techniques & Innovations

Anesthesia

Prior to the advent of anesthesia, surgeries needed to be performed incredibly quickly and often haphazardly. Many operations were performed in under a minute due to the excruciating pain that was inflicted upon an awake patient. These surgeries were often an absolute last resort for conditions such as gangrene or traumatic injury, with mortality rates exceedingly high. Surgical assistants of that time, "dressers," would aid in holding the screaming patient to a wooden bench [15].

A transformative moment in the field of surgery was in October 1846, when Dr. William Thomas Greene Morton publicly demonstrated his "Ether Dome" on patient Edward Abbott at Massachusetts General Hospital [16]. Using ether as a surgical anesthetic, within minutes, the patient was quiet and still, unaware of the mass being removed from his neck. This moment was followed by further developments from Dr. James Young Simpson. In 1847, Dr. Simpson demonstrated the use of chloroform as another method of anesthesia. Both compounds came with extreme risk; ether is very flammable, and chloroform can be very toxic [16]. However, the use of these substances gave surgeons the luxury of time. This opened the door for more invasive procedures, further exploration of anatomical structures, and development of increasingly complex techniques.

As active innovators, surgeons continued to collaborate with early anesthetists to modify dosages and compounds to strike the ideal balance between unconsciousness and stability. In the late nineteenth and early twentieth centuries, spinal and regional anesthesia were introduced, which allowed for conscious, yet painless procedures with increased physiologic stability [17]. By the mid-twentieth century, the combination of paralytics and endotracheal intubation further advanced the capabilities of surgeons [18]. Surgeons were now able to work in very confined spaces with a completely still patient, without the risk of causing harm to nearby structures.

A continuous loop of feedback and collaboration between surgeons and anesthesiologists drove the development of modern-day anesthesia machines. These machines use live hemodynamic and laboratory data from patients to precisely deliver appropriate drugs at the correct time [19]. The history of anesthesia is not solely a story of pain relief; it is a testament to the surgeon's role as a catalyst for progress, constantly pushing the boundaries of what's possible in the operating room.

Antiseptic & Aseptic Technique

It's hard to imagine surgery without thinking of the cold, bright operating room, the steady beeping of monitors, and the surgical team dressed head to toe in blue sterile gowns and gloves. This meticulously curated environment, to ensure patient safety and minimize infection risk, is a relatively new development in the history of surgeons. Prior to the mid-1800s, operations were performed with surgeons in blood-stained coats, unwashed hands, and unsterilized instruments [20]. At the time, postoperative infections were so common that it was considered an expected complication of surgery.

In the mid-1800's, French chemist, Louis Pasteur, began performing experiments on spoiling wine, proving his theory of fermentation [21]. This led to the germ theory of disease, challenging the long-held belief of spontaneous generation of microorganisms. While this fundamental science was discovered in a lab, British surgeon, Joseph Lister would take these discoveries further, when he theorized that microbes in the air and on tools were responsible for the high rates of infections during surgery [22].

In the 1860s, Lister applied Pasteur's work to his surgical procedures and theorized that sterilizing surgical instruments, the patient's skin, and the surgeon's hands with carbolic acid would decrease the rate of surgical infections. He also advocated for spraying this carbolic acid into the air in the operating room, in attempt to kill the airborne microbes. These techniques were known as antiseptic technique, with the goal of killing the existing microorganisms in the air and on the patient and surgeon [22]. This technique decreased the postoperative infection rate dramatically, and its impact could not be ignored.

Lister's innovations and development of antiseptic techniques laid the framework for modern day aseptic techniques [23]. Rather than eliminating germs after the patient has already been exposed, the entire operating room staff now focuses on maintaining an entirely sterile field from the time the patient enters the room, until the wound is completely closed and dressed. This goal gave rise to even larger innovations such as surgical gloves, autoclaving instruments, sterile drapes, and strict handwashing, "scrubbing," protocols.

While all modern-day surgeons follow this aseptic technique, it is crucial to acknowledge the centuries of innovation by historical surgeons who were determined to improve outcomes. Surgical infections are no longer an unavoidable consequence, but a very preventable complication. Even today, the pursuit of complete sterility continues, with continuous ongoing research on prevention of surgical infections.

The Great Turning Point

Throughout most of history, surgery was a last resort. Operations were brutal, dangerous, and painful, and often reserved for the most desperate of patients. Without anesthesia, antiseptic technique, or reliable forms of hemostasis, surgeries had to be performed in mere minutes, with frequent complications including bleeding and infection.

The advent of anesthesia to prevent pain and patient movement and antiseptic techniques made surgery something a patient was increasingly likely to survive past the initial days to weeks. At some point during the late nineteenth century, the cumulative effect of these breakthroughs fundamentally changed the risk–benefit ratio of surgical innovations. Many historians cite this time as the point when the likelihood of survival of surgery began to outweigh the likelihood of death [24].

As techniques improved and mortality declined, operations that were previously avoided entirely, due to fear of death, began to be explored as possibilities. During this time, the public perception of surgery also changed. People began to see surgery as a field driven by scientific rigor and something that patients could truly benefit from. Through the twentieth and twenty-first centuries, surgeons continued to do the once unimaginable and cure patients of ailments that were largely considered unsurvivable.

The Firsts of the Future

What now may be considered staples of the operating room and the surgical field were once unimaginable and unobtainable—as developments such as anesthesia and endoscopy opened doors, the surgical field innovations flourished. Deemed simple procedures and everyday operations and tools each had their firsts in the field, of which all continue to lead us forward toward the future.

Born from the developments of endoscopy, the transition to laparoscopic surgery emerged in the early twentieth century [25]. Surgeons began experimenting with introducing endoscopic instruments into the abdominal cavity via small incisions. Initially used for diagnostic purposes such as evaluating abdominal pain or infertility, laparoscopy evolved with improvements in optics, camera technology, and insufflation techniques that allowed the abdomen to be safely expanded with gas for better visualization and space to operate [7]. By the 1980s and 1990s, laparoscopic techniques had been adapted for therapeutic surgeries, most famously the laparoscopic appendectomy and cholecystectomy, transforming the landscape of surgical practice.

The first laparoscopic appendectomy, performed in 1981 by German gynecologist Kurt Semm, marked a turning point in surgical history [26]. Building on his background in minimally invasive gynecologic procedures, Semm applied laparoscopic principles to general surgery—a bold step that was initially met with skepticism and considered significantly dangerous [26]. He successfully used specially designed laparoscopic instruments, including a needle for insufflation and endoscopic coagulation devices. His innovation demonstrated that complex abdominal operations, although much to the doubt of the field of general surgery at this time, could be performed with minimal trauma, setting the stage for a paradigm shift in surgical technique and recovery. Following Semm's groundbreaking innovations, the first laparoscopic cholecystectomy was performed in 1985 by German general surgeon Dr. Erich Muhe utilizing Semm's instruments and techniques [26]. The success of these early laparoscopic "firsts" reimagined the limits of surgical precision and patient recovery, proving that less could truly be more.

Following along the lines of minimally invasive surgery, the first use of robots in surgery on human patients was in 1985 [27]. This device, the Programmable Universal Machine for Assembly 200 (PUMA), was used alongside a CT scanner and improved accuracy and speed of neurological biopsies [28]. The PUMA was later adapted for use in common urologic procedures, such as transurethral resections of the prostate [29]. Since then, many iterations of surgical robots have been developed, which brought us to the most well-known system today, the da Vinci [27]. The first da Vinci robot was approved by the FDA in 2000. This model was composed of three arms, two with laparoscopic tools and one with an endoscope [27]. Two years later, in 2002, a version with a fourth arm was created, as surgeons saw a need for an extra tool [27]. Throughout the years, continuous improvements have been made to the da Vinci system, allowing for its widespread use. As of 2020, there are more than 5700 da Vinci systems worldwide, and despite competitors' efforts, the da Vinci remains the leading system today [27].

Organ Transplantation

Similarly, the first successful organ transplant represented another pivotal step forward in the evolution of modern surgery and what we consider to be a common expectation in the field. In 1950, Dr. Richard H. Lawler performed first intraabdominal kidney transplant in the at Little Company of Mary Hospital in Illinois, marking a new frontier in surgical innovation [30, 31]. The operation, completed between a patient with polycystic kidney disease and a recently deceased donor, proved that organ replacement could be surgically achieved and that vascular and ureteral connections between humans were technically feasible. Though the transplanted kidney functioned for only several months before removal due to rejection, the patient's extended survival demonstrated the procedure's promise. Lawler's pioneering work laid the foundation for the future of transplant surgery, transforming the idea of replacing failed organs from a distant hope into a clinical reality of which we consider to be a staple of surgery now.

The Future of Surgery

Organ Transplantation—Moving Forward

Since the first successful human kidney transplant over 70 years ago, both the science and art of transplantation have evolved at a staggering pace [31]. What began as a bold experiment in surgical technique and immunologic control has now become a standard, life-saving therapy for patients with end-stage organ failure. Over the decades, improvements in organ preservation, immunosuppressive therapy, and microsurgical precision have expanded the boundaries of what is possible—transforming once-fatal conditions into treatable diseases.

Today, the frontier of transplantation continues to advance into previously unimaginable territory. Surgeons and scientists are now exploring transplants of organs that were once thought to be too complex or too ethically challenging to attempt, including the face, uterus, penis, and even the entire eye. These procedures not only restore physical function but also profoundly impact patients' sense of identity, dignity, and quality of life. Parallel to these achievements, the field of bioprinting and regenerative medicine is redefining the concept of organ replacement altogether. The development of 3D-printed tissues and organs, built from a patient's own cells, holds the promise of reducing transplant waiting lists, minimizing rejection risk, and 1 day creating a limitless supply of personalized grafts.

Together, these innovations represent more than technological milestones—they embody the enduring spirit of surgical creativity and compassion. The modern transplant surgeon stands at the crossroads of biology, engineering, and ethics, leading the next great revolution in the history of surgery: one in which the replacement of human organs may no longer depend on donation, but on design.

When most people think of organ transplants, they think of kidneys, livers, hearts, and maybe even lungs, which were some of the first organs to be transplanted in humans. However, advances in organ preservation, immunosuppression, and medical care have all allowed for a much wider variety of organs to be successfully transplanted. At the University of Gothenburg, researchers noted that there were over 2000 women of childbearing age in Sweden with missing or nonfunctional uteri, which led to the question of whether a uterus could be transplanted and if these transplanted uteri could successfully carry a pregnancy [32]. In September 2012, the first uterus transplantation was performed. Just 2 years later, a healthy male infant was born from a woman with a transplanted uterus. In the US, the first uterus transplant was performed in 2016. Over the next 5 years, 33 transplants were performed with a 74% graft survival at 1 year [33]. Of the women whose graft survived past 1 year, 80% were able to achieve at least 1 live birth [33]. This incredible innovation is giving great opportunity to women with uterine factor infertility and may continue to be used as treatment for other conditions.

Another current area of exploration is research being conducted on whole eye transplantation. Blindness affects about 43 million people worldwide and is an irreversible condition in most cases [34]. Whole eye transplantation has been proposed as a potential solution; however, studies to date have not shown much promise. A very large challenge with this type of procedure relates to the innervation of the eyes. For proper functioning of the eye and eyelid, cranial nerves II, III, IV, VI, and VII need to be working appropriately. Although structural anastomosis of donor and recipient nerves is technically possible, restoration of these central nerve functions is difficult to achieve [34]. The unique ocular immune privilege also creates challenges in prevention of rejection [35]. Despite these challenges, an advisory council at the National Eye Institute concluded in 1978 that "the subject [of eye transplant] is of such overriding clinical importance that it merits research attention" [36]. Despite the fact that this statement is nearly 50 years old, scientists and surgeons have held firmly that this is an important area of research and are striving to create life-changing outcomes.

Another innovation at the forefront of many surgeons' minds is the development of three-dimensional (3D) printed organs, also known as bioprinted *tissues*. This emerging technology has the potential to transform the landscape of transplantation by addressing two of its greatest challenges: the chronic shortage of donor organs and the risk of immune rejection. By using a patient's own cells as the "ink" to build functional tissues layer by layer, 3D bioprinting could 1 day allow for the creation of fully compatible, personalized grafts [37].

Current applications have already demonstrated success in the printing of simpler structures such as skin matrices, cartilage, and vascular grafts, which are being explored for use in burn victims, wound reconstruction, and orthopedic repair [38]. These early successes highlight both the promise and the complexity of bioprinting. For more intricate organs—such as the heart, lungs, liver, or intestines—replicating the precise vascular networks, tissue architecture, and functional integration required for survival remains a significant challenge [39]. Achieving this will likely demand the use of multiple bioprinting modalities, advanced biomaterials, and rigorous quality control measures to ensure both safety and functionality.

Despite these obstacles, the rapid pace of innovation in this field is remarkable. Collaborative efforts among surgeons, biomedical engineers, and material scientists are already pushing the boundaries of what was once considered science fiction. The eventual ability to bioprint transplantable, fully functional organs would not only revolutionize surgical practice but could also redefine the very meaning of organ donation—transforming it from an act of altruism to a process of regeneration and personalized medicine.

Telesurgery

Telesurgery, or remote robotic surgery is a rapidly emerging way for surgeons in one area of the world to operate on patients in an entirely different location. The first telesurgery was performed in 2001, when a surgeon in New York performed a robotic cholecystectomy on a patient in France [40]. Since then, however, only a single randomized control trial has been performed studying percutaneous access to the kidney [40]. Telesurgery, although in its early stages, is expected to have significant impacts on the care of patients in underserved areas.

Several barriers limit the success of robotic telesurgery, which need to be further explored in order to ensure patient safety and surgical safety. These surgical operations require very fast rates of information transfer, with 300 milliseconds being considered safe, but ideally under 100 milliseconds [40, 41]. In order to maintain these incredibly short latency times, many technicians must be available to monitor equipment and troubleshoot any issues that may arise.

Additionally, there are legal issues that must be sorted out before telesurgery becomes common practice. Within the United States, physicians are licensed by their state governing body [42]. Zooming out further to international telesurgery, licensing and regulation varies even more widely between countries. Questions of liability also arise in robotic telesurgery [41]. Who should be held accountable in the case of errors due to technology failure? What kind of consent needs to be obtained from the patient? Should special insurance be required for physicians performing these operations? Experts on the topic advise that international committees form and come together to begin addressing these concerns, so that as technology advances, surgeons are ready to begin operating.

What once seemed like only science fiction is now becoming reality as some surgeons begin performing robotic surgeries across international borders. While much work has to be done to make telesurgery a common practice, each and every day surgeons are breaking down barriers and using these innovations to improve lives.

Innovations in Surgical Education

As surgical practice has transformed dramatically through breakthroughs detailed here such as anesthesia, aseptic technique, minimally invasive approaches, and robotics, so too has the way the next generation of surgeons is being taught. Just as technological innovation has reshaped the operating room, it has also revolutionized the surgical classrooms, skills labs, and the path from intern year to graduation. No longer confined to only the apprenticeship model of "see one, do one, teach one," modern training has shifted to include competency goals, simulation, and immersive learning. Surgical innovation is not solely in the operating room—educational innovations are ever present and are redefining how surgical expertise is developed, assessed, and maintained.

Competency-Based Curricula

For over a century, surgical education has been structured around time-based training models, where residents progress through fixed rotations and case quotas [43]. This traditional framework was born from an era when surgical training was largely modeled after apprenticeship systems, emphasizing time spent rather than skills mastered [44]. However, this designated amount of time for surgical residency has never been shown to be the "right" amount of time for each individual surgical resident to achieve competency [45].

The emergence of competency-based residency training represents a paradigm shift toward outcomes-oriented learning, in which progression is determined by demonstrated ability rather than duration of training. This model encourages programs to focus on *what* residents can do, rather than *how long* they have been doing it. It introduces a structured, transparent approach to assessing readiness for independent practice, while maintaining the flexibility to support learners who progress more rapidly or who may require additional time to reach key milestones.

Competency-based medical education is an outcomes-based training model in which regulatory and accrediting bodies have established key competencies that residency programs may use to reshape their curricula [46]. These competencies exist in the form of Competency-based assessments (CBAs) and Entrustable Professional Activities (EPAs). CBAs and EPAs serve as the building blocks of this new framework—clearly defined, observable acts of clinical work that reflect the essential duties of a surgeon.

Integrating CBAs and EPAs into surgical education provides both structure and accountability, aligning assessment with real-time performance [47, 48]. Rather than relying on each resident having "seen one, done one, and taught one" in an abstract number of hours logged or number of cases completed, EPAs require them to physically show they can perform core surgical tasks safely and effectively under supervision before gaining autonomy [47].

The shift toward competency-based surgical education is ever-growing and continues to be adopted throughout the field [48]. This shift represents more than a structural reform—it marks a cultural transformation and innovation in how surgical mastery is defined and achieved. The emergence of such a curriculum, one centered around demonstrated mastery rather than assumed proficiency, reflects the dynamic and self-improving nature of surgical education itself.

Telesimulation

The evolution of surgical training has been punctuated by innovations that expand access, enhance scalability, and ensure standardization—and none perhaps more so than telesimulation. In essence, telesimulation allows trainees and expert educators to engage in hands-on skill development despite geographic separation, using simulators, video linkups, and real-time feedback. It is a major leap beyond the traditional paradigm of in-person teaching sessions and simulation labs, which were once thought to be impossible as well.

Originally developed in the broader context of medical and emergency training, telesimulation has been applied to medical education widely [49]. Telesimulation has been implemented in fields such as pediatrics, emergency medicine, anesthesia, general surgery, and neurosurgery—for procedures, simple skills, and even advanced tasks and operations [49]. Recent work has demonstrated that trainees who participated in telesimulation-based laparoscopic training achieved equivalent or superior skill acquisition compared with those who trained in person [49]. Participants rated telesimulation highly for its convenience, instructor feedback, and ability to reproduce the psychomotor demands of live procedures. Notably, the study also found that telesimulation reduced overall faculty time per learner, suggesting that remote instruction may enhance both efficiency and reach.

Telesimulation has proven particularly valuable in resource-limited and rural settings where access to formal simulation centers is restricted. Several reports have demonstrated the promise of telesimulation in developing surgical skills in low resource areas. Multiple studies have shown successful utilization of telesimulation to remotely improve the surgical skills of surgeons in Botswana, Africa, a resource-restricted area in which these participants successfully completed a Fundamentals of Laparoscopic Surgery program by the direction of remote instructors [50]. Further, telesimulation has been shown to be an effective and reproducible educational tool for remote teaching during resource-limited situations like the COVID-19 pandemic as well [51]. All in all, whether across the world or across the street, telesimulation has opened doors for surgical education.

Virtual and Augmented Reality

As the technology of extended reality continues to progress, opportunities to innovate surgical training are as well. At the forefront of the newest innovations in surgical education are both virtual reality (VR) and augmented reality (AR).

From the earliest simulators and box trainers emerged a vision of rehearsal: trainees could perform, repeat, receive feedback, and refine without the risks that accompany actual patients. VR takes this vision to the next level, placing the trainee inside a three-dimensional, responsive scenario of surgical anatomy, instruments, and workflow. Studies across multiple specialties show that learners who train with immersive systems complete tasks more rapidly, with fewer errors and greater accuracy, compared to traditional methods [52–54]. The repeated practice, immediate feedback, and safe failure space that VR offers mirror the deliberate-practice principles that underpin mastery in other high-performance fields.

Meanwhile, AR bridges the gap between simulation and the operating room by blending digital overlays with tactile reality. Imagine donning a head-mounted display that projects holographic anatomical landmarks on a cadaver or phantom model, or using eyewear that visualizes hidden structures during a simulated operation in real time. AR enables trainees to engage with layered anatomy, visualize unseen aspects of surgical fields, and practice the cognitive mapping that experienced surgeons still rely upon. Early reviews document that AR modules lead to measurable improvements in spatial orientation, task performance, and trainee confidence, especially when combined with structural feedback and deliberate repetition [55, 56].

The pragmatic appeal of VR and AR in surgical education lies not only in performance metrics but in scalability and adaptability. These platforms allow uniform training experiences across institutions, reduce dependence on rare visits to advanced simulation centers, and support remote learning in an era of geographic dispersion and resource constraints. The immersive and augmented environments also appeal to the new generation of learners—digital natives who are comfortable navigating complex interactive worlds.

In summary, the convergence of VR and AR in surgical education marks a profound shift in how surgeons are trained. It moves the learning process from passive observation to immersive rehearsal, from variability to standardization, and from reliance on case volume to readiness defined by precision and performance. As surgical education continues to mirror the broader evolution of surgery itself, first through technological breakthroughs, then through new techniques, and now through transformative methods of training, these immersive modalities promise to strengthen the surgical mindset long before a scalpel ever touches the skin.

Conclusion

From the first ancient healers performing trepanations to rid people of evil, to the modern techniques of robotic operations, the story of surgery is one of innovation and ingenuity. Each generation of surgeons has learned from its predecessors and pushed forward with new tools, techniques, and technology. What was initially only used as a desperate, and often unsuccessful, lifesaving measure has evolved into a precise science grounded in science, ethics, and innovation.

The innovations explored in this chapter, including aseptic technique, anesthesia, laparoscopy, and more, were all driven by leaders who had one goal in mind: improving the lives of their fellow humans. This devotion and dedication to their work should not be forgotten.

Equally, if not more important than the physical tools used are the educational tools. Over time, surgical education has changed from an apprenticeship model to complex curricula, aiming to create the best providers possible. Competency based education, telesimulation, and the always improving virtual models strive to create the next generation of surgical innovators.

As we look toward the future, innovators continue to push the boundaries of surgery. From printed organs and remote operations to the integration of artificial intelligence and personalized care, concepts that once seemed impossible are becoming a reality. Yet amid these revolutions, one truth remains unchanged: the essence of surgery lies not in the tools we use, but in the minds and hands of those who wield them. The history of surgical innovation is, above all, a testament to the creativity, courage, and compassion of those who have consistently dared to imagine a better way to heal.

References

1. Sachs M, Bojunga J, Encke A. Historical evolution of limb amputation. World J Surg. 1999;23:1088–93.
2. Verano JW. Differential diagnosis: trepanation. Int J Paleopathol. 2016;14:1–9.
3. Hobert L, Binello E. Trepanation in ancient China. World Neurosurg. 2017;101:451–6.

4. Kushner DS, Verano JW, Titelbaum AR. Trepanation procedures/outcomes: comparison of prehistoric peru with other ancient, medieval, and American civil war cranial surgery. World Neurosurg. 2018;114:245–51.
5. Endoscopy noun – Definition, pictures, pronunciation and usage notes. Oxford Advanced American Dictionary at OxfordLearnersDictionaries.com, https://www.oxfordlearnersdictionaries.com/us/definition/american_english/endoscopy. Accessed 26 Oct 2025.
6. Staff. GI endoscopies make up 68% of all endoscopies in U.S.: 5 market trends. Becker's ASC, https://www.beckersasc.com/gastroenterology-and-endoscopy/gi-endoscopies-make-up-68-of-all-endoscopies-in-u-s-5-market-trends/. 2019. Accessed 26 Oct 2025.
7. Rudiman R. Advances in gastrointestinal surgical endoscopy. Ann Med Surg (Lond). 2021;72:103041.
8. Lapeña JF. Mirrors and reflections: the evolution of indirect laryngoscopy. Ann Saudi Med. 2013;33:177–81.
9. The History of the Light Bulb. Energy.gov, https://www.energy.gov/articles/history-light-bulb. Accessed 26 Oct 2025.
10. Otterness K, J Singer A. Updates in emergency department laceration management. Clin Exp Emerg Med. 2019;6:97–105.
11. Mackenzie D. The history of sutures. Med Hist. 1973;17:158–68.
12. Dave T, Habte A, Vora V, et al. Sushruta: the father of Indian surgical history. Plast Reconstr Surg Glob Open. 2024;12:e5715.
13. Muffly TM, Tizzano AP, Walters MD. The history and evolution of sutures in pelvic surgery. J R Soc Med. 2011;104:107–12.
14. Nutton V. Ancient medicine. Taylor & Francis; 2004.
15. How agonising surgery paved the way for anaesthetics. https://www.bbc.com/future/article/20200624-how-agonising-surgery-paved-the-way-for-anaesthetics. 2020. Accessed 26 Oct 2025.
16. Abhyankar RS, Jessop KM. From craft to profession: the development of modern anesthesiology. Mo Med. 2022;119:14–20.
17. Olawin AM, Das JM. Spinal anesthesia. In: StatPearls. Treasure Island: StatPearls Publishing. http://www.ncbi.nlm.nih.gov/books/NBK537299/. 2025. Accessed 26 Oct 2025.
18. Raghavendra T. Neuromuscular blocking drugs: discovery and development. J R Soc Med. 2002;95:363–7.
19. Romero-Ávila P, Márquez-Espinós C, Cabrera Afonso JR. Historical development of the anesthetic machine: from Morton to the integration of the mechanical ventilator. Braz J Anesthesiol (English Edition). 2021;71:148–61.
20. Fulton A. 'The Butchering Art': how a 19th century physician made surgery safer. NPR, 13 October 2017. https://www.npr.org/sections/health-shots/2017/10/13/557367840/the-butchering-art-how-a-19th-century-physician-made-surgery-safer. 13 October 2017. Accessed 26 Oct 2025.
21. Louis Pasteur. Science History Institute, https://www.sciencehistory.org/education/scientific-biographies/louis-pasteur/. Accessed 26 Oct 2025.
22. Michaleas SN, Laios K, Charalabopoulos A, et al. Joseph Lister (1827–1912): a pioneer of antiseptic surgery. Cureus. 2022;14:e32777.
23. Nakayama DK. Antisepsis and asepsis and how they shaped modern surgery. Am Surg. 2018;84:766–71.
24. Brock C. Risk, responsibility and surgery in the 1890s and early 1900s. Med Hist. 2013;57:317–37.
25. Alkatout I, Mechler U, Mettler L, et al. The development of laparoscopy—a historical overview. Front Surg. 2021;8:799442.
26. Litynski GS. Kurt Semm and the fight against skepticism: endoscopic hemostasis, laparoscopic appendectomy, and Semm's impact on the "Laparoscopic revolution". JSLS. 1998;2:309–13.
27. Morrell ALG, Morrell-Junior AC, Morrell AG, et al. The history of robotic surgery and its evolution: when illusion becomes reality. Rev Col Bras Cir. 2021;48:e20202798.

28. Kwoh YS, Hou J, Jonckheere EA, et al. A robot with improved absolute positioning accuracy for CT guided stereotactic brain surgery. IEEE Trans Biomed Eng. 1988;35:153–60.
29. Davies BL, Hibberd RD, Ng WS, et al. The development of a surgeon robot for prostatectomies. Proc Inst Mech Eng H. 1991;205:35–8.
30. Lawler RH, West JW, McNulty PH, et al. Homotransplantation of the kidney in the human. JAMA. 1950;144:844–5.
31. Dash SC, Nair R, Behera V. Kidney transplantation: the journey across a century. Med J Armed Forces India. 2023;79:631–7.
32. Research on uterus transplant. University of Gothenburg, https://www.gu.se/en/research/research-on-uterus-transplant. 2020. Accessed 26 Oct 2025.
33. Johannesson L, Richards E, Reddy V, et al. The first 5 years of uterus transplant in the US: a report from the United States uterus transplant consortium. JAMA Surg. 2022;157:790–7.
34. Bradley EA, Woog JJ. Whole eye transplant-the journey begins. JAMA Ophthalmol. 2024;142:897–9.
35. Zhou R, Caspi RR. Ocular immune privilege. F1000 Biol Rep. 2010;2:3.
36. Scientists urged to hold firm to eye transplant goal. JAMA. 1978;240:1227.
37. Aimar A, Palermo A, Innocenti B. The role of 3D printing in medical applications: a state of the art. J Healthc Eng. 2019;2019:5340616.
38. Weng T, Zhang W, Xia Y, et al. 3D bioprinting for skin tissue engineering: current status and perspectives. J Tissue Eng. 2021;12:20417314211028574.
39. Panja N, Maji S, Choudhuri S, et al. 3D bioprinting of human hollow organs. AAPS PharmSciTech. 2022;23:139.
40. Choi PJ, Oskouian RJ, Tubbs RS. Telesurgery: past, present, and future. Cureus. 2018;10:e2716.
41. Marescaux J, Leroy J, Rubino F, et al. Transcontinental robot-assisted remote telesurgery: feasibility and potential applications. Ann Surg. 2002;235:487–92.
42. Licensing and board certification: What residents need to know. American Medical Association. https://www.ama-assn.org/medical-residents/transition-resident-attending/licensing-and-board-certification-what-residents. 2025. Accessed 26 Oct 2025.
43. Nguyen VT, Losee JE. Time- versus competency-based residency training. Plast Reconstr Surg. 2016;138:527.
44. Camison L, Brooker JE, Naran S, et al. The history of surgical education in the United States: past, present, and future. Ann Surg Open. 2022;3:e148.
45. Long DM. Competency-based residency training: the next advance in graduate medical education. Acad Med. 2000;75:1178–83.
46. Wentzell DD, Chung H, Hanson C, et al. Competency-based medical education in ophthalmology residency training: a review. Can J Ophthalmol. 2020;55:12–9.
47. Skjold-Ødegaard B, Søreide K. Competency-based surgical training and entrusted professional activities—perfect match or a procrustean bed? Ann Surg. 2021;273:e173.
48. Mitchell EL. Assessment in the era of competency-based surgical education. Semin Vasc Surg. 2025;38:122–31.
49. McCoy CE, Sayegh J, Alrabah R, et al. Telesimulation: an innovative tool for health professions education. AEM Educ Train. 2017;1:132–6.
50. Okrainec A, Smith L, Azzie G. Surgical simulation in Africa: the feasibility and impact of a 3-day fundamentals of laparoscopic surgery course. Surg Endosc. 2009;23:2493–8.
51. Falcioni AG, Yang HC, Maricic MA, et al. Effectiveness of telesimulation for pediatric minimally invasive surgery essential skills training. J Pediatr Surg. 2022;57:1092–8.
52. Dorey T, Nicholas J, Leydorf SD, et al. Assessing immersive virtual reality as learning tool for surgical trainees. JSLS. 2025;29:e2025.00021.
53. Mao RQ, Lan L, Kay J, et al. Immersive virtual reality for surgical training: a systematic review. J Surg Res. 2021;268:40–58.
54. Yuan W, Zhou X, Meng X, et al. Anterior cervical discectomy and fusion training with virtual reality: enhance cognition, attitudes, self-efficacy and performance in residents. Eur Spine J. 2025;34:2227–38.

55. Suresh D, Aydin A, James S, et al. The role of augmented reality in surgical training: a systematic review. Surg Innov. 2023;30:366–82.
56. The Role of Augmented Reality in Surgical Training: A Narrative Review. Cureus. https://www.cureus.com/articles/419642-the-role-of-augmented-reality-in-surgical-training-a-narrative-review#!/. Accessed 26 Oct 2025.

An Introduction of Lifestyle Medicine

Caitlin Tremewan, Berrin Ergun-Longmire, Dilip R. Patel, and Mark Goetting

Introduction

According to the American College of Lifestyle Medicine,

> Lifestyle medicine is a medical specialty that uses therapeutic lifestyle interventions as a primary modality to treat chronic conditions, including, but not limited to, cardiovascular diseases, type 2 diabetes, and obesity. Lifestyle medicine-certified clinicians are trained to apply evidence-based, whole-person, prescriptive lifestyle changes to treat and, when used intensively, often reverse such conditions. [1].

Lifestyle medicine is distinct in its approach, focusing on evidence-based lifestyle therapeutic interventions for preventing and treating lifestyle-related diseases. This includes a range of chronic conditions, such as cardiovascular diseases, type 2 diabetes, and obesity. The methodology involves personalized lifestyle changes, which become the first line of treatment, with traditional pharmaceutical, medical, and surgical interventions being secondary or adjunctive measures. The field integrates aspects of behavioral medicine, including biobehavioral mechanisms and public health strategies, emphasizing prevention and health promotion. The interdisciplinary nature of lifestyle medicine requires collaboration among various health professionals to develop a comprehensive understanding and integration of biomedical, psychological, and environmental knowledge [2].

The ACLM describes the following six pillars of lifestyle medicine [1].

C. Tremewan · B. Ergun-Longmire · D. R. Patel (✉) · M. Goetting
Western Michigan University Homer Stryker MD School of Medicine, Kalamazoo, MI, USA
e-mail: Caitlin.tremewan@wmed.edu; Berrin.ergun-longmire@wmed.edu; Dilip.patel@wmed.edu; Mark.goetting@wmed.edu

S. S. Chahin et al. (eds.), *Innovation in Medical Education and Clinical Practice*, https://doi.org/10.1007/978-3-032-19116-8_22

"Optimal Nutrition

Poor overall diet quality is the leading cause of premature death in America. Optimal nutrition is essential for the root-cause treatment of chronic conditions. The American College of Lifestyle Medicine recommends an eating pattern based predominantly on a variety of minimally processed vegetables, fruits, whole grains, legumes, nuts, and seeds.

Physical Activity

Regular physical activity is essential for offsetting a sedentary lifestyle, managing chronic conditions, and supporting overall health. Adults should aim for at least 150 min of moderate aerobic and muscle-strengthening activity per week to help prevent issues such as osteoporosis and cardiovascular disease.

Restorative Sleep

Unhealthy sleep is associated with the most common causes of premature death and disability and can lead to an increased risk of impaired memory, dementia, and cardiovascular disease. Quality sleep powerfully supports chronic disease treatment and overall well-being. Adults should strive to create the right conditions to get 7–9 h of quality sleep every night to allow their bodies to rest and repair.

Stress Management

Chronic stress can exacerbate health issues, such as cardiovascular disease, depression, and insulin resistance. Stress management strategies are crucial for overall health and the treatment of chronic diseases.

Connectedness

Meaningful interactions are a key factor in human happiness, longevity, and the treatment of chronic diseases. Strong social connections, as well as a sense of purpose and meaning affect physical, mental, and emotional health and can even reduce the risk of depression and dementia.

Risky Substance Avoidance

Risky substances such as alcohol, tobacco, and other drugs dramatically increase the risk of death and chronic disease and exacerbate the ill effects of disease. Other risky behaviors and exposures can negatively affect mental and physical health. Addressing these behaviors using evidence-based approaches is essential for health restoration."

Rationale for Lifestyle Medicine

The ACLM has described several tenets of lifestyle medicine as rationale for its integration into clinical practice; these include, recognition by professional societies, evidence for lifestyle interventions in preventing and managing several chronic diseases, comprehensive, intentional care, integrated, multidisciplinary and collaborative model of health care delivery and high-value and cost-effective care.

Clinical Applications

In the United States, increasing expenses associated with disease management, preventable hospital admissions, clinician exhaustion, and overuse of medications are indicators of a healthcare system in turmoil. Tackling these issues requires more than just minor adjustments; it necessitates a fundamental transformation in the way we deliver and prioritize healthcare. A high percentage of Americans, including an alarmingly high number of children, suffer from at least one chronic illness, which contributes substantially to annual healthcare expenses shouldered by taxpayers, despite the fact that most of these conditions are manageable.

In the field of lifestyle medicine, a diverse range of clinical practices is primarily focused on tackling chronic illnesses associated with lifestyle decisions. Healthcare practitioners employ strategies such as plant-based nutrition, exercise routines, stress reduction methods such as mindfulness meditation, and education on sleep hygiene to effectively manage these conditions. These strategies often lead to significant improvements in patient outcomes, particularly when combined with traditional treatments. For instance, adopting a plant-based diet has shown promise in reversing conditions such as coronary artery disease (CAD). Exercise programs are advised not only for weight management but also for mental health concerns, such as depression and anxiety, where physical activity has proven to have antidepressant effects. Stress management, including cognitive behavioral techniques, is essential for handling chronic diseases by addressing the emotional and psychological aspects of health that medications alone may not resolve. This discipline also investigates the integration of traditional medicine with complementary approaches, for example, the use of honey for its therapeutic benefits owing to its antibacterial and anti-inflammatory properties. This underscores the field's openness to combining historical practices with modern scientific validation to offer comprehensive patient care.

Clinically, lifestyle medicine is used to prevent, manage, and sometimes reverse chronic illnesses by focusing on changeable health behaviors and environmental influences. It is primarily used in the treatment of cardiovascular conditions, obesity, type 2 diabetes, hypertension, and other non-communicable diseases, while also promoting general health and wellness [3–11]. The interventions in lifestyle medicine emphasize six key areas: nutrition (often plant-based), physical activity, restorative sleep, stress management, avoiding harmful substances, and fostering positive social interactions [1, 3, 4, 12]. These strategies are recommended as the initial treatment for individuals at metabolic risk and are integral to chronic disease management guidelines, such as those from the Endocrine Society and American Heart Association [6, 7].

Intensive lifestyle changes can lower both morbidity and mortality rates, playing a crucial role in cardiac rehabilitation and preventive cardiology [6, 7, 11]. Despite the introduction of anti-obesity drugs and metabolic surgery, lifestyle medicine remains vital and is endorsed in top-tier guidelines for weight loss and maintenance [8]. For managing type 2 diabetes and metabolic syndrome, lifestyle modification is the primary approach for reducing risks and managing the disease [7]. Interventions involving diet, physical activity, stress reduction, and sleep improvement are effective for preventing and complementing the treatment of hypertension [11]. Research also indicates that lifestyle interventions offer benefits in preventing cancer, stroke, dementia, and Parkinson's disease [10, 13]. Furthermore, lifestyle medicine is gaining recognition for its importance in medical education, workplace health, and transforming health systems, with the goal of addressing the underlying causes of diseases and reducing healthcare expenses [3, 14].

In various clinical environments, lifestyle medicine is used to tackle the root behaviors contributing to chronic diseases, enhance patient outcomes, and decrease dependence on medications and procedures [15–23]. Interventions in lifestyle medicine, which include dietary changes, physical exercise, and behavioral counseling, are well supported by randomized controlled trials and meta-analyses for both preventing and managing type 2 diabetes and cardiovascular disease [15–23]. These interventions are recommended as either primary or supplementary treatments in key clinical guidelines [15–18]. For prevention type 2 diabetes, significant RCTs, such as the Da Qing, Finnish Diabetes Prevention Study, and US Diabetes Prevention Program, have consistently demonstrated that structured lifestyle changes can lower the incidence of T2D by 30–58% over 3–6 years in individuals at high risk. Long-term follow-up indicates ongoing reductions in diabetes and atherosclerotic cardiovascular disease (ASCVD) events for many years after the intervention [15, 16]. The American Diabetes Association endorses programs based on the National Diabetes Prevention Program, aiming for a weight loss of ≥7% and at least 150 min of moderate-intensity exercise weekly [16]. Regarding cardiovascular disease risk reduction, meta-analyses and systematic reviews have verified that behavioral counseling and lifestyle changes decrease composite CVD events in adults with risk factors such as hypertension, dyslipidemia, or metabolic syndrome [19–21]. The PREDIMED RCT and other studies support the Mediterranean diet and similar eating patterns for primary prevention [15]. Prospective cohort data reveal a dose-response relationship: each additional healthy lifestyle behavior further diminishes the risk of CVD and mortality [22, 23]. Lifestyle changes also enhance intermediate outcomes, such as reducing blood pressure, LDL cholesterol, weight, and fasting glucose, within 12–24 months of follow-up. In type 2 diabetes, the Look AHEAD trial discovered that intensive lifestyle changes resulted in more significant weight loss, better glycemic control, and certain cardiovascular benefits, particularly in those who achieved notable weight loss or fitness improvements [21, 24]. Sustained weight loss of ≥5% enhances glycemic control, and a reduction of ≥15% can lead to diabetes remission in several patients [18]. The most compelling evidence supports lifestyle medicine as a fundamental approach for preventing and managing type 2 diabetes and cardiovascular disease, with significant and lasting benefits shown in high-quality trials and meta-analyses.

Challenges

There are several limitations in applying the principles of lifestyle medicine in clinical practice, including uncertainty regarding the best dietary composition, difficulties in maintaining long-term adherence, and inconsistent evidence concerning the reduction of all-cause mortality. More research is necessary in various US populations and on methods to sustain lifestyle changes over time [18, 21].

Lifestyle medicine often encounters the difficulty of integrating its methods into conventional healthcare systems, which predominantly rely on pharmaceutical, medical and surgical approaches. To bolster the evidence supporting lifestyle interventions, expanded research and more stringent clinical trials are required. As the discipline progresses, there is an increasing demand for standardized guidelines and protocols to ensure the uniform application of practices across various environments and to aid in the training of healthcare professionals in this specialized field. Lifestyle medicine is steadily advancing as an essential component of healthcare, offering the promise of a more sustainable preventive health model that focuses on empowering patients to adopt healthier lifestyles. Although the field is making progress with innovations in patient care delivery models, it also necessitates a paradigm shift among healthcare professionals and patients in their perceptions and management of health and wellness. This all-encompassing approach not only results in improved health outcomes but also aligns with the growing focus on holistic and patient-centered care in contemporary healthcare [25]. Compared to traditional medical methods, lifestyle medicine provides several benefits in terms of cost-effectiveness and long-term results, especially for chronic conditions such as diabetes and cardiovascular diseases.

Cost-effective lifestyle medicine interventions are typically cost-effective because they emphasize prevention and long-term lifestyle changes, which can decrease the necessity for expensive medical treatments and hospital stays. For instance, lifestyle interventions aimed at preventing diabetes, which involve changes in diet and physical activity, have proven cost-effective, with certain programs showing favorable cost-effectiveness ratios [26]. In managing diabetes, lifestyle changes have shown improvements in cardiovascular risk factors and are expected to lower lifetime cardiovascular morbidity, often at a reasonable cost [27]. Moreover, a lifestyle intervention program based on primary care, which included supervised exercise and dietary counseling, demonstrated enhancements in quality of life and was found to be highly cost-effective compared to standard care, with notable gains in quality-adjusted life-years (QALYs) [28].

In context of long-term results, lifestyle medicine focuses on maintaining behavioral changes that result in lasting health improvements. Strategies that include health coaching and positive psychology have been demonstrated to boost outcomes by facilitating behavior modification, which in turn enhances physical, social, and emotional well-being [29, 30]. Additionally, interventions aimed at lifestyle-related illnesses frequently report enduring advantages in terms of quality of life and reduced health care expenses. For example, senior gatherings and preventive home visits for the elderly have proven cost-effective, yielding QALY gains and decreasing societal costs over a span of 4 years [31].

Adherence to lifestyle medicine, which focuses on behavioral changes such as diet and physical activity, often encounters adherence challenges. Achieving successful adherence in this area largely depends on patient involvement and self-management. For example, interventions for type 2 diabetes (T2D) that involve strict lifestyle changes can lead to remission but necessitate adherence to low-calorie diets for meaningful results [32]. Despite these limitations, lifestyle interventions can be highly effective if patients adhere to them. Programs frequently include health coaching, nutritional education, and support networks to enhance their adherence. For instance, kitchen-based nutrition education significantly boosted adherence to the Mediterranean dietary pattern among medical trainees by combining dietary education with practical experience [33]. In contrast, traditional medical treatments, especially those involving medications, often face nonadherence issues due to factors such as side effects, complicated regimens, and cost. Medication adherence is a well-known challenge, with many patients not consistently following prescribed regimens, leading to less-than-optimal outcomes [33]. Additionally, adherence to mental health treatments, such as antidepressants, is often poor, with factors such as patient readiness and collaboration with healthcare providers affecting adherence rates [34]. Telemedicine and telehealth platforms provide continuous care and help overcome barriers related to distance and time. They support routine follow-ups and allow providers to monitor patients remotely, thereby promoting adherence by offering accessible and timely health intervention [35, 36]. Mobile health applications serve various purposes, such as sending medication reminders, tracking symptoms, and providing educational information. These apps assist patients in adhering to lifestyle changes and managing chronic conditions effectively by gamifying health tasks and offering real-time feedback [37].

Fitness trackers and smartwatches, among other wearable devices, are used to track physical activity, sleep habits, and various health metrics. These gadgets offer users immediate insights into their health and behaviors, promoting adherence through consistent feedback and goal setting [38]. Devices such as activity trackers, continuous glucose monitors, and smartwatches deliver instant feedback on exercise, nutrition, sleep, and physiological data. This feedback aids patients in self-monitoring and modifying their behaviors, which is linked to increased physical activity, better dietary practices, and improved cardiometabolic health [40, 41]. Meta-analyses indicate that interventions using wearables can significantly boost daily step counts, lower systolic blood pressure, reduce waist size, and decrease LDL cholesterol in individuals with chronic conditions such as diabetes and cardiovascular disease [40, 41]. Wearable devices enhance adherence to lifestyle medicine interventions for chronic illnesses, such as type 2 diabetes and cardiovascular disease, by facilitating real-time self-monitoring, personalized feedback, goal-setting, and increased patient involvement. Wearable technology and digital health tools improve adherence to lifestyle medicine interventions by empowering self-management, offering actionable feedback, and supporting personalized and scalable care for the prevention and management of chronic diseases [39–45].

Remote patient monitoring systems collect health data from patients at home and transmit them to healthcare providers. These systems enhance adherence by ensuring consistent monitoring and enabling early interventions when necessary [35]. Digital therapeutics utilize mobile applications and digital platforms to provide evidence-based therapeutic interventions. They emphasize lifestyle changes, such as mindfulness, meditation, and self-care practices, often in conjunction with traditional pharmacological treatments to boost adherence [39]. Customizing treatment plans based on genetic profiles and individual health traits ensures more effective treatment, thereby improving adherence. Digital health technologies can facilitate personalized interventions by integrating various patient data to optimize treatment plans [36]. Patient portals and electronic health record platforms offer patients easy access to their health information, promoting better communication with healthcare providers and empowering patients to take an active role in managing their health [37].

The integration of mobile health applications and digital platforms enhances adherence by providing personalized recommendations, reminders, and behavioral coaching. For instance, digital health programs that combine wearable data with behavioral insights and goal setting have shown improvements in glycemic control, weight loss, and healthy eating habits in both diabetic and non-diabetic populations [42, 43] The American Diabetes Association emphasizes that incorporating technology into comprehensive care models—such as telehealth and remote monitoring—can enhance diabetes self-management and outcomes, particularly when paired with education and coaching [44]. Technology helps address adherence barriers by improving accessibility, supporting remote care, and facilitating communication between patients and healthcare teams. The American Heart Association has pointed out that technology-enabled interventions can help reduce disparities in cardiovascular health by offering scalable and affordable solutions for populations with limited healthcare access [45, 46]. The success of technology depends on its integration with educational support, personalized feedback, and continuous engagement strategies. Not all studies show consistent benefits, and challenges such as digital literacy, cost, and sustained engagement persist [43, 46, 47].

Children and Adolescents

Lifestyle factors are modifiable elements that influence the overall health of children and adolescents. Health-related lifestyle choices will have the greatest impact in the prevention of chronic diseases when such interventions are implemented in childhood and adolescence.

Obesity is a widely used measure of health in children and adolescents, and studies have consistently shown that it is associated with lifestyle factors. Across studies, low physical activity and sedentary lifestyle were most related to obesity regardless of gender or geographic location [48–51]. Nutrition as a lifestyle factor has a more varied association with obesity. For example, a 2024 study conducted on U.S. children aged 6–15 years old found no statistically significant difference in caloric or nutritional intake between normal weight and overweight/obese children [1]. Further statistical analysis with Lasso regression however, showed a positive association between higher protein intake and higher caffeine intake and being overweight or obese [48]. Another study conducted in Indonesia in 2021 found that high-fat diets were associated with increased risk of adolescent obesity, and the intake of more fruits or vegetables and fewer sweets was not protective against obesity if a high-fat diet was consumed [50]. Other studies found Mediterranean diets to be negatively associated with obesity, while low vegetable intake and high red meat and soda intake were positively associated with obesity [49, 52, 53]. Thus, each study found associations between obesity and nutrition, despite using different dietary measures. Alternatively, a 2024 study by H. Lim and H. Lee focused on how eating habits relate to childhood obesity [51]. This study found that in South Korean children aged 5–6 years, slow eaters had the lowest BMI, whereas fast eaters had the highest BMI. Therefore, both nutrition and eating habits are associated with childhood obesity. Although lifestyle factors are often associated with lower risk for obesity in the literature, in a 2024 study, lifestyle factors were found not to moderate the association between early-life stress exposure and psycho-physical comorbidities in adolescence [54]. Therefore, although lifestyle factors are widely found to independently contribute to improved health outcomes, they do not appear to attenuate the negative effects of early life stress.

In addition to the strong association between lifestyle factors and obesity, other measures of physical health are similarly affected. In a small study out of Japan, physical activity and health awareness were associated with higher bone density in female high school students [55]. Health awareness included knowledge of bone density and self-reported consciousness of personal health. The overall nutritional intake status was not significantly different between the groups; however, participants in the high bone density group reported significantly higher intake of green leafy vegetables, calcium, and vitamin D. Although the study found a statistically significant difference in weight between the high and low bone density groups, the mean BMI in both groups was within the normal range. Therefore, although weight often affects bone density, the statistical difference found in this study may be due to the limited study size. Overall, this study highlights the importance of physical activity as a lifestyle factor that impacts bone health in adolescent females. The association between lifestyle factors and dry eye disease in children was examined in a 2022 study [56]. The study found that increased screen exposure was associated with increased odds of dry eye disease, whereas increased sleep each day was associated with decreased odds. Other lifestyle factors, including physical activity, diet quality, and mental health status, were not associated with pediatric dry eye disease in this study.

Mental health is integral to the overall health of children and adolescents. Studies consistently show that poor sleep quality and short sleep duration are significantly associated with mental health problems or stress in the pediatric population [57–59]. Healthy diet and eating breakfast 5–7 days per week were negatively associated with mental health problems [10, 11]. In a 2021 study on Mongolian elementary school children, no physical activity and long screen time were associated with increased risk of mental health problems [58]. In contrast, a 2022 study focusing on Norwegian adolescents found no statistically significant association between leisure physical activity level and mental health problems [57]. Mental health is both a measure of health and a lifestyle factor that contributes to overall health. Consequently, causality versus effect is difficult to discern in this research. Does a lack of healthy lifestyle factors lead to problems with mental health, or is poor mental health the cause of an unhealthy lifestyle? The answer is likely to be nuanced.

Emerging research highlights the significant role of lifestyle factors in shaping children's overall health. In a study examining the health status of children from various Chinese provinces, children with tobacco use, alcohol use, poor sleep quality and duration, high stress, unhealthy diet, and low exercise had a higher prevalence of suboptimal health status [60]. Another study from 2023 found that adolescents aged 11–20 years old were more likely to have improved health-related quality of life if they had higher lifestyle scores based on a composite of lifestyle factors such as smoking, drinking, sleep duration, internet use, and physical activity [61]. Thus, the presence of multiple healthy lifestyle factors is associated with better health than the presence of one. Sociodemographic factors such as income level, parental educational level, geographic location, ethnicity, and sex also play a major role in overall health outcomes. These factors have substantial interplay with health promoting lifestyle choices.

Addressing modifiable lifestyle factors rather than sociodemographic characteristics presents a more practical opportunity for early health intervention. Bernardo et al. evaluated the efficacy of school-based wellness programs on physiological health of middle-schoolers in Michigan [62]. Prior to beginning the Project Healthy

Schools curriculum, students with abnormal blood pressure were more likely to be obese, have worse cardiometabolic health, drink more soda, and spend more time watching TV or playing video games. The consumption of fruits, vegetables, and fried foods, as well as the physical activity levels, were similar between the normal and abnormal blood pressure groups. Following a curriculum of ten lessons focusing on a healthy diet, regular physical exercise, and reduced screen time, all students showed improvements in cardiometabolic health and physical activity levels, regardless of their initial blood pressure readings. Additionally, students with initial abnormal blood pressures had significant improvements in systolic and diastolic pressures, with over half of these individuals improving to normal blood pressure. Ultimately, this study suggests that programs targeting lifestyle interventions are effective in improving certain health measures in the pediatric population. Increased research with larger sample sizes in pediatric populations will be important in strengthening our understanding of the contribution of lifestyle factors to human health and disease; however, there is significant evidence to suggest that the contribution is notable.

Conclusion

Although lifestyle medicine requires significant initial buy-in and a sustained commitment to change, it often results in more holistic and long-term health benefits. Online and digital health interventions have begun to enhance adherence by providing more accessible and convenient support. These technologies help maintain patient engagement and adherence over time, potentially surpassing traditional methods in terms of effectiveness. Conversely, traditional medical treatments may offer more structured plans with clearer, immediate expectations, which may be easier for some patients to follow but may lack the comprehensive benefits of lifestyle interventions. In summary, while both lifestyle medicine and traditional treatments have adherence challenges, lifestyle medicine may offer better long-term outcomes by promoting sustained behavioral changes and patient empowerment, particularly when supported by innovative interventions such as health coaching and digital health solutions. Patient adherence rates to lifestyle medicine interventions compared to traditional medical treatments present a nuanced picture, influenced by factors such as personal motivation, accessibility, and the nature of the interventions.

Acknowledgements Online PubMed database was used for literature search. Paperpal tool was used for additional search and editing the manuscript.

References

1. https://lifestylemedicine.org/about-lifestyle-medicine/. Accessed 26 Nov 2025.
2. Dekker J, Stauder A, Penedo FJ. Proposal for an update of the definition and scope of behavioral medicine. Int J Behav Med. 2017;24(1):1–4.
3. Hymel PA, Stave GM, Burton WN, et al. Incorporating lifestyle medicine into occupational medicine practice: ACOEM guidance statement. J Occup Environ Med. 2025;67(1):e72–84.
4. Parkinson MD, Stout R, Dysinger W. Lifestyle medicine: prevention, treatment, and reversal of disease. Med Clin North Am. 2023;107(6):1109–20.
5. Kushner RF, Sorensen KW. Lifestyle medicine: the future of chronic disease management. Curr Opin Endocrinol Diabetes Obes. 2013;20(5):389–95.
6. Hivert MF, Arena R, Forman DE, et al. Medical training to achieve competency in lifestyle counseling: an essential foundation for prevention and treatment of cardiovascular diseases and other chronic medical conditions: a scientific statement from the American Heart Association. Circulation. 2016;134(15):e308–27.
7. Rosenzweig JL, Bakris GL, Berglund LF, et al. Primary prevention of ASCVD and T2DM in patients at metabolic risk: an endocrine society* clinical practice guideline. J Clin Endocrinol Metab. 2019;104(9):3939–85.
8. Sannidhi D, Abeles R, Andrew W, et al. Lifestyle medicine for obesity in the era of highly effective anti-obesity treatment. Nutrients. 2025;17(14):2382.
9. Rozanski A, Blumenthal JA, Hinderliter AL, Cole S, Lavie CJ. Cardiology and lifestyle medicine. Prog Cardiovasc Dis. 2023;77:4–13.
10. Katz DL, Frates EP, Bonnet JP, et al. Lifestyle as medicine: the case for a true health initiative. Am J Health Promot. 2018;32(6):1452–8.
11. Valenzuela PL, Carrera-Bastos P, Gálvez BG, et al. Lifestyle interventions for the prevention and treatment of hypertension. Nat Rev Cardiol. 2021;18(4):251–75.
12. Phillips EM, Frates EP, Park DJ. Lifestyle medicine. Phys Med Rehabil Clin N Am. 2020;31(4):515–26.
13. Süß P, Regensburger M, Gassner H, Winkler J. Lifestyle medicine in Parkinson's disease. J Neural Transm (Vienna, Austria: 1996). 2025:10.1007/s00702-025-03059-y. https://doi.org/10.1007/s00702-025-03059-y.
14. Trilk J, Nelson L, Briggs A, Muscato D. Including lifestyle medicine in medical education: rationale for American College of Preventive Medicine/American Medical Association resolution 959. Am J Prev Med. 2019;56(5):e169–75. https://doi.org/10.1016/j.amepre.2018.10.034.
15. Brennan J, Phelps K, McGrady A, Schultz P. Introducing lifestyle medicine into family medicine: theory and applications. Int J Psychiatry Med. 2024;59(4):415–23.
16. Stancic S, Cullimore J, Barnard N. Six applications of plant based diets for health promotion. Am J Lifestyle Med. 2022;16(4):434–8.
17. Joseph JJ, Deedwania P, Acharya T, et al. Comprehensive management of cardiovascular risk factors for adults with type 2 diabetes: a scientific statement from the American Heart Association. Circulation. 2022;145(9):e722–59.
18. Ahmad E, Lim S, Lamptey R, Webb DR, Davies MJ. Type 2 diabetes. Lancet (London, England). 2022;400(10365):1803–20.
19. O'Connor EA, Evans CV, Rushkin MC, Redmond N, Lin JS. Behavioral counseling to promote a healthy diet and physical activity for cardiovascular disease prevention in adults with cardiovascular risk factors: updated evidence report and systematic review for the US Preventive Services Task Force. JAMA. 2020;324(20):2076–94.
20. Demissie GD, Birungi J, Shrestha A, et al. The effectiveness of lifestyle interventions in reducing cardiovascular risk and risk factors in people with prediabetes: a systematic review and meta-analysis. Nutr Metab Cardiovasc Dis. 2025:104130. https://doi.org/10.1016/j.numecd.2025.104130.
21. US Preventive Services Task Force, Krist AH, Davidson KW, et al. Behavioral counseling interventions to promote a healthy diet and physical activity for cardiovascular disease

prevention in adults with cardiovascular risk factors: US preventive services task force recommendation statement. JAMA. 2020;324(20):2069–75.
22. Wu J, Feng Y, Zhao Y, et al. Lifestyle behaviors and risk of cardiovascular disease and prognosis among individuals with cardiovascular disease: a systematic review and meta-analysis of 71 prospective cohort studies. Int J Behav Nutr Phys Act. 2024;21(1):42.
23. Liu G, Li Y, Hu Y, et al. Influence of lifestyle on incident cardiovascular disease and mortality in patients with diabetes mellitus. J Am Coll Cardiol. 2018;71(25):2867–76.
24. Mangione CM, Barry MJ, Nicholson WK, et al. Behavioral counseling interventions to promote a healthy diet and physical activity for cardiovascular disease prevention in adults without cardiovascular disease risk factors: US preventive services task force recommendation statement. JAMA. 2022;328(4):367–74.
25. Hashim MJ. A definition of family medicine and general practice. J Coll Physicians Surg Pak. 2018;28(1):76–7.
26. Saha S, Gerdtham U-G, Johansson P. Economic evaluation of lifestyle interventions for preventing diabetes and cardiovascular diseases. Int J Environ Res Public Health. 2010;7(8):3150–95.
27. Jacobs-Van Der Bruggen MAM, Van Baal PH, Hoogenveen RT, Feenstra TL, Briggs AH, Lawson K, Feskens EJM, Baan CA. Cost-effectiveness of lifestyle modification in diabetic patients. Diabetes Care. 2009;32(8):1453–8.
28. Eriksson MK, Malmgren-Olsson E-B, Österlind J, Hagberg L, Lindholm L, Eliasson M. Quality of life and cost-effectiveness of a 3-year trial of lifestyle intervention in primary health care. Arch Intern Med. 2010;170(16) https://doi.org/10.1001/archinternmed.2010.301.
29. Conn S, Curtain S. Health coaching as a lifestyle medicine process in primary care. Aust J Gen Pract. 2019;48(10):677–80.
30. Lianov LS, Krishnaswami J, Wallace A, Barron C, Fredrickson BL. Positive psychology in lifestyle medicine and health care: strategies for implementation. Am J Lifestyle Med. 2019;13(5):480–6.
31. Zingmark M, Norström F, Lindholm L, Dahlin-Ivanoff S, Gustafsson S. Modelling long-term cost-effectiveness of health promotion for community-dwelling older people. Eur J Ageing. 2019;16(4):395–404.
32. Kelly J, Karlsen M, Steinke G. Type 2 diabetes remission and lifestyle medicine: a position statement from the American College of Lifestyle Medicine. Am J Lifestyle Med. 2020;14(4):406–19.
33. Razavi AC, Ross A, Schlag E, Akhiwu O, Mccormack IG, Harlan TS, Sarris L, Sapin A, Schradle K, Dyer A, Hamilton L, Dotson K, Mcwhorter JW, Stauber Z, Gagen B, Monlezun DJ. Multisite culinary medicine curriculum is associated with cardioprotective dietary patterns and lifestyle medicine competencies among medical trainees. Am J Lifestyle Med. 2020;14(2):225–33.
34. Gonzalez J, Williams JW, Lee S, Noel PH. Adherence to mental health treatment in a primary care clinic. J Am Board Fam Med. 2005;18(2):87–96.
35. Liu J-C, Cheng C-Y, Cheng T-H, Liu C-N, Chen J-J, Hao W-R. Unveiling the potential: remote monitoring and telemedicine in shaping the future of heart failure management. Life (Basel, Switzerland). 2024;14(8):936. https://doi.org/10.3390/life14080936.
36. Sugandh F, Khatri M, Raveena F, Bai K, Varrassi G, Kumar S, Chandio M, Kashif M, Memon UA, Kumar L, Karishma F, Khuwaja S. Advances in the management of diabetes mellitus: a focus on personalized medicine. Cureus. 2023;15(8) https://doi.org/10.7759/cureus.43697.
37. Heudel PE, Ait Ichou M, Favier B, Crochet H, Blay J-Y. Can digital health improve therapeutic compliance in oncology? JCO Clin Cancer Inform. 2024;8(8) https://doi.org/10.1200/cci-24-00205.
38. Thacharodi A, Singh P, Meenatchi R, Tawfeeq Ahmed ZH, Kumar RRS, V N, Kavish S, Maqbool M, Hassan S. Revolutionizing healthcare and medicine: the impact of modern technologies for a healthier future-a comprehensive review. Health Care Sci. 2024;3(5):329–49.

39. Bulaj G, Clark J, Ebrahimi M, Bald E. From precision metapharmacology to patient empowerment: delivery of self-care practices for epilepsy, pain, depression and cancer using digital health technologies. Front Pharmacol. 2021;12(10) https://doi.org/10.3389/fphar.2021.612602.
40. Franssen WMA, Franssen GHLM, Spaas J, Solmi F, Eijnde BO. Can consumer wearable activity tracker-based interventions improve physical activity and cardiometabolic health in patients with chronic diseases? A systematic review and meta-analysis of randomized controlled trials. Int J Behav Nutr Phys Act. 2020;17(1):57.
41. Hodkinson A, Kontopantelis E, Adeniji C, et al. Interventions using wearable physical activity trackers among adults with cardiometabolic conditions: a systematic review and meta-analysis. JAMA Netw Open. 2021;4(7):e2116382.
42. Zahedani AD, McLaughlin T, Veluvali A, et al. Digital health application integrating wearable data and behavioral patterns improves metabolic health. NPJ Digit Med. 2023;6(1):216.
43. Kamei T, Kanamori T, Yamamoto Y, Edirippulige S. The use of wearable devices in chronic disease management to enhance adherence and improve telehealth outcomes: a systematic review and meta-analysis. J Telemed Telecare. 2022;28(5):342–59.
44. Davies MJ, Aroda VR, Collins BS, et al. Management of hyperglycemia in type 2 diabetes, 2022. A consensus report by the American Diabetes Association (ADA) and the European Association for the Study of Diabetes (EASD). Diabetes Care. 2022;45(11):2753–86.
45. Powell-Wiley TM, Brewer LC, Burke LE, et al. Role of technology in promoting heart healthy behavior change to increase equity in optimal cardiovascular health: a scientific statement from the American Heart Association. Circulation. 2025;151(18):e972–85.
46. Alipour P, El-Aghil M, Foo A, Azizi Z. Leveraging mobile health and wearable technologies for the prevention and management of atherosclerotic cardiovascular disease. Curr Atheroscler Rep. 2025;27(1):31.
47. Mattison G, Canfell O, Forrester D, et al. The influence of wearables on health care outcomes in chronic disease: systematic review. J Med Internet Res. 2022;24(7):e36690. https://doi.org/10.2196/36690.
48. Qu Y, Xu W, Guo S, Wu H. Association of sociodemographic and lifestyle factors and dietary intake with overweight and obesity among U.S. children: findings from NHANES. BMC Public Health. 2024;24(1):2176.
49. Francisco López-Gil J, Chen S, López-Bueno R, Gutiérrez-Espinoza H, Angelo Duarte Junior M, Galan-Lopez P, et al. Prevalence of obesity and associated sociodemographic and lifestyle factors in Ecuadorian children and adolescents. 2025; https://doi.org/10.1038/s41390-024-03342-w.
50. Agustina R, Meilianawati, Fenny, Atmarita, Suparmi, Susiloretni KA, et al. Psychosocial, eating behavior, and lifestyle factors influencing overweight and obesity in adolescents. Food Nutr Bull. 2021;42(1_suppl):S72–91.
51. Lim H, Lee H. Eating habits and lifestyle factors related to childhood obesity among children aged 5-6 years: cluster analysis of panel survey data in Korea. JMIR Public Health Surveill. 2024;10:e51581. https://pmc.ncbi.nlm.nih.gov/articles/PMC11031700/
52. Pavlidou E, Papadopoulou SK, Alexatou O, Voulgaridou G, Mentzelou M, Biskanaki F, et al. Childhood Mediterranean diet adherence is associated with lower prevalence of childhood obesity, specific sociodemographic, and lifestyle factors: a cross-sectional study in pre-school children. Epidemiologia. 2024;5(1):11–28.
53. Parra KL, Alaofe HS, Ehiri JE, Nuño VL, Mazariegos M, Garcia B, et al. Prevalence and determinants of underweight, overweight, and obesity: a cross-sectional study of sociodemographic, dietary, and lifestyle factors among adolescent girls in Jutiapa, Guatemala. Food Nutr Bull. 2021;42(4):502.
54. Defina S, Woofenden T, Baltramonaityte V, Tiemeier H, Fairchild G, Felix JF, et al. The role of lifestyle factors in the association between early-life stress and adolescent psycho-physical health: moderation analysis in two European birth cohorts. Prev Med Baltim. 182. https://pubmed.ncbi.nlm.nih.gov/38447658/

55. Yoshihara K, Kawasaki H, Cui Z, Nakaoka S. Lifestyle factors and health awareness for improving bone density acquisition in adolescent girls: a pilot study with secondary data. Cureus. 2024;16(1) https://pubmed.ncbi.nlm.nih.gov/38344566/
56. Wang MTM, Craig JP, Vidal-Rohr M, Menduni F, Dhallu S, Ipek T, et al. Impact of digital screen use and lifestyle factors on dry eye disease in the paediatric population. Ocul Surf. 2022;24:64–6.
57. Barene S, Ruud-Tronsmoen A, Johansen PF. Associations between demographic characteristics, lifestyle factors and school-related conditions and symptoms of mental health problems in Norwegian upper secondary school students. Int J Environ Res Public Health. 2022;19(15):9575.
58. Lee J, Ko YH, Chi S, Lee MS, Yoon HK. Impact of the COVID-19 pandemic on Korean adolescents' mental health and lifestyle factors. J Adolesc Health [Internet]. 2022;71(3):270.
59. Aoki A, Togoobaatar G, Tseveenjav A, Nyam N, Zuunnast K, Lkhagvasuren G, et al. Socioeconomic and lifestyle factors associated with mental health problems among Mongolian elementary school children. Soc Psychiatry Psychiatr Epidemiol. 2021;57(4):791.
60. Xu T, Liu J, Zhu G, Han S. Prevalence and associated lifestyle factors of suboptimal health status among Chinese children using a multi-level model. Int J Environ Res Public Health. 2020;17(5):1497.
61. Xiang H, Feng X, Lin L, Luo S, Liu X, Chen D, et al. Association between healthy lifestyle factors and health-related quality of life among Chinese adolescents: the moderating role of gender. Health Qual Life Outcomes. 2023;21(1):119.
62. Bernardo S, Krallman R, Kline-Rogers E, Montgomery D, Brown AM, DuRussel-Weston J, et al. Physiological and lifestyle factors associated with abnormal blood pressure in adolescents before and after a school-based wellness program in Michigan: a report from project healthy schools. J Adolesc Health. 2021;69(1):127–33.

Technological or Treatment Innovation in Medical Subspecialties

Matthew Krinock, Bradley Christensen, and Lisa Miller

Introduction

Across surgical subspecialties, innovation is redefining how we diagnose, treat, and care for patients. Orthopedics, obstetrics and gynecology, cardiothoracic surgery, ophthalmology, otolaryngology, and urology each illustrate the broader shift toward care that is less invasive, more precise, and increasingly personalized. Advances in robotics are expanding the boundaries of what surgeons can safely achieve, while new imaging tools and digital health platforms are transforming the way diseases are detected and monitored. Breakthroughs in biomaterials, gene therapy, and regenerative medicine are creating opportunities not only to repair but to restore function. These developments emerge in response to long-standing challenges, such as implant durability, diagnostic delays, surgical morbidity, and limited access to specialized care, and are reshaping both the operating room and the clinic. Taken together, they point toward a future in which surgical practice is defined not just by technical skill, but by the integration of technology, biology, and patient-centered innovation.

Orthopedics

The field of orthopedics has experienced particular benefit in moving toward a more patient-specific approach to care. Key advancements in additive manufacturing promise the potential for personalized implant design, while rapid discoveries in materials science support better long-term implant viability. Robotic systems

M. Krinock · B. Christensen · L. Miller (✉)
Western Michigan University Homer Stryker MD School of Medicine, Kalamazoo, MI, USA
e-mail: matthew.krinock@wmed.edu; bradley.christensen@wmed.edu; lisa.miller@wmed.edu

S. S. Chahin et al. (eds.), *Innovation in Medical Education and Clinical Practice*, https://doi.org/10.1007/978-3-032-19116-8_23

continue to enhance surgical accuracy while expanding use cases. Additionally, emerging biologic treatments in the studies of gene and stem cell therapy are opening new treatment pathways promoting natural healing in degenerative joint diseases.

Additive manufacturing (AM), also known as 3D printing, is transforming how orthopedic implants are designed and fabricated. Utilizing AM allows for unique, patient-specific implant design which contributes to improved biomechanical integration of implants for patients. Additionally, the process of AM allows for improved microscopic structures of implants, allowing them to more closely follow the natural porous architecture of bone. Lattice structures provide better osteointegration compared to solid implants [1, 2]. These factors contribute to better implant integration, biological adoption, new bone growth, and implant longevity [3].

The search for better materials is also driven by the limitations of conventional options. Traditional implant materials such as metals such as stainless steel or titanium can cause long-term adverse effects including metal-on-metal wear, consequent inflammatory responses, swelling, and discomfort [1, 4]. Polymers such as polylactic acid (PLA) or polyether ether ketone (PEEK) and ceramics are increasingly used to reduce these adverse effects [5, 6]. Additionally, new surface coatings, such as diamond-like carbon and hydroxyapatite, facilitate osteointegration, improve bacteriostatic properties, and promote osteogenesis. These materials may directly benefit the long-term viability of implants and reduce the need for reoperation [7].

Complementing material and AM innovations are advancements in robotic surgical technology. Robot-assisted platforms for total knee arthroplasty (TKA) and shoulder arthroplasty offer improved surgical performance, efficiency, and accuracy through mapped feedback mechanisms [8]. These platforms have been shown to offer better component alignment, prosthesis positioning, and lower pain scores with improved physical function post-operatively [9, 10].

The ROSA robotic system was recently approved for shoulder arthroplasty in February of 2024, potentially bringing the benefits of robotic assisted TKA to another common orthopedic procedure. This technology is still in its infancy, and adoption across institutions, as well as review of emerging clinical data, is required before widespread adoption [11].Recent implementation of artificial intelligence within these systems potentially offers further benefit by providing higher diagnostic accuracy and more efficient surgical planning. AI models can analyze a surgeon's operative patterns to create predictive models that adjust implant planning, significantly reducing the number of corrections necessary in a patient- and surgeon-specific manner [12].

Alongside technological innovations, emerging biologic treatments offer promise toward promoting tissue regeneration and modulating the inflammatory response in certain disease processes. For osteoarthritis, a recent Phase 1 clinical trial found that a single affected-joint injection of an adeno-associated virus (scAAV) vector delivering IL-1RA, a natural anti-inflammatory protein, resulted in sustained local expression of IL-1RA for over a year with reported improvements in pain and function scores [13].

Mesenchymal stem cells (MSCs) also offer immense potential for orthopedic applications. MSCs possess the ability to differentiate into specific host tissue-lines, such as chondrocytes and osteoblasts, while also having direct paracrine effects on neighboring cells promoting local tissue growth and healing. When incorporated into patient-specific 3D-printed implants, these attributes of MSCs offer strong promise of improved recovery and patient outcomes [14–16]. Additionally, an early phase randomized controlled trial demonstrated the safety and efficacy of MSC injections in the management of knee osteoarthritis, revealing statistically significant and reproducible treatment effects over placebo in the domains of knee pain and function [17].

In summary, innovations in orthopedics are creating a new standard of care where patient-specific 3D-printed implants enhance osteointegration, robotic systems provide unparalleled surgical precision, and biologic options like gene therapy and MSCs offer the potential to regenerate tissue and treat the underlying causes of degenerative joint disease.

Obstetrics and Gynecology

Innovations in obstetrics and gynecology over the last few years include emerging technologies transforming clinical care, diagnostics, and surgical planning. Digital health tools, including telehealth, mobile health applications, and wearable sensors, are expanding access to antenatal care and enabling personalized monitoring outside the clinic. In reproductive medicine, artificial intelligence is refining morphokinetic embryo assessment in IVF, improving prediction of viability and pregnancy outcomes. AI applications in ultrasound and MRI are also enhancing the detection and characterization of gynecologic pathologies such as endometriosis, fibroids, and malignancies, supporting earlier diagnosis and tailored treatment planning. Meanwhile, 3D printing is reshaping surgical preparation and education through patient-specific anatomical models, oncologic planning aids, and realistic training simulations, with ongoing exploration of custom prostheses. These innovations are transforming women's health by driving more precise, accessible, and personalized care.

Advances in digital health technologies are transforming antenatal care through telehealth, mobile health (mHealth) applications, and wearable devices that enable remote monitoring, patient education, and care coordination. Telehealth platforms now support virtual consultations and monitoring of maternal parameters, with emerging tools like tele-ultrasound and continuous wearable sensors showing feasibility and high satisfaction without compromising outcomes [18, 19]. Health interventions like apps, SMS reminders, and interactive helpdesks, have improved visit attendance, education, and preparedness, particularly in low-resource settings [20, 21]. Wearable sensors capable of tracking maternal vitals and fetal heart rate outside clinics are advancing, though there are still challenges with adherence, data reliability, and privacy [19]. Overall, these technologies are enhancing accessibility and personalization of antenatal care, but continued research is needed to optimize safety, efficacy, and integration into routine practice [18, 19].

Parallel to advances in maternal care, innovations in reproductive medicine are reshaping the field of assisted reproduction. In vitro fertilization (IVF) has benefited from integration of time-lapse imaging, artificial intelligence (AI), and developmental markers to refine morphokinetic embryo assessment and improve outcome prediction. Time-lapse systems now provide continuous, non-invasive monitoring of embryo growth, with validated morphokinetic parameters such as time to expanded blastocyst (tEB), time to eight cells (t8), and synchrony of cell divisions (S3) serving as strong predictors of blastocyst quality, chromosomal status, and pregnancy success. Embryos reaching these milestones more rapidly are more likely to be euploid and achieve implantation [22, 23]. Building on this, some AI-based tools can analyze morphokinetic data alongside patient factors like age and oocyte source to generate embryo quality scores that closely correlate with live birth and clinical pregnancy rates, while also clarifying the influence of variables such as maternal age and use of fresh versus frozen oocytes on embryo development and miscarriage risk [23]. Together, these innovations are enhancing precision, personalization, and efficiency in IVF embryo selection.

Beyond reproductive medicine, AI is increasingly being used for ultrasound and MRI to enhance the detection and characterization of gynecologic disease, particularly endometriosis. In transvaginal ultrasound (TVUS), AI models using deep learning and radiomics have improved accuracy for diagnosing deep endometriosis and endometriomas, though superficial disease remains more difficult to detect. Updated pelvic ultrasound protocols endorsed by major societies now integrate dynamic and positional assessments, with AI tools further assisting image interpretation and segmentation. These strategies have significantly increased sensitivity and specificity for deep disease, although generalizability and external validation remain important limitations [24–26]. MRI-based AI approaches have improved lesion segmentation, diagnostic accuracy, and workflow efficiency, with particular value for patients who cannot undergo TVUS or who have complex or extrapelvic disease. Reported sensitivities and specificities for deep and ovarian endometriosis with AI-enhanced MRI now exceed 90% in some studies [24, 27].

In addition to endometriosis, AI applications in MRI and ultrasound are transforming the evaluation of uterine fibroids and gynecologic cancers. Radiomics and multimodal AI fusion techniques enable more accurate differentiation between benign and malignant lesions, such as distinguishing fibroids from leiomyosarcoma or endometrial carcinoma. These methods improve diagnostic accuracy, automate lesion segmentation, and predict histopathology, allowing for more precise patient stratification and individualized management [28–30]. AI-driven imaging innovations hold strong potential to reduce diagnostic delays, enhance noninvasive characterization, and optimize treatment planning across many gynecologic conditions.

Complementing advances in imaging and diagnostics, 3D printing is emerging as a powerful tool in both obstetrics and gynecology for surgical planning, education, and patient engagement. In obstetrics, 3D printing is being used to generate fetal anatomical models from high-resolution ultrasound and MRI data, enhancing preoperative planning for complex interventions such as ex utero intrapartum treatment (EXIT) procedures and fetoscopic repair of spina bifida. These models allow surgical teams to anticipate intraoperative challenges, improve precision, and optimize neonatal outcomes, while also serving as valuable tools for parental counseling by illustrating fetal anatomy in a tangible form [31–33]. In gynecology, individualized 3D-printed anatomical models are increasingly used for oncologic surgical planning, such as advanced ovarian carcinoma, by clarifying tumor boundaries, vascular supply, and organ relationships to support R0 resections and reduce risk [34].

Educational and training applications are rapidly expanding, with 3D-printed models enabling rehearsal of complex cases and providing hands-on learning opportunities for trainees. Advances in artificial intelligence and 4D printing are driving the development of tissue-mimicking constructs and automated model generation, broadening the scope and realism of simulations. These innovations are reshaping both surgical planning and medical education in obstetrics and gynecology, with ongoing work aimed at improving accessibility, standardization, and integration into routine clinical practice [31, 33, 35].

Cardiothoracic Surgery

Similar to the previously discussed subspecialties, cardiothoracic surgery has seen rapid innovation across robotics, advanced imaging, and device engineering. Robotic-assisted surgery has expanded into increasingly complex thoracic and cardiac procedures, including lung transplantation, esophagectomy, mitral valve repair, and coronary revascularization, offering improved dexterity, visualization, and recovery outcomes, with single-port systems further reducing invasiveness. Electromagnetic navigated bronchoscopy–guided microwave ablation has emerged as a safe, effective option for managing multiple pulmonary nodules, supported by advances in imaging integration and workflow efficiency. Major breakthroughs in cardiac support devices include the first successful human implantation of the BiVACOR artificial heart, demonstrating feasibility as a bridge-to-transplant, and engineering progress toward fully wireless LVADs using magnetic and transcutaneous energy transfer systems, which hold promise for reducing infection risk and improving quality of life. These breakthroughs underscore the growing integration of robotics, imaging, and device innovations, pointing toward a future where cardiothoracic surgery is increasingly technology-driven.

Robotic-assisted cardiothoracic surgery has expanded significantly over the past 2 years, with growing adoption across both thoracic and cardiac procedures. In thoracic surgery, robotic platforms are now used for complex operations such as sleeve lobectomy, tracheal and chest wall resections, lung transplantation, and esophagectomy. Compared with video-assisted thoracoscopic surgery (VATS) and open techniques, robotic surgery offers enhanced dexterity, superior visualization, and improved lymph node access, allowing for better pain control, faster recovery, and similar or lower morbidity [36–38]. The introduction of single-port robotic systems further advances minimally invasive approaches, demonstrating safety and feasibility in pulmonary resections and esophagectomy with low conversion rates, shorter hospital stays, and reduced postoperative pain [38, 39].

In cardiac surgery, robotic techniques have become increasingly routine for mitral valve repair, coronary revascularization, and selected intracardiac procedures. Recent data show that robotic mitral valve surgery achieves lower morbidity, shorter ICU stays, and fewer readmissions compared with sternotomy, even in redo cases and elderly patients. Robotic coronary artery bypass and atrial procedures continue to expand, benefiting from precise visualization and instrument control [40, 41].

Similarly benefiting from more precise visualization and instrument control, electromagnetic navigated bronchoscopy (ENB)-guided microwave ablation (MWA) has advanced as a safe and effective minimally invasive option for managing multiple pulmonary nodules, including ground-glass opacities and suspected multiple primary lung cancers. Retrospective studies demonstrate low complication rates, even in patients with limited pulmonary function, with outcomes comparable between unilateral and bilateral ablations or between ablation alone and combined approaches with video-assisted thoracoscopic surgery (VATS). Combining ENB-guided MWA with VATS allows maximal parenchymal preservation and comprehensive treatment of multiple lesions in a single or staged session, showing favorable short-term outcomes and no early local recurrence [42–44].

Technical innovations have further optimized ENB-guided ablation, including the integration of cone-beam CT and digital tomosynthesis for real-time confirmation of ablation zones, enhancing accuracy and procedural confidence. The learning curve is relatively short, with 30 to 50 cases needed to achieve proficiency. Emerging adjuncts such as robotic bronchoscopy, CT-to-body divergence correction software, and alternative ablation modalities such as radiofrequency and pulsed electric field, are under investigation, with MWA remaining the most established technique [45–47].

In the field of cardiac device engineering, the BiVACOR artificial heart stands out as a key pivotal milestone. This device was used in its first successful human implantation at Baylor St. Luke's Medical Center in 2024, where the patient survived for 8 days before undergoing heart transplantation. This demonstrated its feasibility as a bridge-to-transplant option for end-stage biventricular heart failure [48]. This achievement is thanks to extensive preclinical work, including anatomical fitting studies confirming compatibility with a wide range of patient morphologies [49]. In vitro studies have further shown that the device maintains hemocompatibility comparable to clinically approved total artificial hearts, generating a meaningful pulse pressure while keeping hemolysis low, even at the extremes of clinical flow requirements [50]. The BiVACOR system's single magnetically levitated centrifugal rotor, capable of modulating pulsatile flow, is unique among total artificial hearts, and the combination of successful human implantation and supportive hemocompatibility data represents a critical step toward broader clinical trials and potential regulatory approval [48–50].

As another achievement in cardiac device engineering, wireless left ventricular assist devices (LVADs) have seen significant advances recently by focusing on eliminating the percutaneous driveline, a major source of infection and morbidity. Recent engineering developments include prototypes using magnetic torque transmission and transcutaneous energy transfer systems (TETS) to wirelessly power the pump, with hybrid designs capable of operating in both a magnetic mode driven by extracorporeal rotating magnets and an electric mode powered by an intracorporeal battery that is wirelessly charged during magnetic operation. Bench-top testing has demonstrated sustained pump performance and sufficient battery charging for several hours of daily use, though further miniaturization and in vivo testing are needed [51, 52]. Advances are also underway in device miniaturization, biocompatibility, and smart control algorithms, including the integration of artificial intelligence and remote monitoring to optimize pump speed and hemodynamic support in real time [53, 54]. While no fully wireless LVAD has yet reached routine clinical use, these innovations represent a major future direction, with the potential to reduce infection rates, improve patient quality of life, and expand long-term applicability once technical challenges such as heat generation, downsizing, and reliable energy transfer are overcome [51–54].

These innovations highlight how cardiothoracic surgery is increasingly defined by the integration of robotics, imaging, and advanced device engineering. With progress spanning minimally invasive procedures, real-time image-guided interventions, and next-generation cardiac support systems, the specialty is steadily moving toward more precise, efficient, and reliable care. Continued refinement of these technologies will likely expand surgical capabilities and improve outcomes across the full spectrum of cardiothoracic disease.

Ophthalmology

Ophthalmology has similarly embraced technological innovation to enhance microsurgical precision and develop novel therapeutics. Robot-assisted surgical systems are pushing the boundaries of delicate intraocular procedures, while breakthroughs in gene therapy offer hope of restoring vision in patients with inherited diseases. Other innovations in drug delivery have eased the burden of treatment for common conditions, like age-related macular degeneration.

The implementation of robotic-assisted ophthalmologic surgery represents a significant technological leap. Though in its infancy, robotic ophthalmologic surgery has the potential to rapidly become commonplace as technology continues to advance. Surgical systems, such as the da Vinci (Intuitive Surgical, Sunnyvale, CA), Preceyes surgical system (Preceyes BV, Eindhoven, Netherlands), and the Intraocular Robotic Interventional Surgical system (IRISS—Stein Eye Institute, Los Angeles, CA) offer enhanced control and manipulation of multiple instruments. Furthermore, platforms such as IRISS possess integrated optical coherence tomography (OCT) imaging for preoperative and intraoperative planning.

These surgical platforms have been used in successful intraocular and cataract procedures [55–57]. Comparative studies between manual versus robotic retinal peeling procedures showed that robotic procedures reduced retinal hemorrhages and eliminated retinal injuries when compared to manual peeling. Both groups had similar visual outcomes [58, 59].

In parallel with surgical systems, treatment innovations are addressing underlying genetic and chronic conditions. Tailored gene editing therapy is an emerging frontier. Following a single patient FDA approval, a novel gene therapy utilizing Beremagene Geperpavec (B-VEC) was used to treat ocular scarring from dystrophic epidermolysis bullosa. A replication-defective HSV1 viral vector was used to transfect wildtype COL7A1 genes into epithelial cells. Prior to surgical removal of scar tissue and this novel treatment, the patient had visual acuity rated as "hand motion." Eight months following surgery, an exam revealed no evidence of corneal scarring and the patient's vision improved to 20/25 [60].

Finally, the anti-VEGF implantable Port Delivery System (PDS) is a novel drug delivery device recently approved by the FDA for treatment of neovascular age-related macular degeneration (nAMD). This system eliminates the need for frequent intravitreal injections of anti-VEGF medications while maintaining more stable intraocular drug levels to help control disease progression [61–63].

While the advances seen in ophthalmology may be in their early stages, the implications or treatment are exciting. Robotic systems are enhancing surgical safety and precision, gene therapies are offering transformative and potentially curative treatments for devastating genetic eye diseases, and innovative drug delivery technologies are improving the management of chronic conditions affecting millions of patients worldwide.

Otolaryngology

Advancements in the field of otolaryngology have notably brought about refinement in minimally invasive surgery techniques, improvement in intraoperative precision, and restoration of sensory function. Transoral robotic surgery continues to evolve as new robotic surgical systems are developed and tested. Innovations in intraoperative imaging and navigation provide surgeons with real-time guidance for perioperative decision-making. Finally, breakthroughs in cochlear implant technology and gene therapy have allowed for greater hearing restoration for patients with significant hearing loss.

Minimally invasive and robotic approaches have refined surgical techniques. Transoral robotic surgery (TORS) has historically been completed using the Davinci Multi Port Xi (MP) system in the United States. Now, the new da Vinci Single Port (SP) system (Intuitive Surgical, USA) is being employed for TORS which helps reduce instrument clashing, improve oropharyngeal instrument maneuverability, and reduce console time. Studies have shown no significant differences between the daVinci SP and MP systems in terms of safety profile, measured by duration of hospitalization, enteral feeding, and complications. However, the SP demonstrates improved docking and console times when compared with MP [64, 65].

Additionally, intraoperative imaging and navigation provide enhanced surgical precision. Image guidance for endoscopic sinus surgery allows for real-time determination of a surgical instrument's location in relation to anatomical landmarks, reducing complications to other skull base structures and providing a more complete surgery with reduced revision rates [66]. Other intraoperative imaging modalities, such as fluorescence-guided surgery, are aiding surgeons in better visualizing tumor margins during resection, potentially leading to more complete tumor removal and improved oncological outcomes [67, 68].

Furthermore, treatment innovations are focused on restoring function and utilizing biologics. Totally implantable cochlear implants (TICIs) eliminate the need for external components and daily charging, offering a more discrete and convenient solution for individuals with severe to profound hearing loss. Three clinical trials have demonstrated comparable hearing performance between TICIs and traditional cochlear implants [69]. Concurrently, gene therapy has shown remarkable success in treating specific genetic forms of hearing loss, most notably caused by mutations in the OTOF gene. One early clinical trial involving adeno-associated virus gene transfer resulted in marked hearing restoration for children with prelingual deafness due to the OTOF mutation, promising a strong future for similar treatments [70].

In summary, the field of otolaryngology is being driven forward by less invasive and more precise surgical techniques like single-port TORS and image-guided surgery, alongside life-changing innovations in sensory restoration. Advances in cochlear implants and the success of gene therapy for genetic deafness highlight a future where function can be restored, not just managed.

Urology

Urology exemplifies how surgical subspecialties are being transformed by technological and diagnostic innovation. Like other fields highlighted in this chapter, it has embraced robotics and advanced imaging to deliver more precise, less invasive, and increasingly personalized care. What makes urology distinct is the breadth of conditions it addresses, from kidney stones to prostate and kidney cancer, where innovations in instrumentation and visualization can rapidly translate into meaningful improvements in patient outcomes.

One significant example of this innovation can be seen in endourology, where flexible and navigable suction ureteral access sheaths (FANS) have revolutionized retrograde intrarenal surgery (RIRS) by combining steerability with integrated suction channels to improve stone clearance [71–73]. Their active bending and flexible tips enable navigation into the renal pelvis and calyces, while suction connected to vacuum systems facilitates evacuation of stone dust and fragments through continuous or intermittent aspiration using the Venturi effect [71–73].

Compared to traditional access sheaths, FANS are associated with higher stone-free rates, reduced infectious complications, shorter operative times, and improved visualization [71, 73].

Controlled vacuum aspiration systems extend this concept by integrating steerable catheters or sheaths with vacuum-assisted aspiration, alternating irrigation and suction to optimize fragment clearance under fluoroscopic guidance [74–76]. Clinical studies show these systems are safe and effective, with device choice tailored to stone size, location, and anatomy. Larger sheath diameters and digital occlusion provide faster suction, while flexible tips improve access to challenging locations such as lower pole calyces [73, 77, 78].

As device design in endourology continues to optimize control and access, robotic technology has evolved to achieve similar goals in the realms of reconstructive and oncologic surgery. Single-port (SP) robotic surgery in urology has advanced rapidly over the past 3 years with the refinement of the da Vinci SP platform, enabling complex procedures such as radical prostatectomy, partial nephrectomy, nephroureterectomy, and reconstructive surgeries through a single incision [79–81]. Recent studies confirm its safety and feasibility across diverse indications, with perioperative outcomes comparable to multi-port systems, while offering benefits such as shorter hospital stays, reduced blood loss, less opioid use, and improved cosmesis, though there is no proven oncologic or functional superiority [81–83]. Technical innovations, such as transvesical and supine anterior retroperitoneal approaches, have expanded surgical access and efficiency, supporting same-day discharge and enhanced recovery pathways [79, 84, 85]. Despite ongoing challenges with cost and learning curve, single-port robotic surgery is increasingly regarded as a transformative step in minimally invasive urology [79, 80, 85].

While single-port robotic systems are redefining the operative landscape, new innovations in imaging are reshaping diagnostics. Prostate cancer diagnostics have established high-resolution micro-ultrasound (microUS, 29 MHz) as a viable alternative to MRI fusion-guided biopsy within the last few years. The 2025 OPTIMUM randomized clinical trial showed that microUS-guided biopsy is noninferior to MRI fusion-guided biopsy for detecting clinically significant prostate cancer (Gleason Grade Group ≥ 2) in biopsy-naïve men, with similar detection rates across approaches [86]. Meta-analyses and systematic reviews further confirm that microUS achieves detection rates comparable to MRI-targeted biopsy, while offering the advantages of real-time lesion visualization, simplified workflow, and greater accessibility in settings with limited MRI availability or high costs [87–89].

Beyond its use as a stand-alone modality, microUS has also shown value when combined with MRI fusion. Studies demonstrate that microUS can detect MRI-invisible lesions, including some clinically significant cancers, and may upgrade a small subset of patients otherwise missed by MRI-targeted or systematic biopsy alone [90, 91]. The evidence supports microUS as a validated, cost-effective, and accessible alternative to MRI fusion, while ongoing research is focused on refining its integration into prostate cancer diagnostic pathways [86–90].

Recent developments in the field of urology reflect an intersection of surgical precision and diagnostic progress. Flexible and navigable suction ureteral access sheaths (FANS) and controlled vacuum aspiration systems have improved retrograde intrarenal surgery by enhancing stone clearance, visualization, and pressure control. Single-port robotic surgery, driven by the da Vinci SP platform, has expanded minimally invasive options with outcomes comparable to multi-port systems and added benefits in recovery and cosmesis. Meanwhile, high-resolution micro-ultrasound has emerged as a validated, accessible alternative to MRI fusion biopsy in prostate cancer, with ongoing research exploring combined approaches for even greater diagnostic accuracy. Together, these innovations demonstrate how urology is rapidly evolving toward safer, more efficient, and patient-centered care.

References

1. Cong B, Zhang H. Innovative 3D printing technologies and advanced materials revolutionizing orthopedic surgery: current applications and future directions. Front Bioeng Biotechnol. 2025;13:1542179. https://doi.org/10.3389/fbioe.2025.1542179.
2. Suryawanshi CM, Bhallamudi R, Mishra S. Design and additive manufacturing of metamaterials for orthopedic implants and its mechanical characterization. Mech Adv Mater Struct. 2025; https://doi.org/10.1080/15376494.2025.2471033.
3. Gharibshahian M, Salehi M, Beheshtizadeh N, Kamalabadi-Farahani M, Atashi A, Nourbakhsh MS, Alizadeh M. Recent advances on 3D-printed PCL-based composite scaffolds for bone tissue engineering. Front Bioeng Biotechnol. 2023; https://doi.org/10.3389/FBIOE.2023.1168504.
4. Rajaeirad M, Fakharifar A, Posti MHZ, Khorsandi M, Watts DC, Elraggal A, Ouldyerou A, Merdji A, Roy S. Evaluating the effect of functionally graded materials on bone remodeling around dental implants. Dent Mater. 2024;40:858–68. https://doi.org/10.1016/j.dental.2024.04.002.
5. Al-Shalawi FD, Mohamed Ariff AH, Jung DW, Mohd Ariffin MKA, Seng Kim CL, Brabazon D, Al-Osaimi MO. Biomaterials as implants in the orthopedic field for regenerative medicine: metal versus synthetic polymers. Polymers. 2023;15:2601. https://doi.org/10.3390/polym15122601.
6. Ashish Daniel S, Suya Prem Anand P, Naveen J, Khan T, Khahro SH. Advancement in biomedical implant materials—a mini review. Front Bioeng Biotechnol. 2024; https://doi.org/10.3389/FBIOE.2024.1400918.
7. Nikam N, Shenoy BS, K NC, Keni LG, Shetty S, Bhat NS. Advancements in surface coatings for enhancing longevity in hip implants: a review. Prosthesis. 2025;7:21. https://doi.org/10.3390/prosthesis7010021.
8. Chen X, Deng S, Sun ML, He R. Robotic arm-assisted arthroplasty: the latest developments. Chin J Traumatol. 2022;25:125–31. https://doi.org/10.1016/j.cjtee.2021.09.001.
9. Kolessar DJ, Hayes DS, Harding JL, Rudraraju RT, Graham JH. Robotic-arm assisted technology's impact on knee arthroplasty and associated healthcare costs. J Health Econ Outcomes Res. 2022;9:57–66. https://doi.org/10.36469/001c.37024.
10. Inabathula A, Semerdzhiev DI, Srinivasan A, Amirouche F, Puri L, Piponov H. Robots on the stage: a snapshot of the American robotic total knee arthroplasty market. JBJS Open Access. 2024; https://doi.org/10.2106/JBJS.OA.24.00063.
11. Sperling JW. Zimmer Biomet announces successful completion of world's first robotic-assisted shoulder replacement surgery with ROSA® Shoulder System. 2024. https://investor.zimmerbiomet.com/news-and-events/news/2024/04-25-2024. Accessed 4 Nov 2025.

12. Lambrechts A, Wirix-Speetjens R, Maes F, Van Huffel S. Artificial intelligence based patient-specific preoperative planning algorithm for total knee arthroplasty. Front Robot AI. 2022; https://doi.org/10.3389/FROBT.2022.840282.
13. Evans CH, Ghivizzani SC, Robbins PD. The 2024 OREF clinical research award: progress toward a gene therapy for arthritis. J Am Acad Orthop Surg. 2024;32:1052–60. https://doi.org/10.5435/JAAOS-D-24-00831.
14. Mao AS, Mooney DJ. Regenerative medicine: current therapies and future directions. Proc Natl Acad Sci USA. 2015;112:14452–9. https://doi.org/10.1073/pnas.1508520112.
15. Chang C, Yan J, Yao Z, Zhang C, Li X, Mao HQ. Effects of mesenchymal stem cell-derived paracrine signals and their delivery strategies. Adv Healthc Mater. 2021; https://doi.org/10.1002/ADHM.202001689.
16. Liang W, Zhou C, Bai J, et al. Current advancements in therapeutic approaches in orthopedic surgery: a review of recent trends. Front Bioeng Biotechnol. 2024;12:1328997. https://doi.org/10.3389/fbioe.2024.1328997.
17. Freitag J, Chamberlain M, Wickham J, et al. Safety and efficacy of an allogeneic adipose-derived mesenchymal stem cell preparation in the treatment of knee osteoarthritis: a phase I/IIa randomised controlled trial. Osteoarthr Cartil Open. 2024; https://doi.org/10.1016/j.ocarto.2024.100500.
18. Mohamed H, Ismail A, Sutan R, Rahman RA, Juval K. A scoping review of digital technologies in antenatal care: recent progress and applications of digital technologies. BMC Pregnancy Childbirth. 2025; https://doi.org/10.1186/S12884-025-07209-8.
19. Stricker K, Radan AP, Surbek D. Continuous remote home monitoring solutions for mother and fetus: a scoping review. Eur J Obstet Gynecol Reprod Biol. 2025;305:170–7. https://doi.org/10.1016/J.EJOGRB.2024.12.018.
20. Hsieh MF, Slavin V, Huang MZ, Wang HH, Hsieh HF. mHealth use during pregnancy: a systematic review. Int J Gynaecol Obstet. 2025; https://doi.org/10.1002/IJGO.70205.
21. Vatsa R, Chang W, Akinyi S, et al. Impact evaluation of a digital health platform empowering Kenyan women across the pregnancy-postpartum care continuum: a cluster randomized controlled trial. PLoS Med. 2025; https://doi.org/10.1371/JOURNAL.PMED.1004527.
22. Jiang R, Yang G, Wang H, et al. Exploring key embryonic developmental morphokinetic parameters that affect clinical outcomes during the PGT cycle using time-lapse monitoring systems. BMC Pregnancy Childbirth. 2024; https://doi.org/10.1186/S12884-024-07080-Z.
23. Ten J, Tio MC, Pini P, et al. Decoding embryo development: the effect of clinical variables in morphokinetics and artificial intelligence quality scoring. Reprod Biomed Online. 2025; https://doi.org/10.1016/J.RBMO.2025.104866.
24. Avery JC, Deslandes A, Freger SM, et al. Noninvasive diagnostic imaging for endometriosis part 1: a systematic review of recent developments in ultrasound, combination imaging, and artificial intelligence. Fertil Steril. 2024;121:164–88. https://doi.org/10.1016/J.FERTNSTERT.2023.12.008.
25. Mittal S, Tong A, Young S, Jha P. Artificial intelligence applications in endometriosis imaging. Abdom Radiol. 2025; https://doi.org/10.1007/S00261-025-04897-W.
26. Moro F, Giudice MT, Ciancia M, Zace D, Baldassari G, Vagni M, Tran HE, Scambia G, Testa AC. Application of artificial intelligence to ultrasound imaging for benign gynecological disorders: systematic review. Ultrasound Obstet Gynecol. 2025;65:295–302. https://doi.org/10.1002/UOG.29171.
27. Alonzo L, Cannella R, Gullo G, et al. Magnetic resonance imaging of endometriosis: the role of advanced techniques. J Clin Med. 2024;13:5783. https://doi.org/10.3390/JCM13195783.
28. Cai C, Hu W, Zhou H, Zhang X, Ren R, Liu Y, Ye F. Artificial intelligence–assisted radiation imaging pathways for distinguishing uterine fibroids and malignant lesions in patients presenting with cancer pain: a literature review. Front Oncol. 2025; https://doi.org/10.3389/FONC.2025.1621642.

29. Moro F, Ciancia M, Zace D, et al. Role of artificial intelligence applied to ultrasound in gynecology oncology: a systematic review. Int J Cancer. 2024;155:1832–45. https://doi.org/10.1002/IJC.35092.
30. Shrestha P, Poudyal B, Yadollahi S, et al. A systematic review on the use of artificial intelligence in gynecologic imaging—background, state of the art, and future directions. Gynecol Oncol. 2022;166:596–605. https://doi.org/10.1016/J.YGYNO.2022.07.024.
31. Fils AJ, Kasmirski J, Okpaise O, Reynolds JM, Tonni G, Werner H, Ruano R. The use of 3D printing in fetal surgery for surgical planning: a scoping review. J Clin Med. 2024; https://doi.org/10.3390/JCM13174999.
32. De Paredes JG, Gosnell J, Strug M, Giuliani E, Thakur M, Romero VC, Cordoba M. Antenatal three-dimensional printing for ex utero intrapartum treatment procedures. Obstet Gynecol. 2022;139:313–6. https://doi.org/10.1097/AOG.0000000000004650.
33. Wolder D, Blazuk-Fortak A, Góra T, Michalska A, Kaczmarek P, Świercz G. The role of three-dimensional printed models of fetuses obtained from ultrasonographic examinations in obstetrics: clinical and educational aspects. Eur J Obstet Gynecol Reprod Biol. 2025; https://doi.org/10.1016/J.EJOGRB.2025.114538.
34. Xi H, Liu C, Tian N, Geng M, Hu J, Li H, Pan W, Sun X, Cai Z, Bai S. Application of 3D printing technology in the surgical management of advanced ovarian serous carcinoma: a case report. Front Oncol. 2025; https://doi.org/10.3389/FONC.2025.1541919.
35. Tripathi S, Ansari AA, Singh M, et al. Transforming surgical planning and procedures through the synergistic use of additive manufacturing, advanced materials and artificial intelligence: challenges and opportunities. Mater Horiz. 2025; https://doi.org/10.1039/D5MH00501A.
36. Odeh AM, Wyant K, Freeman RK, Abdelsattar ZM. Tackling complex thoracic surgical operations with robotic solutions: a narrative review. J Thorac Dis. 2024;16:1521–36. https://doi.org/10.21037/JTD-23-1570.
37. Pan JM, Watkins AA, Stock CT, Moffatt-Bruce SD, Servais EL. The surgical renaissance: advancements in video-assisted thoracoscopic surgery and robotic-assisted thoracic surgery and their impact on patient outcomes. Cancers (Basel). 2024; https://doi.org/10.3390/CANCERS16173086.
38. Tung KH, Yendamuri S, Seastedt KP. Adoption of the robotic platform across thoracic surgeries. J Clin Med. 2024; https://doi.org/10.3390/JCM13195764.
39. Lee JH, Park TH, Kim HK. Robotic thoracic surgery using the single-port robotic system: initial experience with more than 100 cases. J Thorac Cardiovasc Surg. 2024;168:1513–1522.e2. https://doi.org/10.1016/J.JTCVS.2024.03.005.
40. Hibino M, Murphy DA, Halkos ME. Robotic mitral surgery: recent advances and outcomes. Curr Opin Cardiol. 2024;39:543–50. https://doi.org/10.1097/HCO.0000000000001174.
41. Tasoudis PT, Caranasos TG, Doulamis IP. Robotic applications for intracardiac and endovascular procedures. Trends Cardiovasc Med. 2024;34:110–7. https://doi.org/10.1016/J.TCM.2022.10.002.
42. Qu R, Tu D, Hu S, Wang Q, Ping W, Hao Z, Cai Y, Zhang N, Wang J, Fu X. Electromagnetic navigation bronchoscopy-guided microwave ablation combined with Uniportal video-assisted thoracoscopic surgery for multiple ground glass opacities. Ann Thorac Surg. 2022;113:1307–15. https://doi.org/10.1016/J.ATHORACSUR.2021.04.061.
43. Wang S, Su C, Li J, et al. The use of electromagnetic navigation bronchoscopy-guided microwave ablation in patients with multiple bilateral pulmonary nodules: a retrospective study of 26 cases. J Thorac Dis. 2024;16:6347–56. https://doi.org/10.21037/JTD-24-1052.
44. Zeng C, Fu X, Yuan Z, Hu S, Wang X, Ping W, Cai Y, Wang J. Application of electromagnetic navigation bronchoscopy-guided microwave ablation in multiple pulmonary nodules: a single-centre study. Eur J Cardiothorac Surg. 2022; https://doi.org/10.1093/EJCTS/EZAC071.
45. Chan JWY, Siu ICH, Chang ATC, Li MSC, Lau RWH, Mok TSK, Ng CSH. Transbronchial techniques for lung cancer treatment: where are we now? Cancers (Basel). 2023; https://doi.org/10.3390/CANCERS15041068.

46. Folch E, Guo Y, Senitko M. Therapeutic bronchoscopy for lung nodules: where are we now? Semin Respir Crit Care Med. 2022;43:480–91. https://doi.org/10.1055/s-0042-1749368.
47. Huang Y, Zhou L, Wang Y, Wang J, Hao Z, Fu X. Learning curve for electromagnetic navigation bronchoscopy-guided microwave ablation: a cumulative sum analysis. J Thorac Dis. 2025;17:3971–80. https://doi.org/10.21037/JTD-2024-2162.
48. Shah AM. First successful implant of BiVACOR's total artificial heart. Artif Organs. 2024;48:1075–6. https://doi.org/10.1111/AOR.14844.
49. Emmanuel S, Jansz P, McGiffin D, Kure C, Watson A, Connellan M, Granger E, Iyer A, Timms D, Hayward C. Anatomical human fitting of the BiVACOR total artificial heart. Artif Organs. 2022;46:50–6. https://doi.org/10.1111/AOR.14077.
50. Mee APM, Timms D, Nestler F, Bartnikowski N, Tansley GD, Wu E, Simmonds MJ. In vitro hemocompatibility of the BiVACOR total artificial heart near the boundaries of clinical operation. ASAIO J. 2025; https://doi.org/10.1097/MAT.0000000000002536.
51. Horie H, Isoyama T, Ishiyama K. Design of an innovative wireless left ventricular assist device driven by either extracorporeal magnets or an Intracorporeal battery pack. ASAIO J. 2023;69:E73–9. https://doi.org/10.1097/MAT.0000000000001874.
52. Horie H, Isoyama T, Ishiyama K. Design of a hybrid left ventricular assist device with a new wireless charging system. Artif Organs. 2024;48:309–14. https://doi.org/10.1111/AOR.14666.
53. Kozakov K, Provaznik Z, Schmid C, Camboni D. Advancing LVAD technology: overcoming challenges and shaping the future of mechanical circulatory support. J Clin Med. 2024; https://doi.org/10.3390/JCM13247813.
54. Moeller CM, Valledor AF, Oren D, Rubinstein G, Sayer GT, Uriel N. Evolution of mechanical circulatory support for advanced heart failure. Prog Cardiovasc Dis. 2024;82:135–46. https://doi.org/10.1016/J.PCAD.2024.01.018.
55. De Smet MD, Naus GJL, Faridpooya K, Mura M. Robotic-assisted surgery in ophthalmology. Curr Opin Ophthalmol. 2018;29:248–53. https://doi.org/10.1097/ICU.0000000000000476.
56. Wilson JT, Gerber MJ, Prince SW, Chen CW, Schwartz SD, Hubschman JP, Tsao TC. Intraocular robotic interventional surgical system (IRISS): mechanical design, evaluation, and master–slave manipulation. Int J Med Robot Comput Assist Surg. 2018; https://doi.org/10.1002/RCS.1842.
57. Chen CW, Lee YH, Gerber MJ, et al. Intraocular robotic interventional surgical system (IRISS): semi-automated OCT-guided cataract removal. Int J Med Robot Comput Assist Surg. 2018; https://doi.org/10.1002/RCS.1949.
58. Maberley DAL, Beelen M, Smit J, Meenink T, Naus G, Wagner C, de Smet MD. A comparison of robotic and manual surgery for internal limiting membrane peeling. Graefes Arch Clin Exp Ophthalmol. 2020;258:773–8. https://doi.org/10.1007/s00417-020-04613-y.
59. Chatzimichail E, Feltgen N, Motta L, Empeslidis T, Konstas AG, Gatzioufas Z, Panos GD. Transforming the future of ophthalmology: artificial intelligence and robotics' breakthrough role in surgical and medical retina advances: a mini review. Front Med (Lausanne). 2024;11:1434241. https://doi.org/10.3389/fmed.2024.1434241.
60. Vetencourt AT, Sayed-Ahmed I, Gomez J, Chen H, Agostini B, Carroll K, Parry T, Krishnan S, Sabater AL. Ocular gene therapy in a patient with dystrophic epidermolysis bullosa. N Engl J Med. 2024;390:530–5. https://doi.org/10.1056/NEJMoa2301244.
61. Ghoraba HH, Do DV, Nguyen QD. Port delivery system with Ranibizumab: as always—risks versus benefits for the recipients. Ophthalmic Surg Lasers Imaging Retina. 2022;53:416–7. https://doi.org/10.3928/23258160-20220713-01.
62. Khanani AM, Callanan D, Dreyer R, et al. End-of-study results for the ladder phase 2 trial of the port delivery system with Ranibizumab for neovascular age-related macular degeneration. Ophthalmol Retina. 2021;5:775–87. https://doi.org/10.1016/j.oret.2020.11.004.
63. Ribeiro L, Oliveira J, Kuroiwa D, Kolko M, Fernandes R, Junior O, Moraes N, Vasconcelos H, Oliveira T, Maia M. Advances in vitreoretinal surgery. J Clin Med. 2022; https://doi.org/10.3390/JCM11216428.

64. Sampieri C, Pirola F, Costantino A, Kim D, Ho JJ, Lee K, De Virgilio A, Park YM, Kim SH. Single-port versus multiport da Vinci system for Transoral robotic surgery of hypopharyngeal and laryngeal carcinoma. Otolaryngol Head Neck Surg. 2023;169:548–55. https://doi.org/10.1002/ohn.287.
65. Oberhelman N, Bruening J, Jackson RS, et al. Comparison of da Vinci single port vs Si systems for Transoral robotic-assisted surgery: a review with technical insights. JAMA Otolaryngol Head Neck Surg. 2024;150:165–71. https://doi.org/10.1001/jamaoto.2023.3994.
66. Nobre ML, Sarmento ACA, de Paula Bedaque H, Medeiros KS, Cobucci RN, Júnior JD, Gonçalves AK. Image guidance for endoscopic sinus surgery: systematic review and meta-analysis. Rev Assoc Med Bras. 2023;69:e20230633. https://doi.org/10.1590/1806-9282.20230633.
67. de Wit JG, Vonk J, Voskuil FJ, et al. EGFR-targeted fluorescence molecular imaging for intraoperative margin assessment in oral cancer patients: a phase II trial. Nat Commun. 2023;14(1):1–10. https://doi.org/10.1038/s41467-023-40324-8.
68. Keith BA, Marrero-Gonzalez AR, Chau IJ, Nguyen SA, Albergotti WG, Kejner AE, Newman JG. Intraoperative fluorescence in solid head and neck cancer: a scoping review. Eur Arch Oto-Rhino-Laryngol. 2025; https://doi.org/10.1007/S00405-025-09442-5.
69. Dubey P, Vasisht S, Chatterjee I. Advancements in cochlear implant technology: a comprehensive overview. IP J Otorhinolaryngol Allied Sci. 2025;8:5–11. https://doi.org/10.18231/j.ijoas.2025.003.
70. Lv J, Wang H, Cheng X, et al. AAV1-hOTOF gene therapy for autosomal recessive deafness 9: a single-arm trial. Lancet. 2024;403:2317–25. https://doi.org/10.1016/S0140-6736(23)02874-X.
71. Chen Y, Li C, Gao L, Lin L, Zheng L, Ke L, Chen J, Kuang R. Novel flexible vacuum-assisted ureteral access sheath can actively control intrarenal pressure and obtain a complete stone-free status. J Endourol. 2022;36:1143–8. https://doi.org/10.1089/END.2022.0004.
72. Edmonds VS, Ballantyne CC, Cabo JJ, Ostergar AS, Humphreys MR, Stern KL. First prospective, in vivo experience using a novel steerable suction ureteral access sheath in North America. Urology. 2025; https://doi.org/10.1016/j.urology.2025.07.064.
73. Gauhar V, Traxer O, Castellani D, Ragoori D, Heng CT, Chew BH, Somani BK, Bin HS. A feasibility study on clinical utility, efficacy and limitations of 2 types of flexible and navigable suction ureteral access sheaths in retrograde Intrarenal surgery for renal stones. Urology. 2023;178:173–9. https://doi.org/10.1016/j.urology.2023.05.032.
74. Geavlete P, Multescu R, Mares C, Buzescu B, Iordache V, Geavlete B. Retrograde Intrarenal surgery for Lithiasis using suctioning devices: a shift in paradigm? J Clin Med. 2024; https://doi.org/10.3390/JCM13092493.
75. Ostergar A, Wong D, Shiang A, Ngo S, Venkatesh R, Desai A, Sands K. Intrarenal pressure with vacuum-assisted ureteral access sheaths using an in situ cadaveric porcine model. J Endourol. 2023;37:353–7. https://doi.org/10.1089/END.2022.0573.
76. Wang D, Xu Y, Liu Z, Liang J, Lai D, Guan W, Xu G. Using vacuum-assisted ureteral access sheath in the treatment of complex steinstrasse. Urolithiasis. 2023; https://doi.org/10.1007/S00240-023-01462-2.
77. Law YXT, Tan YQ, Htoo EEA, et al. In vitro suction comparison of 3 flexible and navigable suction ureteral access sheaths (FANS) of 2 sizes using a 7.5Fr single-use flexible ureteroscope: an AUSET-EAU endourology collaboration. World J Urol. 2025; https://doi.org/10.1007/S00345-025-05812-0.
78. Madden A, Altez C, Lueza JP, Cabrera J, Quarà A, Moretto S, Popescu RI, Corrales M, Traxer O. Size matters: an in vitro evaluation of flexible vacuum-assisted ureteral access sheaths. Urolithiasis. 2025; https://doi.org/10.1007/S00240-025-01710-7.
79. Biasatti A, Soputro NA, Porpiglia F, et al. The current landscape of single-port robotic surgery in urology. Nat Rev Urol. 2025; https://doi.org/10.1038/S41585-025-01081-Z.
80. Nguyen TT, Basilius J, Ali SN, Dobbs RW, Lee DI. Single-port robotic applications in urology. J Endourol. 2023;37:688–99. https://doi.org/10.1089/END.2022.0600.

81. Ren S, Zheng Y, Hu X, Bao Y, Wang D, Chang Y. Recent advances in single-site/incision robotic-assisted radical prostatectomy. Eur J Surg Oncol. 2023;49:1341–50. https://doi.org/10.1016/J.EJSO.2023.03.213.
82. Ge S, Zeng Z, Li Y, Gan L, Meng C, Li K, Wang Z, Zheng L. Comparing the safety and efficacy of single-port versus multi-port robotic-assisted techniques in urological surgeries: a systematic review and meta-analysis. World J Urol. 2024; https://doi.org/10.1007/S00345-023-04711-6.
83. Xu MC, Hemal AK. Single-port vs multiport robotic surgery in urologic oncology: a narrative review. J Endourol. 2025;39:271–84. https://doi.org/10.1089/END.2024.0528.
84. Kaouk J, Beksac AT, Zeinab MA, Duncan A, Schwen ZR, Eltemamy M. Single port Transvesical robotic radical prostatectomy: initial clinical experience and description of technique. Urology. 2021;155:130–7. https://doi.org/10.1016/J.UROLOGY.2021.05.022.
85. Pellegrino AA, Chen G, Morgantini L, Calvo RS, Crivellaro S. Simplifying retroperitoneal robotic single-port surgery: novel supine anterior retroperitoneal access. Eur Urol. 2023;84:223–8. https://doi.org/10.1016/J.EURURO.2023.05.006.
86. Kinnaird A, Luger F, Cash H, et al. Microultrasonography-guided vs MRI-guided biopsy for prostate cancer diagnosis: the OPTIMUM randomized clinical trial. JAMA. 2025;333:1679–87. https://doi.org/10.1001/JAMA.2025.3579.
87. Dias AB, Ghai S. Prostate cancer diagnosis with micro-ultrasound: what we know now and new horizons. Radiol Clin North Am. 2024;62:189–97. https://doi.org/10.1016/J.RCL.2023.06.014.
88. Dias AB, O'Brien C, jean Michel Correas, Ghai S. Multiparametric ultrasound and micro-ultrasound in prostate cancer: a comprehensive review. Br J Radiol. 2022; https://doi.org/10.1259/BJR.20210633.
89. Sountoulides P, Pyrgidis N, Polyzos SA, Mykoniatis I, Asouhidou E, Papatsoris A, Dellis A, Anastasiadis A, Lusuardi L, Hatzichristou D. Micro-ultrasound-guided vs multiparametric magnetic resonance imaging-targeted biopsy in the detection of prostate cancer: a systematic review and meta-analysis. J Urol. 2021;205:1254–62. https://doi.org/10.1097/JU.0000000000001639.
90. Rakauskas A, Peters M, Martel P, van Rossum PSN, La Rosa S, Meuwly JY, Roth B, Valerio M. Do cancer detection rates differ between transperineal and transrectal micro-ultrasound mpMRI-fusion-targeted prostate biopsies? A propensity score-matched study. PLoS One. 2023; https://doi.org/10.1371/JOURNAL.PONE.0280262.
91. Socarrás MER, Rivas JG, Rivera VC, Elbers JR, González LL, Mercado IM, Del Alamo JF, Del Dago PJ, Sancha FG. Prostate mapping for cancer diagnosis: the Madrid protocol. Transperineal prostate biopsies using multiparametric magnetic resonance imaging fusion and micro-ultrasound guided biopsies. J Urol. 2020;204:726–32. https://doi.org/10.1097/JU.0000000000001083.

The Advantages of Telehealth in Clinical Medicine

W. Ethan Coleman and Yong Li

Introduction

This chapter aims to provide an overview of telehealth's evolution, clarify its advantages, and outline its role in shaping the future of healthcare delivery within modern medicine. Telehealth first started as a tool to reach patients in rural and underserved areas or those who had challenges with in-person appointments, but it has since grown into a key driver of accessibility and convenience in healthcare [1]. The COVID-19 pandemic was a significant turning point in the use of telehealth, making virtual healthcare an integral part of modern medicine [2]. In the wake of the pandemic and current medical services, telehealth and telemedicine have become necessary parts of care and are seen almost ubiquitously among healthcare providers, with up to 74% of physicians working in practices that offer telehealth [3].

The traditional framework of healthcare access has been defined through availability, accessibility, accommodation, affordability, and acceptability [4]. Telehealth and its adoption have managed to reshape each dimension directly and indirectly. Availability and accessibility were extended through virtual reach. Accommodation and affordability grew through flexible scheduling and cheaper visits, and COVID-19 brought its acceptance to the forefront of healthcare [5]. However, despite these

W. E. Coleman
Western Michigan University, Homer Stryker MD School of Medicine (WMed), Kalamazoo, MI, USA

Y. Li (✉)
Division of Medical Engineering, Department of Surgical Sciences, Western Michigan University, Homer Stryker MD School of Medicine (WMed), Kalamazoo, MI, USA

Division of Orthopedic Surgery, Western Michigan University, Homer Stryker MD School of Medicine (WMed), Kalamazoo, MI, USA
e-mail: Yong.li@wmed.edu

S. S. Chahin et al. (eds.), *Innovation in Medical Education and Clinical Practice*, https://doi.org/10.1007/978-3-032-19116-8_24

recent changes, questions remain regarding equity. Not all populations can or want to receive digital healthcare.

Distinguishing between telehealth and telemedicine is important. Although the two terms are closely related, they refer to different aspects of healthcare delivery. Telehealth refers to the use of digital technology to deliver and support healthcare services, including education and system management. Telemedicine refers to the remote delivery of care through diagnoses, treatments, and consultations, making telemedicine a subset of telehealth. Every telemedicine encounter is telehealth, but not all involve direct patient care. Modern definitions, including those from governmental agencies, increasingly favor the term "telehealth" to capture its wider role in prevention, education, and healthcare coordination beyond clinical encounters [6]. Accordingly, this chapter focuses on telehealth as a system-wide transformation of healthcare delivery.

COVID-19: Rapid Adoption

During the COVID-19 pandemic, telehealth transformed from a supplementary option to an essential component of medical care. In early 2020, after the pandemic began to change daily lives both within and outside medicine, telehealth visits skyrocketed. The CDC reported a 50% increase in telehealth use in the first quarter compared with 2019, and by late March, there was a 154% increase [7]. Originally, these visits were not related to COVID-19, but in the last 3 weeks of March, COVID-related visits increased from 5.5% to 16.2% of telehealth visits. These changes were set in motion through CDC recommendations for the use of virtual services in February 2020, and CMS emergency waivers and the CARES Act in March 2020. This leads to better reimbursement for providers and opportunities for out-of-state care [7]. Insurance data from private companies also showed a 766% increase in virtual visits between spring 2019 and spring 2020 [8]. Medicare numbers show the same change in healthcare practices and a jump in the usage of telehealth. Data estimates there were under a million visits in 2019 and approximately 52.7 million in 2020 [9], peaking with almost half of the primary care visits (43.5%) using telehealth in April compared with 0.1% in February 2020 [10].

Beyond these statistics, telehealth's rise during COVID-19 revealed how quickly healthcare systems can adapt when cultural barriers are lowered. Before 2020, skepticism among clinicians and patients often stemmed from unfamiliarity, reimbursement concerns, and uncertainty regarding quality [11]. The pandemic normalized virtual care and showed that regulatory flexibility and cultural change matter as much as technical capacity.

Increased Usage

The Centers for Medicare and Medicaid (CMS) provided a telemedicine coverage waiver in March 2020 in the wake of COVID that allowed everyone to be eligible for insurance reimbursement for telehealth visits. One study of 30 million Americans found that once the waivers went into effect, telehealth usage jumped from less than half a percent of visits to nearly 10% thereafter. With the increase in telehealth usage following waivers, minority populations showed the greatest increase, suggesting that telehealth did not widen racial disparities but may even have helped. [12].

While usage surged across all demographics during this time, utilization data alone cannot capture whether access has improved equitably. Many patients used telehealth because in-person care was unavailable, but not necessarily because telehealth was superior or accessible to all. Researchers have cautioned against conflating with access. Structural barriers such as Internet or data coverage, device ownership, and digital literacy can hide exclusion, even within apparently growing numbers [13]. Consequently, the apparent statistical reach of telehealth during COVID-19 may overstate its social inclusivity.

Clinical Adaptations

Before the pandemic, telehealth use among most advanced practice nurses (APRNs) was minimal. One study found that only 6% of APRNs used telehealth daily, but this number jumped to 49% during the pandemic. Before 2020, 73% of the APRNs had never used telehealth services. [14]. This shift shows how quickly providers had to adjust to the new standards of healthcare. Although usage has since declined from its peak during the pandemic, many providers keep telehealth incorporated with their practices.

The shift to telehealth has redefined professional competencies. Clinicians needed new skills, such as digital communication, virtual examination, and technology troubleshooting, which were not focused on in traditional medical training. Several training programs have now incorporated telemedicine modules, focusing on virtual bedside methods and remote diagnostics [15].

Remote Monitoring

Remote patient monitoring (RPM) is becoming increasingly important. During the COVID-19 pandemic, it was used to track patients at home, helping hospitals save beds for the sickest patients. In one trial, RPM reduced hospitalization without increasing patient risk [16]. The Mayo Clinic also reported that patients enrolled in the RPM had better outcomes than those who were not, including improved costs, mortality, and fewer hospital or ICU admissions [17]. Without RPM, many hospitals may have had larger issues with resource allocation, especially the limited number of beds available during the pandemic.

Remote monitoring has also introduced the concern of "data deluge." Continuous streams of information from wearables and home sensors can overwhelm clinicians and create liability concerns when alerts are missed [18]. Artificial intelligence offers potential triage solutions but comes with its own concerns. The ethical question becomes whether convenience might unintentionally harm continuity of care.

Psychiatric Care

Psychiatry and psychotherapy were among the first specialties to move online almost entirely at the start of the pandemic. In some clinics, nearly every patient was transferred from in-person to virtual care during lockdown. In one clinic from UCSD, 98% of patients were in person prior to the lockdown, but they were able to convert all of them to telehealth visits within 3 days [19]. Many chose to continue with telehealth after they were allowed to go in person because of convenience. Both patients and clinicians enjoy the benefits of telehealth, with clinicians stating that it helped with their workflow [20, 21].

While telepsychiatry dramatically increased continuity of care, particularly during lockdowns, it also revealed the strengths and limitations of virtual rapport. Patients appreciated privacy and convenience, yet some reported reduced emotional connection or "screen fatigue" [22, 23]. Clinicians expressed concern about missed non-verbal cues and limited ability to assess home environments safely [24]. These mixed outcomes suggest that telehealth excels when communication and monitoring are the main goals of care, but they may struggle when nuanced observation or therapies are central. This variation emphasizes the importance of hybrid models, such as the use of virtual models for maintenance and in-person models for complex or high acuity concerns.

International Acceptance

Telehealth use has expanded rapidly in medical clinics worldwide during the COVID-19 pandemic, although the degree of growth varies by country. In Argentina, for example, online medical visits more than doubled in 2020 compared with before the pandemic, especially in areas hit hardest by COVID-19 [25]. Other countries saw similar increases as health systems adapted to social distancing and clinical closures.

The rise in telehealth has not been limited to primary care. Specialties, such as oncology, obstetrics, and mental health, have also turned to virtual care and remote monitoring to maintain contact with patients [26]. In India, large-scale programs used phone calls and text messages to reach millions of pregnant women and new mothers with prenatal and postnatal health information [27]. In Kenya, telemedicine platforms have been developed to connect rural mothers with nurses and midwives when travel is restricted [28].

High-income countries were able to expand telehealth more rapidly because of well-developed Internet infrastructure, widespread smartphone access, and insurance systems that support virtual care. In contrast, many low- and middle-income countries face challenges, such as limited connectivity and lower digital literacy. Despite these barriers, these regions often find creative ways to use technology to improve their access.

Telehealth Now

Access

Access remains one of the most transformative achievements in telehealth. Access to healthcare has almost always been a struggle for people with difficulty traveling or for those in rural, remote, and underserved areas. For any people who face barriers to travel or distance to reliable healthcare, telehealth makes it possible to connect with providers without needing transportation or taking time away from work or other obligations [29].

There is a nationwide shortage of healthcare workers, especially among primary care physicians and specialists. Telemedicine allows these physicians to visit the patient and save on travel time, cost, and logistical burdens. Telemedicine has shown a significant benefit in outcomes through increased access, especially among patients with chronic diseases [29]. Not only did the outcomes improve, but these patients also reported better satisfaction with their care. Telemedicine has made it easier to check in more often, improving follow-up and adherence to treatment.

Beyond the difficulties of travel or geographic access, logistical issues, such as timing and continuity of care, have also improved through the implementation of telehealth. Telehealth allows physicians to work outside clinic hours, as they do not have to rely on a physical location's working hours. The ability to see patients through telehealth also reduces waiting times, especially for non-urgent and follow-up issues [3]. Less waiting for the patient means quicker care and a better fit for each patient.

Telehealth provides easier access to physician-to-physician consultation. The increased use of telehealth has paved the way for more e-consultations. Primary care physicians can consult with specialists through e-consultation, and specialists can also consult with each other through these services [30]. These services allow for much more rapid care delivery and avoid further travel to different specialists for patients. E-consultations have allowed these specialty services to be delivered in places where they were previously unavailable or limited [31].

Telehealth can also circumvent legal and logistical barriers in areas where reproductive services are limited or stigmatized. One review found that digital health has significantly expanded access to medication abortions in the United States, particularly for people in remote or restrictive settings [32]. The review reported that telemedicine-based abortion services were highly effective, with 94%–99% of procedures completed successfully without surgical intervention. Both patients and providers found this acceptable. Despite their success, as of 2023, 14 states have passed laws prohibiting telemedicine abortion [32].

Telehealth has made healthcare easier to reach, especially by reducing travel time and scheduling barriers; however, its impact on cost and comfort with use has not been the same for everyone. For some, virtual visits can make care much more available, but for others, such as older adults, foreign language speakers, or those unfamiliar with digital platforms, the process can be confusing or unwelcoming. Designing systems that are culturally aware, multilingual, and easy to use will ensure that access is expanded and reaches those who need it the most.

Financial Benefit

Telehealth offers financial benefits to both patients and the healthcare system. Hospitals and clinics can use less physical space and overhead when visits occur. Remote check-ins also sometimes mean catching problems early, which can prevent expensive ER visits later [10]. For patients, telehealth removes significant financial barriers that are present with work coverage, transportation, and caring for children for the duration of the visit [33]. These costs are often an extra strain for patients and can represent prohibitive challenges in healthcare.

One study found that, on average, telehealth appointments among those less than 65 years with cancer saved between $147 and $186 per visit [34]. In Patel's study, 25,000 visits from 11,700 patients saved a total of $1.6 million between the saved productivity with drive time and visit time. Another study within a neurooncology department showed that patients saved an average of 4.1–5.6 h per visit, with an average financial saving of $223 [35].

One study of UCSD showed that factoring in travel distance, time, and cost of 3 million telehealth encounters saved 53 million miles of traveling, 1.8 million hours of travel time, and a total cost of over $33 million [36]. In addition to these benefits, lack of travel prevented 42 crash-related injuries [36].

The financial aspects of telehealth may seem simple, but they remain complex. For most patients, virtual visits save money; however, even with lower costs in some areas for hospitals and clinics, the picture is not always clear. Setting up secure telehealth platforms and maintaining data systems can be expensive, and reimbursement policies do not always keep up with how care is delivered. Some health systems save money by reducing overhead, while others lose revenue from fewer in-person services such as labs or imaging [37, 38]. The true benefits of telehealth financial outcomes depend on whether there are payment models that can balance affordability for patients while ensuring sustainability for providers.

Effectiveness

Research shows that outcomes with telehealth are similar to those of in-person care, especially for chronic diseases, where monitoring and quick adjustments are the main reasons for a doctor's visit. For example, remote patient monitoring in conditions such as diabetes, heart failure, and COVID-19 has been shown to match or sometimes even improve outcomes compared to in-person visits [39, 40]. In one study, comparing palliative care through telehealth and in-person care, telehealth produced equal QoL outcomes [41].

Evidence shows that telehealth is clinically equivalent for certain conditions, such as hypertension, some endocrine disorders, and mental health, but it remains inadequate for others that rely on tactile or procedural assessment [42, 43] The real advantage lies in continuity for chronic conditions, as remote follow-ups prevent gaps in care and support early interventions. However, when telehealth replaces rather than complements in-person visits, subtle complications may be missed.

Human Factors

Most patients who try telehealth appreciate how easy it is to fit into their lives. Shorter wait times, not having to travel, and being able to check more frequently are all big pluses. For people managing long-term conditions, easier access to providers can also make them feel more in control of their health [44].

It is not just the patients who benefit. Telehealth has helped providers become more flexible, collaborate virtually, and, in some cases, reduce exposure risk [1]. During the pandemic, many clinicians and trainees have also received more exposure to telemedicine, which may improve how the future workforce thinks about digital health.

The long-term success of telehealth depends on how well people accept and adapt. The main appeal for patients is convenience, and many studies report that patients are satisfied with virtual visits overall, especially for follow-ups or managing chronic conditions [45]. Several studies have noted that patients lack personal connections and a sense of empathy that often comes with face-to-face visits [46]. Without nonverbal cues and physical presence, it can be more difficult for both sides to build trust, especially when the relationship is new.

Providers experienced similar mixed feelings. Many appreciate the flexibility of telehealth and the ability to reach patients who might not otherwise come in. Others have described feelings of depersonalization and the pressure to always be available online. Recent research has found that telemedicine can blur the line between work and personal life, contributing to burnout and fatigue [47]. Clinicians report being overwhelmed by electronic messages, technical problems, and expectations of constant responsiveness [48]. As virtual care becomes part of daily practice, these emotional and workload concerns are becoming increasingly important in addressing technical challenges.

Restrictions and Drawbacks

Despite its many advantages, telehealth remains limited by systemic, technical, and ethical barriers. The most pressing challenge is the digital divide, a structural inequity that risks reversing the very access gains telehealth promises. Patients without reliable broadband, smartphones, or digital literacy are excluded from video visits, especially in low-income, elderly, and rural populations [33]. Studies reporting increased access to telehealth often draw from insured or urban cohorts, making it unclear whether the expansion truly reached the most underserved.

Research shows that patients who are older, from racial and ethnic minority groups, or of lower socioeconomic status continue to use virtual visits less often than their wealthier or White counterparts [49]. In resource-limited areas, unreliable broadband access can make virtual appointments difficult to sustain, especially in rural communities that already face healthcare shortages [50]. Effective telehealth participation also depends on owning a capable device and having basic digital literacy requirements that not all patients meet. These barriers mean that although telehealth can reduce some access gaps, it also risks reinforcing the structural inequities it aims to solve.

Telehealth remains a valuable supplement to in-person medicine, particularly for chronic disease follow-up and mental health care, but it cannot yet replace physical examinations, emergency interventions, or diagnostic testing that require direct clinician contact [1]. As telehealth technology evolves, these limitations may lessen, but the current system still depends on integrating virtual and in-person care rather than replacing one with the other.

Another challenge involves the relative novelty of telehealth. Although telehealth existed before 2020, it was not a routine component of most healthcare services until the COVID-19 pandemic made it essential. Studies from that period show a rapid, almost universal surge in adoption across specialties, transforming telehealth from a niche tool into a mainstream practice [2, 51]. However, because most of this data is recent, much of the existing research remains preliminary and still tied to pandemic-era circumstances. Long-term outcomes, quality measures, and cost-effectiveness analyses will require several more years of observation before firm conclusions can be drawn.

Despite its progress, telehealth continues to face important concerns around data security and privacy. Any platform transmitting protected health information over the internet is inherently vulnerable to breaches or unauthorized access [52]. Unlike in-person visits, which confine data within hospital systems, virtual encounters introduce multiple points of entry through personal devices, home networks, and third-party applications. While large-scale telehealth data breaches remain rare, national reports warn that expanding virtual care increases cybersecurity exposure and demands stronger standards and oversight [53].

Future Directions

The next stage of telehealth development must balance innovation with evidence-based governance. Artificial intelligence (AI) and machine learning are being integrated into virtual triage and chronic disease management, yet questions of algorithmic bias and clinical validation remain unresolved [54, 55]. Remote monitoring through wearables, such as continuous glucose and cardiac sensors, can expand preventative care, but these technologies often reinforce inequity by only providing for patients who can afford them.

Policy reform will determine whether telehealth's pandemic-era gains persist. Temporary CMS and state-level licensure waivers dramatically expanded virtual care, but many remain provisional [56]. To make telehealth fair and lasting, healthcare systems need consistent payment for virtual care, easier licensing across states, and reliable broadband for all communities. Without these, telehealth risks becoming a convenience for the privileged rather than helping the underserved.

Future research must move beyond utilization data and measure long-term outcomes, cost-effectiveness, and patient safety across populations. Comparative effectiveness studies, hybrid care models, and environmental impact analyses, such as those showing reductions in travel emissions and healthcare's carbon footprint, should guide policy. Ultimately, telehealth's success depends not on technological capability but on thoughtful integration by ensuring virtual care enhances, rather than skips over, the human relationship at the center of medicine.

Another dimension gaining attention is environmental sustainability. By reducing travel and physical resource use, telehealth may contribute to lowering healthcare's carbon footprint, which is a non-trivial factor as hospitals are among the most energy-intensive institutions globally [57]. Simultaneously, AI-driven triage systems and virtual assistants promise to streamline care but introduce new ethical concerns [58]. The future of telehealth requires a governance model that is as innovative as the technology itself. It requires balanced efficiency, safety, and social justice.

Conclusion

Telehealth has evolved from a necessity during a crisis into a defining feature of modern healthcare delivery. Its rapid expansion during the COVID-19 pandemic demonstrated the potential of virtual care to overcome traditional barriers of distance, cost, and time. Yet the same acceleration revealed how those gains can become smaller if technology, policy, and equity are misaligned.

Evidence shows that telehealth can deliver outcomes comparable to in-person care for many chronic conditions and mental health services, but these findings depend heavily on patient selection, infrastructure, and provider adaptation. Sustained policy reform and investment in digital access will be needed to ensure the benefits go beyond the already connected and insured to help everyone.

As medicine continues to digitize, telehealth's future will be defined less by innovation and more by integration. It will need to complement, instead of replace, in-person care. The challenge is ensuring that virtual medicine strengthens the patient–provider relationship rather than substituting for it. When designed thoughtfully and ethically, telehealth can move from a reactive tool of necessity to a permanent part of twenty-first-century healthcare. Telehealth's greatest advantage is not only convenience but continuity and its capacity to make care a persistent presence rather than an episodic event. Yet, its sustainability will depend on whether innovation remains aligned with equity, empathy, and evidence.

References

1. Wosik J, Fudim M, Cameron B, Gellad Z, Cho A, Phinney D, et al. Telehealth transformation: COVID-19 and the rise of virtual care. J Am Med Inform Assoc. 2020;27(6):957–62. https://doi.org/10.1093/jamia/ocaa067.
2. Monaghesh E, Hajizadeh A. The role of telehealth during COVID-19 outbreak: a systematic review based on current evidence. BMC Public Health. 2020;20:1193. https://doi.org/10.1186/s12889-020-09301-4.
3. Ehrenfeld JM. Permanently expanding telehealth access will improve public health [Internet]. AMA; 2024. [cited 2025 Sept 30]. Available from: https://www.ama-assn.org/about/leadership/permanently-expanding-telehealth-access-will-improve-public-health.
4. Penchansky R, Thomas JW. The concept of access: definition and relationship to consumer satisfaction. Med Care. 1981;19(2):127–40. https://doi.org/10.1097/00005650-198102000-00001.
5. Haj D, Nguyen L, Naqvi K, Jacus N, Li P, Sawyer R, et al. Telemedicine and its application in pandemic. Am J Biomed Sci Res. 2023;18(6):597–601. https://doi.org/10.34297/AJBSR.2023.18.002530.
6. Doarn CR, Pruitt S, Jacobs J, Harris Y, Bott DM, Riley W, et al. Federal efforts to define and advance telehealth—a work in progress. Telemed J E Health. 2014;20(5):409–18. https://doi.org/10.1089/tmj.2013.0336.
7. Koonin LM, Hoots B, Tsang CA, Harris AM, Luther K, Tracy M, et al. Trends in the use of telehealth during the emergence of the COVID-19 pandemic-United States, January–March 2020. MMWR. 2020;69:1595–9. https://doi.org/10.15585/mmwr.mm6943a3.
8. Betancourt JA, Rosenberg MA, Zevallos A, Brown JR, Mileski M. The impact of COVID-19 on telemedicine utilization across multiple service lines in the United States. Healthcare (Basel). 2020;8(4):380. https://doi.org/10.3390/healthcare8040380.
9. Samson L, Tarazi W, Turrini G, Sheingold S. Medicare beneficiaries' use of telehealth services in 2020—trends by beneficiary characteristics and location [Internet]. Washington, DC: Office of the Assistant Secretary for Planning and Evaluation (ASPE), U.S. Department of Health and Human Services; 2021. [cited 2025 Oct 29]. Available from: https://aspe.hhs.gov.

10. Bosworth A, Ruhter J, Samson LW, Sheingold S, Taplin C, Tarazi W, et al. Medicare beneficiary use of telehealth visits: early data from the start of COVID-19 pandemic [Internet]. Washington, DC: ASPE, U.S. Department of Health and Human Services; 2020. [cited 2025 Oct 29]. Available from: https://aspe.hhs.gov.
11. Lee NT, Karsten J, Roberts J. Removing regulatory barriers to telehealth before and after COVID-19 [Internet]. 2020. [cited 2025 Oct 18]. Available from: https://www.brookings.edu/articles/removing-regulatory-barriers-to-telehealth-before-and-after-covid-19/.
12. Bose S, Dun C, Zhang GQ, Walsh C, Makary MA, Hicks CW. Medicare beneficiaries in disadvantaged neighborhoods increased telemedicine use during the COVID-19 pandemic. Health Aff (Millwood). 2022;41(5):635–42. https://doi.org/10.1377/hlthaff.2021.01706.
13. Hernandez K, Faith B. Online but still falling behind: measuring barriers to internet use 'after access'. Internet Pol Rev. 2023;12(2). https://doi.org/10.14763/2023.2.1713.
14. Schorn MN, Myers CR, Barroso J, Hande K, Hudson T, Kim J, et al. Changes in telehealth experienced by advanced practice RNs during COVID-19: US survey results. Comput Inform Nurs. 2023;41(7):507–13. https://doi.org/10.1097/CIN.0000000000000979.
15. Eberly LA, Tennison A, Mays D, Wright J, Bennett C, McCoy R, et al. Telephone-based guideline-directed medical therapy optimization in Navajo nation: the Hózhó randomized clinical trial. JAMA Intern Med. 2024;184(6):681–90. https://doi.org/10.1001/jamainternmed.2024.1523.
16. Joyce D, De Brún A, Symmons SM, Fitzgerald C, Murphy E, McCarthy S, et al. Remote patient monitoring for COVID-19 patients: comparisons and framework for reporting. BMC Health Serv Res. 2023;23:826. https://doi.org/10.1186/s12913-023-09526-0.
17. Haddad TC, Coffey JD, Deng Y, Glasgow AE, Christopherson LA, Sangaralingham LR, et al. Impact of a high-risk, ambulatory COVID-19 remote patient monitoring program on utilization, cost, and mortality. Mayo Clin Proc. 2022;97(12):2215–25. https://doi.org/10.1016/j.mayocp.2022.08.015.
18. Bawa D, Kabra R, Ahmed A, Bansal S, Darden D, Pothineni NVK, et al. Data deluge from remote monitoring of cardiac implantable electronic devices and importance of clinical stratification. Heart Rhythm O2. 2023;4(6):374–81. https://doi.org/10.1016/j.hroo.2023.04.005.
19. Yellowlees P, Nakagawa K, Pakyurek M, Hanson A, Elder J, Kales HC. Rapid conversion of an outpatient psychiatric clinic to a 100% virtual telepsychiatry clinic in response to COVID-19. Psychiatr Serv. 2020;71(7):749–52. https://doi.org/10.1176/appi.ps.202000230.
20. Abrams Z. How well is telepsychology working? Monit Psychol. 2020;51(5) [cited 2025 Oct 19]. Available from: https://www.apa.org/monitor/2020/07/cover-telepsychology.
21. Gentry MT, Puspitasari AJ, McKean AJ, Williams MD, Breitinger S, Geske JR, et al. Clinician satisfaction with rapid adoption and implementation of telehealth services during the COVID-19 pandemic. Telemed J E Health. 2021;27(12):1385–92. https://doi.org/10.1089/tmj.2020.0575.
22. Galvin E, Desselle S, Gavin B, Quigley E, Flear M, Kilbride K, et al. Patient and provider perspectives of the implementation of remote consultations for community-dwelling people with mental health conditions: A systematic mixed-studies review. J Psychiatr Res. 2022;156:668–78. https://doi.org/10.1016/j.jpsychires.2022.10.051.
23. Myronuk L. Effect of telemedicine via videoconference on provider fatigue and empathy: implications for the quadruple aim. Healthc Manage Forum. 2022;35(3):174–8. https://doi.org/10.1177/08404704211059944.
24. Morreale M, Cohen I, Van Wert M, Beccera A, Miller L, Narrow W, et al. Determinants of experience & satisfaction in telehealth psychiatry during the COVID-19 pandemic for patients & providers. Front Psychiatry. 2023;14:1237249. https://doi.org/10.3389/fpsyt.2023.1237249.
25. Busso M, Gonzalez MP, Scartascini C. On the demand for telemedicine: evidence from the COVID-19 pandemic. Health Econ. 2022;31(7):1491–503. https://doi.org/10.1002/hec.4523.
26. Tormen M, Toniolo B, Pecci L, Soraci G, Taliento C, Greco P, et al. Exploring the impact of integrating telehealth in obstetric care: A scoping review. Eur J Obstet Gynecol Reprod Biol. 2024;302:242–8. https://doi.org/10.1016/j.ejogrb.2024.09.031.

27. Lalan A, Verma S, Rodriguez Diaz P, Danassis P, Mahale A, Madhu Sudan K, et al. Improving health information access in the world's largest maternal mobile health program via bandit algorithms. Proc AAAI Conf Artif Intell. 2024;38(21):22913–9. https://doi.org/10.1609/aaai.v38i21.30329.
28. Kim EJ, Moretti ME, Kimathi AM, Chan SY, Wootton R. Use of provider-to-provider telemedicine in Kenya during the COVID-19 pandemic. Front Public Health. 2022;10:1028999. https://doi.org/10.3389/fpubh.2022.1028999.
29. Ezeamii VC, Okobi OE, Wambai-Sani H, Perera GS, Zaynieva S, Okonkwo CC, et al. Revolutionizing healthcare: how telemedicine is improving patient outcomes and expanding access to care. Cureus. 2024;16(7):e63881. https://doi.org/10.7759/cureus.63881.
30. Keely E, Guglani S, Mitchell E, Sethuram C, Afkham A, Liddy C. Specialists accessing specialty advice: evaluating utilization, benefits, and impact of care of an e-consultation service. J Telemed Telecare. 2025;31(5):690–6. https://doi.org/10.1177/1357633X231211352.
31. Vimalananda VG, Orlander JD, Afable MK, Fincke BG, Solch AK, Rinne ST, et al. Electronic consultations (e-consults) and their outcomes: a systematic review. J Am Med Inform Assoc. 2020;27(3):471–9. https://doi.org/10.1093/jamia/ocz185.
32. Kumsa FA, Prasad R, Shaban-Nejad A. Medication abortion via digital health in the United States: a systematic scoping review. npj Digit Med. 2023;6:128. https://doi.org/10.1038/s41746-023-00871-2.
33. Chang E, Penfold RB, Berkman ND. Patient characteristics and telemedicine use in the US, 2022. JAMA Netw Open. 2024;7(3):e243354. https://doi.org/10.1001/jamanetworkopen.2024.3354.
34. Patel KB, Turner K, Alishahi Tabriz A, Gonzalez BD, Oswald LB, Nguyen OT, et al. Estimated indirect cost savings of using telehealth among nonelderly patients with cancer. JAMA Netw Open. 2023;6(1):e2250211. https://doi.org/10.1001/jamanetworkopen.2022.50211.
35. Liu JKC, Kang R, Bilenkin A, Prorok R, Whiting J, Patel KB, et al. Patient satisfaction and cost savings analysis of the telemedicine program within a neuro-oncology department. J Neuro-Oncol. 2022;160(2):517–25. https://doi.org/10.1007/s11060-022-04173-7.
36. Sharma S, Yellowlees PM, Gotthardt CJ, Luce MS, Avdalovic MV, Marcin JP. Environmental impact of ambulatory telehealth use by a statewide university health system during COVID-19. Telemed J E Health. 2023;29(8):1134–42. https://doi.org/10.1089/tmj.2022.0396.
37. NCQA. Taskforce on telehealth policy findings and recommendations—telehealth effect on total cost of care [Internet]. National Committee for Quality Assurance; 2020. [cited 2025 Oct 19]. Available from: https://www.ncqa.org/programs/data-and-information-technology/telehealth/taskforce-on-telehealth-policy/taskforce-on-telehealth-policy-findings-and-recommendations-telehealth-effect-on-total-cost-of-care/.
38. AMA. AMA issue brief: supporting equitable payment for telehealth [Internet]. AMA; 2023. [cited 2025 Oct 19]. Available from: https://www.ama-assn.org/system/files/issue-brief-equitable-payment-for-telehealth.pdf.
39. Umeh CA, Torbela A, Saigal S, Kaur H, Kazourra S, Gupta R, et al. Telemonitoring in heart failure patients: systematic review and meta-analysis of randomized controlled trials. World J Cardiol. 2022;14(12):640–56. https://doi.org/10.4330/wjc.v14.i12.640.
40. SeyedAlinaghi S, Yarmohammadi S, Mirzapour P, Dehghani S, Ahmadi S, Abbaspour F, et al. A systematic review of telehealth applications in endocrinology. Telemed Rep. 2024;5(1):269–89. https://doi.org/10.1089/tmr.2024.0032.
41. Greer JA, Temel JS, El-Jawahri A, Jackson VA, Smith CB, Pirl WF, et al. Telehealth vs in-person early palliative care for patients with advanced lung cancer: a multisite randomized clinical trial. JAMA. 2024;332(14):1153–64. https://doi.org/10.1001/jama.2024.13964.
42. Bulkes NZ, Davis K, Kay B, Riemann BC. Comparing efficacy of telehealth to in-person mental health care in intensive-treatment-seeking adults. J Psychiatr Res. 2022;145:347–52. https://doi.org/10.1016/j.jpsychires.2021.11.003.
43. Jackson TN, Sreedhara M, Bostic M, Spafford M, Popat S, Lowe Beasley K, et al. Telehealth use to address cardiovascular disease and hypertension in the United States: a systematic review

and meta-analysis, 2011–2021. Telemed Rep. 2023;4(1):67–86. https://doi.org/10.1089/tmr.2023.0011.
44. Poghosyan L, Martsolf GR, Liu J, Poghosyan H, Shaffer J, Berkowitz SA. Telehealth use by advanced practice nurses during the COVID-19 pandemic. J Am Assoc Nurse Pract. 2023;35(5):332–41. https://doi.org/10.1097/JXX.0000000000000855.
45. Duffy LV, Evans R, Bennett V, Hady JM, Palaniappan P. Therapeutic relational connection in telehealth: concept analysis. J Med Internet Res. 2023;25:e43303. https://doi.org/10.2196/43303.
46. Ramachandran M, Brinton C, Wiljer D, Shaw J, Sheikh A, Walji M, et al. The impact of eHealth on relationships and trust in primary care: a review of reviews. BMC Prim Care. 2023;24:228. https://doi.org/10.1186/s12875-023-02176-5.
47. Boksa V, Pennathur P. Assessing contributing and mediating factors of telemedicine on healthcare provider burnout. Health Policy Technol. 2024;13(6):100942. https://doi.org/10.1016/j.hlpt.2024.100942.
48. Apaydin EA, Der-Martirosian C, Yoo C, Rose DE, Jackson NJ, Stockdale SE, et al. Secure messages, video visits, and burnout among primary care providers in the Veterans Health Administration: national survey study. J Med Internet Res. 2025;27:e68858. https://doi.org/10.2196/68858.
49. Khoong E, Nouri S, Lyles C, Karliner L. Addressing equity in telemedicine for chronic disease management during the COVID-19 pandemic. NEJM Catal Innov Care Deliv. 2020. https://doi.org/10.1056/CAT.20.0123.
50. Benda N, Veinot TC, Sieck C, Ancker J. Broadband internet access is a social determinant of health! Am J Public Health. 2020;110:1123–5. https://doi.org/10.2105/AJPH.2020.305784.
51. Shaver J. The state of telehealth before and after the COVID-19 pandemic. Prim Care. 2022;49(4):517–30. https://doi.org/10.1016/j.pop.2022.04.002.
52. Kruse CS, Karem P, Shifflett K, Vegi L, Ravi K, Brooks M. Evaluating barriers to adopting telemedicine worldwide: a systematic review. J Telemed Telecare. 2018;24(1):4–12. https://doi.org/10.1177/1357633X16674087.
53. U.S. Government Accountability Office. Telehealth and cybersecurity: increased use highlights need for improved standards [Internet]. Washington, DC: GAO; 2022. [cited 2025 Oct 19]. Available from: https://www.gao.gov/products/gao-22-104454.
54. Seyyed-Kalantari L, Zhang H, McDermott MBA, Chen IY, Ghassemi M, Beede E, et al. Underdiagnosis bias of artificial intelligence algorithms applied to chest radiographs in under-served patient populations. Nat Med. 2021;27:2176–82. https://doi.org/10.1038/s41591-021-01595-0.
55. Challen R, Denny J, Pitt M, Gompels L, Edwards T, Tsaneva-Atanasova K. Artificial intelligence, bias and clinical safety. BMJ Qual Saf. 2019;28(3):231–7. https://doi.org/10.1136/bmjqs-2018-008370.
56. American Hospital Association. Telehealth waivers and flexibilities fact sheet [Internet]. AHA; 2025. [cited 2025 Oct 15]. Available from: https://www.aha.org/fact-sheets/2025-02-07-fact-sheet-telehealth-waivers.
57. Purohit A, Smith J, Hibble A. Does telemedicine reduce the carbon footprint of healthcare? A systematic review. Futur Healthc J. 2021;8(1):e85–91. https://doi.org/10.7861/fhj.2020-0080.
58. Da'Costa A, Teke J, Origbo JE, Osonuga A, Egbon E, Olawade DB. AI-driven triage in emergency departments: a review of benefits, challenges, and future directions. Int J Med Inform. 2025;197:105838. https://doi.org/10.1016/j.ijmedinf.2025.105838.

Index

S. S. Chahin et al. (eds.), *Innovation in Medical Education and Clinical Practice*, https://doi.org/10.1007/978-3-032-19116-8

MIX
Papier aus verantwortungsvollen Quellen
Paper from responsible sources
FSC® C105338

If you have any concerns about our products,
you can contact us on
ProductSafety@springernature.com

In case Publisher is established outside the EU,
the EU authorized representative is:
Springer Nature Customer Service Center GmbH
Europaplatz 3, 69115 Heidelberg, Germany

Printed by Libri Plureos GmbH
in Hamburg, Germany